VOLUME ONE HUNDRED AND THIRTY

Advances in
CANCER RESEARCH

VOLUME ONE HUNDRED AND THIRTY

Advances in
CANCER RESEARCH

Edited by

KENNETH D. TEW

*Department of Cell and Molecular Pharmacology,
Medical University of South Carolina, Charleston,
South Carolina, United States*

PAUL B. FISHER

*Department of Human and Molecular Genetics,
VCU Institute of Molecular Medicine, and VCU Massey
Cancer Center, Virginia Commonwealth University,
School of Medicine, Richmond, Virginia, United States*

AMSTERDAM • BOSTON • HEIDELBERG • LONDON
NEW YORK • OXFORD • PARIS • SAN DIEGO
SAN FRANCISCO • SINGAPORE • SYDNEY • TOKYO
Academic Press is an imprint of Elsevier

ELSEVIER

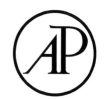

Academic Press is an imprint of Elsevier
50 Hampshire Street, 5th Floor, Cambridge, MA 02139, USA
525 B Street, Suite 1800, San Diego, CA 92101-4495, USA
The Boulevard, Langford Lane, Kidlington, Oxford OX5 1GB, UK
125 London Wall, London, EC2Y 5AS, UK

First edition 2016

ISBN: 978-0-12-804789-7
ISSN: 0065-230X

For information on all Academic Press publications
visit our website at http://store.elsevier.com/

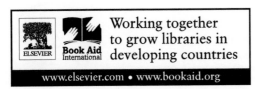

Working together
to grow libraries in
developing countries

www.elsevier.com • www.bookaid.org

CONTENTS

T. Murray-Stewart
The Sidney Kimmel Comprehensive Cancer Center, Johns Hopkins University, Baltimore, MD, United States

B. Peterson
Medical University of South Carolina, Charleston, SC, United States

J. Small
Medical University of South Carolina, Charleston, SC, United States

M. Stone
The Sidney Kimmel Comprehensive Cancer Center, Johns Hopkins University, Baltimore, MD, United States

M. Topper
The Sidney Kimmel Comprehensive Cancer Center, Johns Hopkins University, Baltimore, MD, United States

S. Waxman
The Tisch Cancer Institute, Icahn School of Medicine at Mount Sinai, New York, NY, United States

C.A. Zahnow
The Sidney Kimmel Comprehensive Cancer Center, Johns Hopkins University, Baltimore, MD, United States

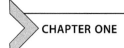

CHAPTER ONE

The Evolving, Multifaceted Roles of Autophagy in Cancer

J. Liu, J. Debnath[1]
Helen Diller Family Comprehensive Cancer Center, University of California, San Francisco, CA, United States
[1]Corresponding author: e-mail address: jayanta.debnath@ucsf.edu

Contents

Abstract

Autophagy is a lysosomal degradation process crucial for adaptation to stress and cellular homeostasis. In cancer, autophagy has been demonstrated to serve multifaceted roles in tumor initiation and progression. Although genetic evidence corroborates a role

Advances in Cancer Research, Volume 130
ISSN 0065-230X
http://dx.doi.org/10.1016/bs.acr.2016.01.005

for autophagy as a tumor suppressor mechanism during tumor initiation, autophagy also sustains metabolic pathways in cancer cells and promotes survival within the harsh tumor microenvironment and in response to diverse anticancer therapies. Moreover, though traditionally viewed as an autodigestive process, more recent work demonstrates that autophagy also facilitates cellular secretion; the importance of these new functions of the autophagy pathway is being increasingly appreciated during cancer progression and treatment. In this review, we discuss how these evolving and diverse roles for autophagy both impede and promote tumorigenesis.

1. INTRODUCTION

Autophagy, literally defined as self-eating, is a conserved catabolic pathway by which cells degrade and recycle cytoplasmic material in the lysosome (Klionsky, 2007). Studies in yeast and higher eukaryotes point to an evolutionarily conserved role for the autophagy pathway as a cellular response to starvation and stress (Reggiori & Klionsky, 2002). Autophagy actually refers to a trio of tightly regulated catabolic processes, all of which deliver cytoplasmic components to the lysosome for degradation—macroautophagy, microautophagy (Li, Li, & Bao, 2012), and chaperone-mediated autophagy (Cuervo & Wong, 2014); this article will focus on macroautophagy (hereafter used interchangeably with autophagy). In mammals, diverse stimuli, including nutrient starvation, infection, hypoxia, oxidative stress, and endoplasmic reticulum (ER) stress, induce autophagy (Kroemer, Mariño, & Levine, 2010). On the single-cell level, autophagy provides a source of biomaterials and metabolites to enable continued cell function and survival in response to these stresses; in addition, basal autophagy plays a homeostatic function by removing damaged or toxic cellular components within cells (Murrow & Debnath, 2013; Rabinowitz & White, 2010). Although generally considered cytoprotective, autophagy may also be involved in programmed cell death under certain conditions (Levine & Yuan, 2005; Liu & Levine, 2015). In humans, autophagy has been implicated in diverse pathologies, including aging (Rubinsztein, Mariño, & Kroemer, 2011), neurodegeneration (Nixon, 2013), cardiovascular disease (Levine & Kroemer, 2008), liver disease (Rautou et al., 2010), myopathy (Levine & Kroemer, 2008), inflammation and infection (Deretic, Saitoh, & Akira, 2013), metabolic diseases (Choi, Ryter, & Levine, 2013), and cancer (Kenific & Debnath, 2015).

In cancer, autophagy has been found to have tumor-suppressive or tumor-promoting effects at various stages of initiation, progression, and metastasis, painting a complex mechanistic picture (Kenific, Thorburn, & Debnath, 2010; White, 2012, 2015). One proposed explanation for these divergent effects is that the homeostatic function of autophagy prevents cancer initiation by clearing cells of oncogenic components, whereas stress-induced autophagy promotes tumor progression in the face of cancer-related stresses (Galluzzi et al., 2015; White, 2012). Moreover, in addition to regulating activity in cancer cells, autophagy may also influence cancer progression via its effects in other cell types that reside in the tumor microenvironment (Maes, Rubio, Garg, & Agostinis, 2013; Tang & Lotze, 2013).

In addition to its canonical degradative functions, autophagy has been found to contribute to secretory pathways in both yeast and mammalian cells (Ponpuak et al., 2015). Elucidating these emerging roles of autophagy-related secretion in cancer will be important for generating a more complete picture by which autophagy contributes to cancer and how autophagy-related pathways may be targeted for therapeutic benefit. Here, we discuss the pleiotropic roles of autophagy in cancer initiation and progression, including its established functions in catabolism, metabolic adaptation, and cell survival, as well as overview its emerging roles in the control of cellular secretion.

2. OVERVIEW OF AUTOPHAGY

Macroautophagy is a multistep process involving the formation of an autophagosome, a double membrane-bound structure that sequesters cytoplasmic components, and the ultimate fusion of this vesicle with a lysosome, resulting in the degradation of engulfed proteins and organelles (Yang & Klionsky, 2009). Studies in yeast have identified over 30 autophagy-related genes (*ATGs*) and proteins (Atgs), and many of their orthologs have also been established in mammals and other higher eukaryotes (Nakatogawa, Suzuki, Kamada, & Ohsumi, 2009; Yang & Klionsky, 2009).

2.1 Molecular Machinery of Autophagosome Biogenesis

Three steps of autophagosome biogenesis—initiation, nucleation, and elongation—have been characterized (Fig. 1). In yeast, this process is proposed to occur at a single location called the phagophore assembly site

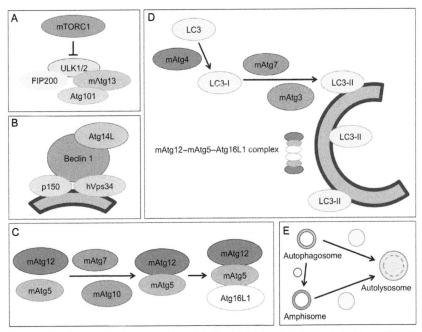

Fig. 1 Autophagosome biogenesis and fusion. (A) Initiation is regulated by mTORC1, which inhibits the ULK complex when nutrients are abundant and dissociates under starvation conditions. (B) Nucleation involves the formation of the class III PI3K complex, which includes the regulatory target Beclin 1. (C, D) Elongation of the growing phagophore membrane and generation of LC3-II require dual ubiquitin-like conjugation systems. The first pathway produces the mAtg12–mAtg5–Atg16L1 complex (C), which then promotes the lipidation of LC3 (a mammalian ortholog of Atg8) to form LC3-II during autophagosome formation. (E) The completed autophagosome can fuse directly with a lysosome to form an autolysosome, or it may first fuse with an endosome to form an amphisome. (See the color plate.)

(Suzuki et al., 2001), whereas in mammals, autophagosomes are thought to form via multiple membrane sites in the cytoplasm (Itakura & Mizushima, 2010). This section will provide an overview of autophagy trafficking from a mechanistic standpoint; more detailed reviews on this topic are available elsewhere (Lamb, Yoshimori, & Tooze, 2013; Parzych & Klionsky, 2014; Weidberg, Shvets, & Elazar, 2011).

2.1.1 Initiation of Autophagosome Biogenesis by the ULK Complex
In mammals, autophagosome biogenesis begins with the initiation complex, which is comprised of unc-51-like kinase 1 or 2 (ULK1 or ULK2, orthologs of yeast Atg1), mAtg13, focal adhesion kinase family-interacting protein of

200 kDa (FIP200), and Atg101 (Mizushima, 2010). When nutrients are abundant, mammalian target of rapamycin complex 1 (mTORC1) associates with and inhibits the ULK complex; under starvation conditions, mTORC1 dissociates, leading to activation of the complex (Yang & Klionsky, 2010). Biochemically, this switch to initiation is mediated by changes in phosphorylation status of the complex members. ULK complex-associated mTORC1 phosphorylates ULK1/2 and mAtg13 to inhibit autophagy; dissociation of mTORC1 leads to dephosphorylation of these proteins, allowing for ULK1/2-mediated phosphorylation of mAtg13 and FIP200 and initiation of autophagy (Hosokawa et al., 2009; Jung et al., 2009).

2.1.2 Nucleation of the Phagophore by the Class III PI3K Complex

Following activation of the ULK complex, additional proteins are recruited to form an initial double membrane structure called the phago-phore (He & Klionsky, 2009). Nucleation requires the activity of the class III phosphatidylinositol 3-kinase (PI3K) complex, which produces the phosphatidylinositol(3)-phosphate necessary for recruiting other autophagy-related proteins (Burman & Ktistakis, 2010). In humans, the class III PI3K complex includes human vacuolar protein sorting-associated protein 34 (hVps34, a lipid kinase), Beclin 1 (an ortholog of yeast Atg6), and p150 (an ortholog of yeast Vps15) (Yang & Klionsky, 2010).

Several key modulators interact with the class III PI3K complex in order to regulate autophagy at this step. Atg14-like protein (Atg14L, a homolog of yeast Atg14), also known as Beclin 1-associated autophagy-related key reg-ulator (Barkor), is believed to promote autophagy by localizing the class III PI3K complex to sites of autophagosome biogenesis via its interaction with Beclin 1 (Itakura, Kishi, Inoue, & Mizushima, 2008; Matsunaga et al., 2009; Sun et al., 2008). Another protein, ultraviolet irradiation resistance-associated gene (UVRAG, an ortholog of yeast Vps38), may also promote autophagy through its interaction with Beclin 1 (Liang et al., 2006), in addi-tion to its roles in the endocytic trafficking pathway (Itakura et al., 2008; Liang et al., 2008). The UVRAG-associated class III PI3K complex also forms a platform for the binding of Bax-interacting factor 1 (Bif-1), which is implicated in curving the phagophore membrane (Takahashi et al., 2007), and RUN domain Beclin 1-interacting and cysteine-rich containing protein (Rubicon), which negatively regulates autophagosome maturation (Matsunaga et al., 2009; Zhong et al., 2009). Other proteins which interact with Beclin 1 have been identified: activating molecule in Beclin

1-regulated autophagy (Ambra 1) promotes autophagy (Fimia et al., 2007), while the apoptosis regulator Bcl-2 (Bravo-San Pedro et al., 2015; Pattingre et al., 2005), serine/threonine-protein kinase Akt (Wang et al., 2012), and epidermal growth factor receptor are inhibitory (Wei et al., 2013).

2.1.3 Elongation of the Phagophore by the mAtg12 and LC3 Conjugation Systems

The nascent phagophore membrane is then elongated by dual interrelated conjugation systems that involve the ubiquitin-like proteins mAtg12 and mammalian orthologs of Atg8 (Nakatogawa, 2013). In one system, mAtg12 is covalently bound to mAtg5 by the E1-like activating enzyme mAtg7 and the E2-like conjugating enzyme mAtg10 (Shpilka, Mizushima, & Elazar, 2012). Next, Atg16-like 1 protein (Atg16L1, an ortholog of yeast Atg16) associates with mAtg5, ultimately forming a dimeric mAtg12–mAtg5–Atg16L1 complex (Nakatogawa, 2013; Shpilka et al., 2012). In the second system, a mammalian Atg8 ortholog is first proteolytically cleaved by a mammalian ortholog of Atg4 (Tanida, Ueno, & Kominami, 2004). Of note, mammals have four Atg4 isoforms, of which mAtg4B has the widest activity against Atg8 orthologs (Li et al., 2011). Additionally, there are at least eight mammalian Atg8 orthologs which can be subdivided into two groups: the microtubule-associated protein 1 light chain 3 (LC3) subfamily is thought to function earlier in the formation of autophagosomes, and the γ-aminobutyric acid receptor-associated protein (GABARAP) subfamily is believed to be important later during maturation (Weidberg et al., 2010). Next, LC3-I, the mAtg4-cleaved version of LC3, is activated by mAtg7 and covalently conjugated to phosphatidylethanolamine (PE) by the E2-like conjugating enzyme mAtg3 to form LC3-II (Tanida et al., 2004). At this step, the mAtg12–mAtg5–Atg16L1 complex can function as an E3-like ligase to aid in the generation of LC3-II at the growing phagophore membrane (Fujita et al., 2008; Hanada et al., 2007). Of note, Atg4 has also been demonstrated to cleave membrane-bound Atg8-PE in yeast, thereby mediating the process of deconjugation (Kirisako et al., 2000; Nair et al., 2012).

2.2 Fusion

Less is known mechanistically about how autophagosomes mature and fuse following their biogenesis. Atg2A and Atg2B are required for closure of the phagophore to form the closed autophagosome (Velikkakath, Nishimura, Oita, Ishihara, & Mizushima, 2012). Other major factors involved in mediating autophagosome maturation and fusion events include the soluble N-ethylmaleimide-sensitive factor attachment protein receptor (SNARE) family member vesicle-associated membrane protein 3 (VAMP-3) (Fader, Sánchez, Mestre, & Colombo, 2009), the small GTPase Rab7 (Gutierrez, Munafó, Berón, & Colombo, 2004; Jäger et al., 2004), and the class C Vps complex (Liang et al., 2008). Importantly, fusion of the mature autophagosome with the lysosome or early endosome is temporally regulated by the SNARE family member syntaxin-17, which is recruited to the closed autophagosome but not the open phagophore (Itakura, Kishi-Itakura, & Mizushima, 2012).

Mammalian autophagosomes may fuse directly with lysosomes to form autolysosomes in which the sequestered cargo is degraded, and/or they may generate intermediate structures called amphisomes by first fusing with endosomes (Mizushima, 2007). Evidence for involvement of the endocytic pathway came from studies in which impairment of the endosomal sorting complex required for transport (ESCRT) system, which facilitates multivesicular body formation, resulted in buildup of autophagosomes (Lee, Beigneux, Ahmad, Young, & Gao, 2007; Rusten et al., 2007) and disruption of autophagy-mediated degradation (Filimonenko et al., 2007). Furthermore, recent work identified an interaction between the ESCRT-associated protein PDCD6IP, also known as Alix, and the core autophagy regulators mAtg12 and mAtg3, which promoted both late endosome and autophagosome trafficking to the lysosome, further highlighting functional interconnections between these pathways (Murrow, Malhotra, & Debnath, 2015).

Finally, the actin and microtubule cytoskeletal networks have been found to uniquely direct autophagosome maturation in a context-dependent manner. Inhibition of actin polymerization by treatment with latrunculin impaired in vitro fusion of autophagosomes with lysosomes under full growth medium conditions but not under starvation conditions, suggesting that actin remodeling is required for autophagosome maturation in basal, but not stress-induced, autophagy (Lee et al., 2010). In addition, the microtubular network has been implicated in mediating autophagosome trafficking (Fass, Shvets, Degani, Hirschberg, & Elazar, 2006; Köchl, Hu, Chan, & Tooze, 2006; Monastyrska, Rieter, Klionsky, & Reggiori, 2009); in particular, the minus end-directed motor protein dynein is thought to facilitate translocation of autophagosomes toward lysosomes (Jahreiss, Menzies, & Rubinsztein, 2008; Kimura, Noda, & Yoshimori, 2008).

2.3 Regulation of Mammalian Autophagy

Autophagy can be modulated by various metabolic and stress signaling pathways. This section will briefly outline several key regulatory systems.

2.3.1 Nutrient and Growth Factor Starvation

Nutrient and growth factor deprivation potently upregulate autophagy through two main signaling mediators: mTORC1 and 5′-adenosine monophosphate-activated protein kinase (AMPK) (Goldsmith, Levine, & Debnath, 2014; Russell, Yuan, & Guan, 2014). mTORC1 is a central sensor of metabolic status in the cell, incorporating signals from various upstream nutrient pathways to govern cellular activity (Howell & Manning, 2011). Amino acids can activate mTORC1 via Ras-related GTP-binding protein (Rag GTPase)-facilitated transport of mTOR to the protein Ras homolog enriched in brain (Rheb), its direct activator (Sancak et al., 2008). hVps34 has also been implicated as an intermediate in amino acid-induced mTOR stimulation (Nobukuni et al., 2005). Additionally, in a colon cancer cell line, amino acids downregulated autophagy by preventing activation of Galpha-interacting protein (GAIP) by the Ras–Raf1–MEK–ERK signaling pathway (Pattingre, Bauvy, & Codogno, 2003). Growth factors can also activate mTORC1 via the class I PI3K–Akt signal transduction pathway, which relieves tuberous sclerosis complex 1/2 (TSC1/2)-dependent inhibition of Rheb activity (He & Klionsky, 2009).

AMPK plays another key metabolic role by sensing cellular energy status and upregulating autophagy in response to decreased glucose (Russell et al., 2014). Low energy states, as determined by increased levels of AMP relative to ATP, lead to activation of AMPK, which promotes TSC1/2-based inhibition of mTOR activity (Inoki, Zhu, & Guan, 2003). Additionally, AMPK may exert its effects by directly phosphorylating other proteins including regulatory-associated protein of mTOR (raptor), a member of mTORC1 (Gwinn et al., 2008), ULK1, a component of the autophagy initiation complex (Kim, Kundu, Viollet, & Guan, 2011), and Beclin 1, when associated with Atg14L in the proautophagy class III PI3K complex (Kim et al., 2013).

Additional studies indicate that starvation-induced autophagy is also tightly controlled at the transcriptional level. The transcription factor EB was shown to upregulate expression of both autophagy-related and lysosomal genes in response to nutrient starvation (Settembre et al., 2011). Moreover, starvation-dependent hepatic autophagy was found to be coordinated through competition of the nuclear receptors peroxisome proliferator-activated receptor-α (PPARα), which upregulates autophagy, and farnesoid X receptor (FXR), which suppresses autophagy, for binding to shared sites on the promoters of *ATGs* (Lee et al., 2014). Finally, Akt signaling may modulate transcriptional regulation of autophagy through Forkhead box protein O3 (FoxO3), which was shown to govern expression of several *ATGs* including *LC3B* and *ATG12* in muscle cells (Zhao et al., 2007).

2.3.2 Hypoxia

Conditions of low oxygen also contribute to regulation of autophagy, although the exact mechanisms are less well understood and may be cell type-dependent (Mazure & Pouysségur, 2010). The transcriptional regulator hypoxia-inducible factor 1 (HIF-1) has been shown to promote autophagy by increasing expression of Bcl-2/adenovirus E1B 19 kDa protein-interacting protein 3 (BNIP3) and the related BNIP3-like protein (BNIP3L), which are thought to displace Beclin 1 from the antiautophagic Bcl-2 (Bellot et al., 2009). The central stress sensor AMPK has also been connected to hypoxia-related autophagy via its regulation of TSC2 (Papandreou, Lim, Laderoute, & Denko, 2008), and platelet-derived growth factor receptor (PDGFR) was shown to modulate HIF-1 activity through autocrine signaling (Wilkinson, O'Prey, Fricker, & Ryan, 2009).

2.3.3 Oxidative Stress

The presence of reactive oxygen species (ROS) has been linked to autophagy induction through several mechanisms. For example, H_2O_2 was shown to directly inhibit mAtg4 via oxidation of its cysteine residues, thus preventing delipidation of LC3 at the growing phagophore membrane (Scherz-Shouval et al., 2007). Additionally, ROS may regulate autophagy through general mediators of the cellular response to oxidative stress. c-Jun-N-terminal kinases (JNKs) are activated under conditions of oxidative stress (Shen & Liu, 2006), and JNK isoform 1 (JNK1) was shown to block antiautophagic Bcl-2 from interacting with Beclin 1 (Wei, Pattingre, Sinha, Bassik, & Levine, 2008). Moreover, tumor suppressor p53 can also be activated by oxidative stress (Liu & Xu, 2010) and was demonstrated to indirectly block mTOR via transcriptional upregulation of Sestrins (Budanov & Karin, 2008).

targeting genes involved in autophagosome biogenesis have also been identified (Füllgrabe et al., 2014), including several which are under the transcriptional control of phosphorylated ΔNp63α (Huang, Guerrero-Preston, & Ratovitski, 2012).

2.4 Selective Capture of Autophagic Cargo in Mammals

Although autophagy was originally proposed to nonselectively degrade cytoplasmic contents, it is now recognized that autophagy is a selective process, resulting in the targeted engulfment of specific cargo such as protein aggregates and organelles. In mammals, selective autophagy is predominantly mediated by autophagy cargo receptors that act as scaffolds between cargo and the developing autophagosome via a motif called the LC3-interacting region (LIR), which mediates their binding to Atg8 isoforms (Birgisdottir, Lamark, & Johansen, 2013). For example, ubiquitinated proteins are targeted to autophagosomes via the LC3-interacting protein p62, also called Sequestosome-1 (SQSTM1) (Komatsu & Ichimura, 2010). In addition, organelles can be selectively degraded by autophagy. In mitophagy, the PTEN-induced putative protein kinase 1 (PINK1) and the E3 ubiquitin ligase Parkin mediate clearance of damaged mitochondria (Ashrafi & Schwarz, 2013). Mechanistically, PINK1-mediated phosphorylation of ubiquitin was recently implicated in activating autophagy at the mitochondria via recruitment of the autophagy receptors NDP52 and optineurin (OPTN); in this model, Parkin-mediated ubiquitination is thought to act by amplifying the phospho-ubiquitin signal (Lazarou et al., 2015). In another setting, maturing red blood cells remove their mitochondria in a process mediated by the LIR-containing protein BNIP3L, also known as NIP3-like protein X (Nix) (Ashrafi & Schwarz, 2013). Under hypoxic conditions, mitophagy is facilitated by the HIF-1-inducible factors BNIP3 and BNIP3L/Nix (Chourasia, Boland, & Macleod, 2015) as well as by another mitochondrial outer membrane protein, FUNDC1 (Liu et al., 2012). Finally, mammalian pexophagy, or peroxisome-specific autophagy, is thought to depend on the LC3-interacting autophagy receptors next to BRCA1 gene 1 protein (NBR1) (Deosaran et al., 2013) and p62/SQSTM1 (Kim, Hailey, Mullen, & Lippincott-Schwartz, 2008).

3. TUMOR-SUPPRESSIVE ROLES FOR AUTOPHAGY IN CANCER

Given the role of autophagy in cellular homeostasis, it is thought that autophagy exerts tumor-suppressive effects in cancer, particularly during

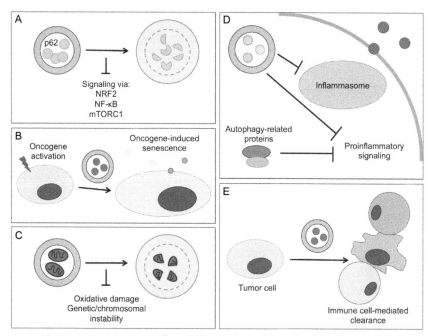

Fig. 2 The tumor-suppressive effects of autophagy. Roles for autophagy in mediating tumor suppression include: (A) degradation of p62/SQSTM1, a multidomain signaling adapter that functions upstream of multiple prosurvival and proinflammatory pathways in cancer cells; (B) facilitation of oncogene-induced senescence, a barrier to cancer progression, by enhancing the senescence-associated secretory phenotype; (C) removal of damaged proteins and mitochondria, which mitigates oxidative DNA damage and genomic instability; (D) turnover of the inflammasome and inhibition of proinflammatory signaling; and (E) maintenance of antitumor immune surveillance. (See the color plate.)

the early stages of tumorigenesis. In this section, we review the tumor-suppressive functions for autophagy and the possible mechanisms underlying these phenotypes (Fig. 2).

3.1 Genetic Basis for the Involvement of Autophagy in Tumor Suppression

Analysis of human cancers and corresponding genetic experimentation in mice have identified several autophagy-related proteins and genes that may act as tumor suppressors. *Beclin 1*, for example, was thought to be a tumor suppressor on the basis that the 17q21 chromosomal locus, where the *beclin 1* gene is located, is estimated to be deleted in up to 40% of prostate cancers, 50% of breast cancers, and 75% of ovarian cancers (Aita et al., 1999). Moreover, decreased Beclin 1 protein expression was detected in both human breast carcinoma cell lines and primary tumor tissue

(Liang et al., 1999). Subsequent genetic studies in mice implicated Beclin 1 as a haploinsufficient tumor suppressor, since *beclin 1*$^{+/-}$ mice developed spontaneous tumors at a higher rate than *beclin 1*$^{+/+}$ mice, and this was not due to loss of the wild-type allele in the tumors (Qu et al., 2003; Yue, Jin, Yang, Levine, & Heintz, 2003). Conversely, exogenous expression of *beclin 1* in *beclin 1*-deficient human MCF7 breast carcinoma cells resulted in decreased tumorigenicity upon injection into nude mice (Liang et al., 1999). Despite this genetic evidence for *beclin 1* as a tumor suppressor, particularly in mouse models, more recent work has called into question the applicability of these studies to human cancer and alternately proposed that observational loss of *beclin 1* in tumors is secondary to loss of *BRCA1*, which is also located at locus 17q21 and may instead constitute the driver mutation in these tumors (Laddha, Ganesan, Chan, & White, 2014).

Nonetheless, other studies have proposed tumor-suppressive functions for other autophagy-related genes. For example, a study of microsatellite instability-high gastric and colorectal carcinomas identified frameshift mutations in *ATG2B*, *ATG5*, and *ATG9B*, suggesting that impairment of autophagy is linked to development of these cancers (Kang et al., 2009). In mice, systemic mosaic deletion of *ATG5* resulted in the development of multiple benign tumors in the liver (Takamura et al., 2011), similar to the phenotype seen in mice with liver-specific *ATG7* deficiency (Inami et al., 2011; Takamura et al., 2011), while conditional *ATG7* deletion in hematopoietic cells in mice resulted in atypical myeloproliferation that appeared similar to human acute myeloid leukemia (Mortensen et al., 2011). Additionally, Ambra 1 was recently implicated as a haploinsufficient tumor suppressor through its ability to promote protein phosphatase 2A (PP2A)-regulated turnover of c-Myc, consistent with the finding that monoallellic *Ambra 1* deletion enhanced spontaneous liver and lung tumorigenesis in mice (Cianfanelli et al., 2015).

3.2 Inhibition of p62-Mediated Signaling Pathways

A key mechanism by which autophagy is thought to exert tumor-suppressive effects is through clearance of its substrate p62/SQSTM1 (Galluzzi et al., 2015). Under conditions of oxidative stress, p62 is transcriptionally upregulated by nuclear factor erythroid 2-related factor 2 (NRF2), a transcription factor, which mediates the cellular antioxidant response (Puissant, Fenouille, & Auberger, 2012). The p62 protein can further enhance NRF2 activity by interacting with kelch-like ECH-associated protein 1 (Keap 1), which inactivates NRF2 (Komatsu et al., 2010; Lau et al., 2010). When autophagy is impaired, however, accumulation of p62 results in overactivation of NRF2 (Komatsu et al., 2010), thereby conferring a prosurvival effect that is no longer under normal regulation. p62 also interacts with other signaling pathways, including TNF receptor-associated factor 6 (TRAF6)-facilitated activation of the prosurvival transcriptional regulator nuclear factor (NF)-κB (Moscat & Diaz-Meco, 2009) and mTORC1-mediated growth and metabolic pathways (Duran et al., 2011). In addition, p62 overexpression can enhance the growth of oncogenic class I PI3K-transformed MCF10A cells in 3D culture; in this model, p62-induced proliferation correlates with activation of mitogenic ERK signaling (Chen, Eritja, Lock, & Debnath, 2013). These studies suggest that p62 accumulation in autophagy-deficient cells may exert pro-tumorigenic effects via the coordinated activation of multiple tumor-promoting signaling pathways.

Indeed, several lines of evidence support a model in which autophagy prevents the tumorigenic effects of excess p62 accumulation. *ATG5* deficiency in Bcl-2-expressing immortalized baby mouse kidney (iBMK) cells was associated with increased stress-induced p62 accumulation relative to autophagy-competent control cells, and exogenous p62 expression resulted in increased tumor growth in an autophagy-impaired setting (Mathew et al., 2009). In a mouse model of hepatocellular adenoma, liver-specific *ATG7* deficiency was associated with p62 accumulation and colocalization with Keap 1, as well as increased NRF2 target gene expression (Inami et al., 2011). Importantly, concurrent deletion of *p62* with *ATG7* deficiency resulted in decreased liver tumor size (Takamura et al., 2011). Additionally, p62 was shown to be necessary for *Ras*-driven tumorigenesis, as *p62* deficiency in oncogenic *HRas*-expressing iBMK cells blocked tumor growth, and exogenous p62 reexpression rescued this effect (Guo et al., 2011). In humans, elevated p62 and NRF2 expression levels were detected in subsets of non-small cell lung cancer (NSCLC) cases and were associated with worse prognosis (Inoue et al., 2012). Mechanistically, besides its regulation of NRF2, p62 was also shown to be important for activation of NF-κB in *Ras*-transformed cells; accordingly, *p62* deficiency resulted in decreased tumor burden in a mouse model of activated *KRas*-induced lung cancer (Duran et al., 2008). Furthermore, while autophagy impairment by genetic deletion of the critical autophagy regulator *FIP200* inhibited tumor growth, the resulting p62 accumulation was proposed to exert tumor-promoting effects via activation of the NF-κB pathway; accordingly, tumor growth

(Coussens & Werb, 2002). One mechanism by which autophagy limits inflammation is through regulation of the inflammasome, a protein complex involved in the activation and release of inflammatory cytokines in response to both pathogen-associated molecular patterns and damage-associated molecular patterns (Deretic et al., 2013). Autophagy is primarily implicated in the control of the inflammasome pathway at two levels: degradation of the inflammasome itself (Shi et al., 2012) and clearance of substances that activate the inflammasome (Nakahira et al., 2011; Zhou, Yazdi, Menu, & Tschopp, 2011). The autophagic machinery may also prevent excessive inflammation by disrupting proinflammatory signaling cascades, such as retinoic acid-inducible gene I (RIG-I) and IFN-β promoter stimulator 1 (IPS-1)-mediated production of type I IFN (Jounai et al., 2007) as well as B-cell CLL/lymphoma 10 (Bcl-10)-regulated activation of NF-κB (Paul, Kashyap, Jia, He, & Schaefer, 2012). Finally, autophagy may limit inflammation associated with necrotic tumor cell death (Degenhardt et al., 2006). Autophagy inhibition by constitutively active *Akt* expression in *Bax/Bak*-deficient iBMK cells or by allelic *beclin 1* loss in *Bcl-2*-expressing iBMK cells led to increased necrosis in tumors formed after injection into nude mice, and a heavy macrophage infiltrate was seen in the activated *Akt*-positive, *Bax/Bak*-deficient tumors (Degenhardt et al., 2006). A proposed clinical example of how autophagy may intersect with cancer-promoting inflammation is Crohn's disease, a manifestation of inflammatory bowel disease that confers an increased risk of colorectal cancer and, in some populations, is associated with a polymorphism of *ATG16L1* that results in a threonine-to-alanine substitution (Brest et al., 2010); however, the exact mechanisms underlying this relationship are unknown.

Increasingly, failure of the immune system to adequately recognize and destroy cancer cells is also understood to be a contributing factor to the development and progression of cancer (Schreiber, Old, & Smyth, 2011). Along these lines, autophagy has been implicated in maintaining cancer immune surveillance (Ma et al., 2013). In a mouse colorectal cancer cell line, *ATG7* and *ATG5* deficiency resulted in decreased release of ATP during chemotherapy-induced cell death, and autophagy-deficient tumor cells failed to recruit dendritic cells and T-cells following chemotherapy in vivo (Michaud et al., 2011). However, when extracellular ATP concentrations were increased by co-treatment with an ecto-ATPase inhibitor, immune cell recruitment following chemotherapy was restored and tumor growth was blunted (Michaud et al., 2011). Moreover, another study found that *ATG5* deficiency in a mouse colon carcinoma cell line resulted in decreased sensitivity to IR, as indicated by greater tumor growth than autophagy-competent controls, in immunocompetent mice, which differed from the increased sensitivity seen in immunodeficient mice (Ko et al., 2014). Treatment with an ecto-ATPase inhibitor promoted lymphocyte infiltration into tumors and ablated the resistance of *ATG5*-deficient tumors in immunocompetent mice to IR, once again suggesting a role for autophagy in immunogenic cell death following cancer therapy (Ko et al., 2014). Additionally, autophagy may contribute to immune surveillance clearance of nascent tumor cells. In an oncogenic *KRas*-driven NSCLC mouse model, *ATG5* deficiency was associated with increased numbers of early hyperplastic foci as well as elevated counts of regulatory T-cells (Tregs), and antibody-mediated inhibition or depletion of Tregs lowered the numbers of hyperplastic lesions to those seen in controls (Rao et al., 2014).

3.5 Clearance of Defective Mitochondria and Maintenance of Genomic Integrity

Exposure to ROS, which can damage DNA, lipids, and proteins, is believed to cause cancer through a variety of pathways, including DNA mutagenesis and activation of pro-proliferative signaling pathways (Waris & Ahsan, 2006). Because mitochondria can serve as an intracellular source of ROS, one mechanism by which autophagy is hypothesized to exert tumor-suppressive effects is through mitophagy (Jin, 2006), although the precise role of mitophagy pathways in cancer progression remains indeterminate. In *Bcl-2*-expressing iBMK cells, heterozygous loss of *beclin 1* was associated with increased aneuploidy and chromosome structure abnormalities as well as metabolic stress-induced histone H2AX phosphorylation, consistent with a role for autophagy in maintaining genetic and/or genomic stability (Mathew et al., 2007). Further studies in these cells under conditions of metabolic stress indicated that *beclin 1* allelic loss was associated with increased levels of ROS, and *ATG5* deficiency was associated with accumulation of abnormal mitochondria (Mathew et al., 2009), supporting a link between autophagy impairment and mitochondrial dysfunction. Separately, other studies which demonstrated that *ATG* deficiencies in *Ras-* and *Braf*-driven mouse tumor models were associated with buildup of defective mitochondria found that genetic inhibition of autophagy resulted in increased tumor formation early on, although there was a protective effect against later tumor progression (Rao et al., 2014; Strohecker et al., 2013). Moreover, knockout of *NRF2* accelerated early tumorigenesis in the *Braf*-induced lung tumor model in both *ATG7*-competent and *ATG7*-deficient mice, suggesting that oxidative damage was responsible for the initial enhanced tumor growth seen in *ATG7*-deficient mice (Strohecker et al., 2013). In these studies, the possibility that the observed phenotypes were due to effects of impaired autophagy other than mitochondrial dysfunction cannot be excluded. For example, p62 aggregates, which accumulate in the absence of normal autophagy, may themselves cause oxidative damage (Komatsu et al., 2007; Mathew et al., 2009).

Tumor-suppressive roles for several of the factors involved in mitochondria-specific autophagy—including Parkin (Fujiwara et al., 2008) and Nix/BNIP3L (Fei et al., 2004)—have also been reported. Additionally, Bif-1 was also identified as a regulator of mitophagy and implicated as a tumor suppressor, as *Bif-1* haploinsufficiency was associated with accumulation of mitochondria, increased aneuploidy, and enhanced tumor development in a mouse model of B-cell lymphoma (Takahashi et al., 2013). Further research will be necessary to determine the extent to which the tumor-suppressive effects of these proteins can be attributed to their specific roles in mitophagy as opposed to their other functions in the cell.

3.6 Autophagy-Inducing Agents in Cancer Therapy

On the basis that autophagy plays multiple tumor-suppressive roles and may have cytotoxic effects, several autophagy inducers have been investigated as potential therapeutic agents in cancer, particularly in combination with other pharmacological agents or radiation therapy. For example, mTORC1 inhibitors, including rapamycin (Palumbo et al., 2012; Takeuchi et al., 2005), temsirolimus (Yazbeck et al., 2008), and everolimus (Crazzolara et al., 2009), which potently induce autophagy in addition to blocking growth and proliferation pathways downstream of mTORC1, were suggested to have therapeutic benefit against cancer cells. However, because autophagy induction can also promote cell survival and resistance to therapy, other studies have indicated that simultaneous autophagy inhibition may be required to prevent resistance to mTORC1 inhibitors (Rosich et al., 2012; Xie, White, & Mehnert, 2013). Other compounds that induce autophagy include vorinostat, a histone deacetylase (HDAC) inhibitor (Shao, Gao, Marks, & Jiang, 2004), and imatinib, a tyrosine kinase inhibitor (Ertmer et al., 2007). Overall, however, the benefit of autophagy induction during cancer therapy is unclear, given that autophagy also has multiple tumor-promoting functions including prosurvival signaling and mediating resistance to therapy.

4. TUMOR-PROMOTING ROLES FOR AUTOPHAGY IN CANCER

As a survival pathway for cells under conditions of stress, autophagy may also have tumor-promoting effects, particularly during later stages of tumor progression. This section outlines the mechanisms by which autophagy promotes tumorigenesis (Fig. 3).

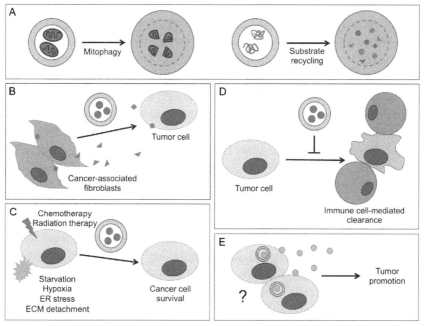

Fig. 3 The tumor-promoting effects of autophagy. Mechanisms by which autophagy contributes to cancer development and progression include: (A) maintenance of cancer cell metabolism through clearance of damaged mitochondria and recycling of metabolic substrates; (B) facilitation of interactions between cancer cells and cancer-associated fibroblasts; (C) induction of prosurvival programs in response to stresses in the tumor microenvironment and following chemotherapy and radiation therapy; (D) escape from immune surveillance; and (E) secretion of cytokines that promote tumor cell invasion and cancer stem cell function. (See the color plate.)

The mechanism by which autophagy deficits lead to mitochondrial dysfunction and impaired tumor growth, however, is unclear and may be context dependent. While some studies have implicated defective mitophagy as the cause (Guo et al., 2011; Rao et al., 2014), other studies point to impaired metabolic substrate recycling as an explanation (Guo et al., 2013; Strohecker et al., 2013; Yang et al., 2011). Indeed, a study focusing on pancreatic cancer found that while autophagy inhibition by chloroquine treatment impaired oxidative phosphorylation in a PDAC cell line, there were no meaningful increases in mitochondrial mass or mitochondrial membrane depolarization (Yang et al., 2011). Instead, pyruvate supplementation decreased the sensitivity of the cells to chloroquine, suggesting that autophagy was maintaining TCA substrate availability (Yang et al., 2011). Other studies demonstrated that glutamine supplementation rescued survival of autophagy-deficient cells under starvation conditions, further highlighting the role of autophagy in maintaining substrate homeostasis (Guo et al., 2013; Strohecker et al., 2013).

The importance of autophagy in supporting cancer metabolism also pertains to its role in facilitating glycolysis (Lock et al., 2011; Wei et al., 2011). Some cancers have been observed to undergo a shift from oxidative phosphorylation to aerobic glycolysis in the production of ATP from glucose, putatively to direct glycolytic metabolites toward biosynthetic pathways, which is known as the "Warburg effect" (Vander Heiden, Cantley, & Thompson, 2009). *ATG5* deficiency in oncogenic *HRas*-expressing mouse embryonic fibroblasts (MEFs) resulted in decreased soft agar colony formation, increased anoikis, and blunted proliferation compared to autophagy-competent controls (Lock et al., 2011). Moreover, autophagy deficiency in transformed cells was associated with decreased uptake of a glucose analog as well as reduced de novo production of lactate, while no changes in lactate production were seen between autophagy-competent and autophagy-impaired nontransformed MEFs, implicating a role for autophagy in *Ras*-associated glycolytic flux (Lock et al., 2011). Importantly, reducing the concentration of glucose in the MEF growth medium dramatically decreased the ability of autophagy-competent oncogenic *HRas*-expressing cells to form colonies in soft agar but did not affect colony formation in autophagy-impaired cells, supporting the idea that autophagy may promote the tumorigenic growth properties of *Ras*-transformed cells through mediating glycolysis (Lock et al., 2011). In addition, a study using the MMTV–PyMT mouse breast cancer model found that *FIP200* deficiency impaired autophagy, inhibited tumor formation and progression, and reduced glycolytic capability, as determined by decreased glucose analog uptake and reduced lactate production (Wei et al., 2011).

Finally, recent work indicates that autophagy-related metabolic changes in cancer are transcriptionally regulated (Perera et al., 2015). In human PDAC cell lines, nuclear import of the microphthalmia/transcription factor E (MiT/TFE) family of transcription factors, which upregulate autophagy-related and lysosomal genes, was found to be uncoupled from their normal nutrient status-dependent regulation, consistent with increased autophagy in PDAC cells compared to nontransformed pancreatic ductal epithelial cells (Perera et al., 2015). Importantly, knockdown of MiT/TFE members by shRNA impaired PDAC colony-forming ability in vitro and tumor-forming ability in vivo, an effect that could be attributed to the prosurvival role of MiT/TFE-induced autophagy in maintaining intracellular amino acid levels (Perera et al., 2015).

4.3 Survival Programs, Therapeutic Resistance, and Tumor Dormancy

Cancer cells face major intra- and extracellular challenges, including limited nutrients (Jones & Thompson, 2009), hypoxia (Höckel & Vaupel, 2001), and ER stress (Yadav, Chae, Kim, & Chae, 2014). In addition, during invasion and metastasis, tumor cells must overcome various environmental stresses including loss of contact with the extracellular matrix (ECM) (Kenific et al., 2010). As a stress-response mechanism, autophagy is thought to facilitate the survival of cancer cells under these conditions. Under ischemia-simulating conditions of low oxygen and glucose depletion, genetic inhibition of autophagy by siRNA-mediated targeting of *beclin 1* reduced survival of both *Bax/Bak*-deficient iBMK cells and *Bcl-x_L*- or *Bcl-2*-expressing HeLa cells, suggesting that autophagy promotes survival of apoptosis-resistant cells during metabolic stress (Degenhardt et al., 2006). Additionally, there is evidence that autophagy is induced in regions of tumors subject to hypoxia, as indicated by the presence of punctate LC3 in the unvascularized central area of early *Bax/Bak*-deficient iBMK cell-derived tumors (Degenhardt et al., 2006) and acinar LC3 membrane translocation in 3D culture of *Bcl-2*-expressing immortalized mouse mammary epithelial cells (Karantza-Wadsworth et al., 2007). Cancer cells are also subject to heavy ER stress due to the increase in protein synthesis and folding required of rapidly proliferating cells (Yadav et al., 2014), and autophagy may play a role in promoting cancer cell survival under these conditions through its involvement in the unfolded protein response

(Hart et al., 2012). PERK-mediated autophagy was found to be important for the survival of cells undergoing c–Myc-induced ER stress, as pharmacologic inhibition of autophagy via bafilomycin A1 and genetic inhibition via *ULK1*-targeting siRNA and *ATG5* deletion in MEFs resulted in increased PARP cleavage relative to autophagy-competent controls upon activation of c–Myc (Hart et al., 2012).

In addition to responding to these metabolic and biosynthetic challenges, autophagy may also promote survival under environmental changes encountered during cancer progression and metastasis. Autophagy was induced when human mammary epithelial cells were cultured in suspension, and inhibition via siRNA knockdown of *ATG5*, *ATG7*, and *beclin 1* led to increased anoikis, or apoptosis of suspended cells, as indicated by greater caspase-3 cleavage and decreased clonogenic replating efficiency (Fung, Lock, Gao, Salas, & Debnath, 2008), suggesting that autophagy may be important for cell survival during ECM detachment and invasion, a crucial event in the progression to metastasis. Moreover, in vivo, autophagy inhibition by *FIP200* deletion was associated with decreased metastases to the lung in the MMTV–PyMT mouse breast cancer model (Wei et al., 2011), consistent with a role for autophagy in metastatic progression.

In addition, cancer therapy constitutes another major source of cellular stressors, including genotoxic and replicative stress, inhibition of growth and proliferative signaling pathways, and induction of metabolic stress. Given its cytoprotective role, autophagy has been implicated in mediating resistance to various types of treatment, including antiangiogenics (Hu et al., 2012), antiestrogens (Schoenlein, Periyasamy-Thandavan, Samaddar, Jackson, & Barrett, 2009), antiandrogens (Nguyen et al., 2014), cytotoxic agents (Ding et al., 2011; Fukuda et al., 2015; Paillas et al., 2012; Zhang et al., 2012), combined PI3K/mTOR (Mirzoeva et al., 2011) and Akt/mTOR (Rosich et al., 2012) inhibitors, protein kinase inhibitors (Bellodi et al., 2009; Han et al., 2011; Levy et al., 2014; Zou et al., 2013), and radiation therapy (Apel et al., 2008). These findings suggest that inhibition of autophagy may sensitize cancer cells to cancer therapy, at least in certain contexts.

An important feature of cancer is tumor dormancy, a period during which disease is clinically undetectable following treatment despite the persistence of cancer cells that may later give rise to relapse and metastatic disease (Yeh & Ramaswamy, 2015). Quiescence, or reversible cell cycle arrest in G0, is thought to permit survival and drug resistance of cancer cells during the dormant state (Aguirre-Ghiso, 2007), and autophagy has been implicated in mediating tumor dormancy (Sosa, Bragado, Debnath, & Aguirre-Ghiso, 2013). In a study of ovarian cancer, aplasia Ras homolog member I (ARHI, also called Di-Ras3) was found to regulate tumor dormancy via activation of autophagy (Lu et al., 2008). Additionally, autophagy was implicated in the quiescence-mediated resistance of gastrointestinal stromal tumors to the tyrosine kinase inhibitor imatinib, which prevents the progression of these tumors but is usually not curative (Gupta et al., 2010). Finally, there is evidence suggesting that autophagy supports the cancer stem cell phenotype (Galluzzi et al., 2015; Gong et al., 2013; Viale et al., 2014), which is thought to contribute to both tumor initiation and relapse (Clarke et al., 2006). Indeed, the role of autophagy in stem cells has been intensively studied; a detailed review of this area is available elsewhere (Guan et al., 2013).

4.4 Interaction with the Tumor Microenvironment

Increasingly, it is understood that cancer progression depends not just on the proliferation of cancer cells alone but also crucially on their interactions with other players in the tumor microenvironment, including fibroblasts, immune cells, pericytes, and endothelial cells (Pietras & Östman, 2010). These stromal components are thought to contribute to cancer progression by promoting angiogenesis, remodeling the ECM, facilitating immune surveillance escape, and secreting growth factors, among other mechanisms (Quail & Joyce, 2013). For example, autophagy is thought to mediate crucial metabolic changes in cancer-associated fibroblasts (CAFs) that promote tumor progression through metabolic coupling of stromal cells and cancer cells (Martinez-Outschoorn, Sotgia, & Lisanti, 2014). In this model, autophagy is induced in CAFs upon oxidative stress from neighboring cancer cells, resulting in a feed-forward loop involving downregulation of caveolin-1 (Cav-1) and generation of oxidative damage that leads to mitochondrial defects and mitophagy (Martinez-Outschoorn, Balliet, et al., 2010; Martinez-Outschoorn, Trimmer, et al., 2010; Pavlides et al., 2012). The subsequent shift to glycolysis in CAFs results in the release of metabolites such as lactate, which can be used by cancer cells for mitochondrial oxidative phosphorylation to support anabolism (Martinez-Outschoorn et al., 2014). Additionally, Cav-1 knockdown in fibroblasts was also shown to protect co-cultured breast cancer cells from apoptosis (Martinez-Outschoorn, Trimmer, et al., 2010), constituting another mechanism by which CAFs may promote cancer cell survival. Loss of stromal

Cav-1 is associated with poor prognosis in several cancer types including breast cancer (Witkiewicz et al., 2009), prostate cancer (Di Vizio et al., 2009), and colorectal cancer (Zhao et al., 2015). Therefore, at least in certain contexts, autophagy is hypothesized to promote tumor progression through the loss of Cav-1 in CAFs. Moreover, because autophagy contributes to senescence (Young et al., 2009) and senescence-associated secretion of extracellular proteases and inflammatory cytokines by fibroblasts may be tumorigenic (Coppé, Desprez, Krtolica, & Campisi, 2010), another tumor-promoting role for autophagy is thought to be the maintenance of senescent stromal cells.

Additionally, autophagy may modulate tumor cell interactions with the immune system to create a protumorigenic environment. Under conditions of hypoxia, lung carcinoma cells displayed decreased killing by cytotoxic T-lymphocytes (CTLs) and increased autophagy, and siRNA knockdown of *ATG5* and *beclin 1* reversed the resistance of these cells to CTL-mediated lysis (Noman et al., 2011), implicating autophagy as a protective mechanism during hypoxic stress. Similarly, induction of epithelial-to-mesenchymal transition (EMT) in a breast cancer cell line was associated with decreased cytotoxic killing by a CTL clone as well as increased autophagic flux, and inhibition of autophagy via siRNA against *beclin 1* partially restored CTL-mediated killing of these cells (Akalay et al., 2013), suggesting that autophagy may facilitate invasion and metastasis by protecting cells undergoing EMT. Furthermore, in an MMTV–PyMT mouse model of breast cancer where *FIP200* deletion was associated with decreased cancer development, an increased IFN-γ^+CD4$^+$ and IFN-γ^+CD8$^+$ T-cell infiltrate was seen in *FIP200*-null tumors, consistent with an increased production of T-cell chemo-attractants including CXCL10 (Wei et al., 2011). Importantly, antibody-mediated depletion of CD8$^+$ T-cells in these mice resulted in earlier tumor formation, suggesting that the tumor-suppressive effects of *FIP200* deletion were at least in part due to increased immune surveillance (Wei et al., 2011). Taken together, these findings suggest that autophagy exerts tumor-promoting effects by facilitating cancer cell escape from immune cell-mediated clearance.

4.5 Autophagy-Inhibiting Agents in Cancer Therapy

Inhibition of autophagy is currently an attractive therapeutic strategy, given the multiple tumor-promoting effects of autophagy in cancer. In vitro studies suggest that the use of antimalarials such as chloroquine and its derivative hydroxychloroquine, both of which block lysosomal acidification, may have therapeutic benefit in cancer (Rahim & Strobl, 2009), and several clinical trials have investigated these agents (Duffy, Le, Sausville, & Emadi, 2015). Antimalarials may be particularly useful in combination with other agents to prevent autophagy-mediated therapeutic resistance, as suggested by phase I studies investigating the use of hydroxychloroquine in combination with bortezomib, a proteasome inhibitor (Vogl et al., 2014), temsirolimus, an mTORC1 inhibitor (Rangwala, Chang, et al., 2014), vorinostat, an HDAC inhibitor (Mahalingam et al., 2014), or temozolomide, a DNA-damaging agent (Rangwala, Leone, et al., 2014). However, a separate phase I/II study found that the addition of hydroxychloroquine at the maximum tolerated dose in combination with temozolomide and radiation therapy did not enhance overall survival, indicating a need for investigating other autophagy inhibitors and/or dosing regimens (Rosenfeld et al., 2014). Additionally, there is also evidence that chloroquine may act on pathways in cancer cells that do not depend on autophagy (Maes et al., 2014; Maycotte et al., 2012). Notably, recent evidence suggests that, in addition to autophagy, the inhibition of the oxidative pentose phosphate pathway may be an important regulator of tumor cell death induced by antimalarials (Salas, Roy, Marsh, Rubin, & Debnath, 2015). Finally, bafilomycin A1, which blocks autophagosome-to-lysosome fusion, was also suggested to have utility in cancer treatment via inhibition of autophagy (Kanematsu et al., 2010; Kanzawa et al., 2004).

5. NEW INTERSECTIONS BETWEEN AUTOPHAGY AND SECRETION

Although autophagy is classically considered a degradative pathway, recent findings suggest that it may also have secretory functions. This section overviews the role of autophagy in protein secretion and discusses emerging research on the contributions of secretory autophagy to cancer.

5.1 Evidence for Autophagy-Dependent Secretion

A growing body of work has identified a nondegradative function for autophagy in both conventional and unconventional protein secretion (Ponpuak et al., 2015). In conventional secretion, proteins containing an N-terminal signal peptide are directed to the ER for folding and subsequently modified in the Golgi apparatus before being released from the cell (Sakaguchi, 1997). Autophagy has been implicated in the secretion of various substances considered to follow the conventional pathway, including IL-6 and IL-8 by senescent fibroblasts (Young et al., 2009), cathepsin K by osteoclasts (DeSelm et al., 2011), and von Willebrand factor by endothelial cells (Torisu et al., 2013). Cells can also utilize unconventional pathways to secrete leaderless proteins, which do not contain a signal peptide, as well as signal peptide–containing proteins that exit the cell by alternate routes (Nickel & Rabouille, 2009).

Two seminal studies in yeast focusing on the secretion of acyl coenzyme A-binding protein (Acb1), which lacks a signal peptide and is released upon starvation conditions, offered early evidence for a genetic link between autophagy and unconventional secretion (Duran, Anjard, Stefan, Loomis, & Malhotra, 2010; Manjithaya, Anjard, Loomis, & Subramani, 2010). In *Saccharomyces cerevisiae* and *Pichia pastoris*, deletion of autophagy-related genes led to impaired Acb1 secretion (Duran et al., 2010; Manjithaya et al., 2010). Because the deletion of genes involved in autophagosome-to-vacuole fusion did not impact Acb1 secretion, these findings suggested that the early autophagosome formation machinery contributes to the secretory rather than degradative handling of Acb1 (Duran et al., 2010; Manjithaya et al., 2010). In mammals, the secretion of the inflammatory cytokine IL-1β was also linked to autophagy (Dupont et al., 2011). The proform of IL-1β lacks a signal peptide, and yet the cleaved, active form of IL-1β is potently secreted by macrophages and monocytes upon activation of the inflammasome (Lopez-Castejon & Brough, 2011). In murine bone marrow–derived macrophage (BMM) cells, IL-1β secretion after inflammasome stimulation was dependent on starvation-induced autophagy, as BMMs from *ATG5*-deficient mice showed decreased secretion (Dupont et al., 2011). The same study found that the release of IL-18 and HMGB1 from cells after inflammasome stimulation was also regulated by autophagy (Dupont et al., 2011).

The biochemical relationship between autophagy and secretion remains unclear. It is not definitively known if the vesicles that traffic secretory cargo are autophagosomes *sensu stricto*, autophagosome-like structures specialized for secretion, or a different class of vesicle altogether. Remarkably, a recent study using a nonmacrophage reconstitution system demonstrated that IL-1β secretion genetically required *ATG*s but proceeded via its translocation into a distinct vesicular intermediate instead of its engulfment and sequestration into a classical autophagosome (Zhang, Kenny, Ge, Xu, & Schekman, 2015). Moreover, while genetic evidence in yeast suggests that endosomal elements are involved in autophagy-dependent unconventional secretion (Duran et al., 2010), the specific fusion and/or engulfment events are unknown. Indeed, the mechanisms underlying unconventional secretion in general are not well understood and, in fact, appear to encompass several trafficking routes which may or may not involve autophagy (Rabouille, Malhotra, & Nickel, 2012; Zhang & Schekman, 2013). Another consideration is whether autophagy can mediate the unconventional secretion of proteins that are typically secreted via conventional pathways and, if so, under what conditions this occurs. For example, although not secreted from the cell per se, the cystic fibrosis transmembrane conductance regulator ion channel was found to traffic to the cell membrane in an autophagy-dependent manner upon ER-to-Golgi blockade (Gee, Noh, Tang, Kim, & Lee, 2011). Finally, it is also possible that autophagy plays an indirect role in secretion, such as by regulating the turnover of other proteins more directly involved in secretory pathways.

5.2 Emerging Roles for Autophagy-Dependent Secretion in Cancer

Tumors are highly secretory entities, a property that is hypothesized to contribute to several pathophysiological processes leading to cancer progression, including recruitment of fibroblasts and immune cells to the tumor microenvironment, stimulation of angiogenesis, development of proinvasive properties, and influencing distant tissues to facilitate metastasis, among others (Paltridge, Belle, & Khew-Goodall, 2013). Interestingly, an analysis of several breast cancer cell lines revealed that a large portion of the proteins detected in the conditioned media from these cells appeared to be secreted unconventionally (Villarreal et al., 2013). Moreover, there is increasing evidence that cancer cells interact with each other via a class of structures collectively termed extracellular vesicles (Vader, Breakefield, & Wood, 2014), constituting another form of cancer-related secretion. Additionally, as discussed earlier, fibroblasts may foster tumor progression through senescence-associated secretion (Coppé et al., 2010). Given the emerging literature surrounding autophagy-dependent secretion, it appears that the effects of autophagy in cancer are not limited to its degradative function in survival and homeostasis but, rather, may also include its secretory function.

Recently, autophagy was shown to be required for the secretion of Ras-associated proinvasive factors (Lock, Kenific, Leidal, Salas, & Debnath, 2014). Mammary epithelial cells expressing oncogenic HRas displayed an invasive phenotype in 3D culture, which was suppressed upon inhibition of autophagy by shRNA knockdown of *ATG7* or *ATG12* (Lock et al., 2014). While autophagy-deficient *HRas*-transformed cells formed spherical structures when cultured alone, they formed invasive protrusions when co-cultured with autophagy-competent *HRas*-transformed cells or when treated with conditioned media from the autophagy-competent cells, suggesting that secreted factors were influencing the invasive morphogenesis of these cells (Lock et al., 2014). Indeed, the proinvasive cytokine IL-6 was found to be secreted from these cells in an autophagy-dependent manner, as *ATG* knockdown reduced detection of IL-6 in conditioned media from *HRas*-transformed cell cultures but did not reduce IL-6 mRNA or protein expression levels in these cells (Lock et al., 2014). In 3D culture, antibody inhibition of IL-6 in conditioned media from autophagy-proficient trans-formed cells blocked the formation of invasive protrusions by autophagy-impaired transformed cells, while addition of recombinant IL-6 was sufficient to induce invasive protrusions by autophagy-deficient cells (Lock et al., 2014). These findings point to a role for secretory autophagy in mediating *Ras*-driven invasion in vitro.

Mechanistically, a distinction should be made between what appears to be autophagy-dependent secretion per se and autophagy-dependent pro-duction of secreted factors. In the same study of *HRas*-transformed mam-mary epithelial cells, matrix metalloproteinase-2 (MMP2) and Wnt-5a were also determined to influence invasive morphology through their release into conditioned media, as treatment of autophagy-competent onco-genic *HRas*-expressing cells with an MMP2 inhibitor blunted protrusion formation, and treatment of autophagy-impaired *HRas*-transformed cells with recombinant Wnt-5a induced their formation (Lock et al., 2014). Importantly, the mRNA and protein expression levels of MMP2 and Wnt-5a in these cells were reduced by *ATG* knockdown, implying that their intracellular production was autophagy-dependent (Lock et al., 2014). Similarly, in a separate study utilizing lung cancer cell lines, autophagy induction via activation of TLRs led to increased detection of proinvasive and promigratory cytokines, including IL-6, CCL2, CCL20, VEGFA, and MMP2, in the supernatants of cultured cells, and treatment with neutralizing antibodies reduced invasion and migration in vitro (Zhan et al., 2014). Pharmacological inhibition of autophagy by treatment with 3-methyladenine reduced mRNA expression of these cytokines (Zhan et al., 2014), suggesting that autophagy was regulating the intracellular pro-duction of these factors as well. A subsequent study found that autophagy modulation also affected the production of IL-6 by breast cancer cells, albeit with somewhat differing results (Maycotte, Jones, Goodall, Thorburn, & Thorburn, 2015). In an autophagy-dependent cancer cell line, *ATG7* and *beclin 1* knockdown decreased extracellular IL-6 detection in the media, while in an autophagy-independent cancer cell line, extracellular IL-6 detection was increased upon autophagy inhibition (Maycotte et al., 2015), indicating that the relationship between autophagy and the production of secreted factors may vary depending on the cellular context. Functionally, IL-6 was found to be important for the formation of mammospheres in the autophagy-dependent cell line, as both IL-6 treatment and conditioned media from autophagy-competent cells partially rescued the decrease in mammosphere formation seen in *ATG7*-deficient cells (Maycotte et al., 2015). Additionally, a separate study found that in cancer stem cells, the release of exosomes, which can mediate intercellular communication, coincided with the activation of autophagy (Kumar, Gupta, Shankar, & Srivastava, 2015). Finally, a recent proteomic study uncovered multiple new secreted factors that may reflect autophagy dynamics in melanoma cells (Kraya et al., 2015). Notably, these experiments did not distinguish whether any of the differentially secreted proteins actually arose from altered autophagy-dependent secretion vs secondary changes in transcriptional or translational programs following autophagy inhibition. Nevertheless, several secreted products identified in this study showed promise as serum biomarkers of autophagic status in human melanoma patients (Kraya et al., 2015). The need for clinical biomarkers to dynamically monitor autophagy during therapy remains a major unmet clinical challenge in targeting autophagy against cancer; accordingly, this study highlighted the promise of autophagy-dependent secreted factors in this regard (Kraya et al., 2015). Overall, these studies indicate that autophagy may influence tumor-promoting secretory phenotypes in cancer cells, although further work will be necessary to better understand the multiple levels at which this occurs.

Although the literature on the role of autophagy-dependent secretion in cancer is limited, it raises important questions for reexamining previous work as well as conducting new experiments. Are the phenotypes seen in autophagy-deficient tumor models, for example, related only to degradative autophagy or can secretory autophagy also explain these effects? Does autophagy have differing roles in secretion in cancer cells vs other components of the tumor microenvironment, such as fibroblasts and immune cells? Attention should be paid to the selective modulation of autophagy in specific cellular compartments, as this may impact the generation of different secretory phenotypes in a cell type-dependent manner. Future studies conducted through this new lens will provide additional insight into the complex relationship between autophagy and cancer.

6. CONCLUDING REMARKS AND PERSPECTIVES

The studies above attest to the complex and, in certain instances, controversial functions of autophagy during cancer initiation and progression. Because of the highly dynamic nature of the autophagy trafficking process and its intricate regulation by diverse stimuli and signals, innumerable pathways have been delineated by which cancer cells can either activate or inhibit autophagy for their benefit. Nevertheless, defining the molecular contexts in which to inhibit vs activate autophagy in cancer remains an active and vibrant area of research. Moreover, these fundamental studies of autophagy in cancer continue to harbor immense clinical significance because of the enormous interest in modulating autophagy in the clinical oncology setting. Indeed, we still have much to learn about how autophagy impacts cancer progression and how to most effectively exploit this pathway for anticancer treatment. For example, for over a decade, we have largely viewed autophagy as a degradation pathway that promotes tumor cell survival and metabolic adaptation during stress; now, studies linking autophagy to secretion have begun to illuminate a completely new non-cell autonomous role for autophagy in tumorigenesis. Elucidating the cellular mechanisms underlying autophagy-dependent secretion may provide insight into new therapeutic strategies for modulating autophagy in cancer. For example, if autophagy-dependent secretion occurs by a mechanism separate from degradative autophagy, then blocking secretion by cancer cells may require pharmacological agents distinct from chloroquine and its derivatives, which inhibit downstream lysosomal activity in canonical degradative autophagy. As we continue to unravel these new facets of the autophagy pathway in both normal and cancerous cells, we may reveal new opportunities for the specific targeting of autophagy-dependent phenotypes in cancer.

ACKNOWLEDGMENTS

J.D. is supported by the NIH (CA126792, CA188404), the DOD BCRP (W81XWH-11-1-0130), and the Samuel Waxman Cancer Research Foundation.

REFERENCES

Abedin, M. J., Wang, D., McDonnell, M. A., Lehmann, U., & Kelekar, A. (2007). Autophagy delays apoptotic death in breast cancer cells following DNA damage. *Cell Death and Differentiation, 14*(3), 500–510. http://www.nature.com/cdd/journal/v14/n3/suppinfo/4402039s1.html.

Aguirre-Ghiso, J. A. (2007). Models, mechanisms and clinical evidence for cancer dormancy. *Nature Reviews. Cancer, 7*(11), 834–846. Retrieved from, http://dx.doi.org/10.1038/nrc2256.

Aita, V. M., Liang, X. H., Murty, V. V. V. S., Pincus, D. L., Yu, W., Cayanis, E., ... Levine, B. (1999). Cloning and genomic organization of beclin 1, a candidate tumor suppressor gene on chromosome 17q21. *Genomics, 59*(1), 59–65. http://dx.doi.org/10.1006/geno.1999.5851.

Akalay, I., Janji, B., Hasmim, M., Noman, M. Z., André, F., De Cremoux, P., ... Chouaib, S. (2013). Epithelial-to-mesenchymal transition and autophagy induction in breast carcinoma promote escape from T-cell–mediated lysis. *Cancer Research, 73*(8), 2418–2427. http://dx.doi.org/10.1158/0008-5472.can-12-2432.

Apel, A., Herr, I., Schwarz, H., Rodemann, H. P., & Mayer, A. (2008). Blocked autophagy sensitizes resistant carcinoma cells to radiation therapy. *Cancer Research, 68*(5), 1485–1494. http://dx.doi.org/10.1158/0008-5472.CAN-07-0562.

Artal-Martinez de Narvajas, A., Gomez, T. S., Zhang, J. S., Mann, A. O., Taoda, Y., Gorman, J. A., ... Billadeau, D. D. (2013). Epigenetic regulation of autophagy by the methyltransferase G9a. *Molecular and Cellular Biology, 33*(20), 3983–3993. http://dx.doi.org/10.1128/MCB.00813-13.

Ashrafi, G., & Schwarz, T. L. (2013). The pathways of mitophagy for quality control and clearance of mitochondria. *Cell Death and Differentiation, 20*(1), 31–42. Retrieved from, http://dx.doi.org/10.1038/cdd.2012.81.

Bellodi, C., Lidonnici, M. R., Hamilton, A., Helgason, G. V., Soliera, A. R., Ronchetti, M., ... Calabretta, B. (2009). Targeting autophagy potentiates tyrosine kinase inhibitor–induced cell death in Philadelphia chromosome positive cells, including primary CML stem cells. *The Journal of Clinical Investigation, 119*(5), 1109–1123. http://dx.doi.org/10.1172/JCI35660.

Bellot, G., Garcia-Medina, R., Gounon, P., Chiche, J., Roux, D., Pouysségur, J., & Mazure, N. M. (2009). Hypoxia-induced autophagy is mediated through hypoxia-inducible factor induction of BNIP3 and BNIP3L via their BH3 domains. *Molecular and Cellular Biology, 29*(10), 2570–2581. http://dx.doi.org/10.1128/mcb.00166-09.

Birgisdottir, Å. B., Lamark, T., & Johansen, T. (2013). The LIR motif—Crucial for selective autophagy. *Journal of Cell Science, 126*(15), 3237–3247. Retrieved from, http://jcs.biologists.org/content/126/15/3237.abstract.

Bravo-San Pedro, J. M., Wei, Y., Sica, V., Maiuri, M. C., Zou, Z., Kroemer, G., & Levine, B. (2015). BAX and BAK1 are dispensable for ABT-737-induced dissociation of the BCL2-BECN1 complex and autophagy. *Autophagy, 11*(3), 452–459. http://dx.doi.org/10.1080/15548627.2015.1017191.

Brest, P., Corcelle, E. A., Cesaro, A., Chargui, A., Belaïd, A., Klionsky, D. J., ... Mograbi, B. (2010). Autophagy and Crohn's disease: At the crossroads of infection, inflammation, immunity, and cancer. *Current Molecular Medicine, 10*(5), 486–502. Retrieved from, http://www.ncbi.nlm.nih.gov/pmc/articles/PMC3655526/.

Bristol, M. L., Di, X., Beckman, M. J., Wilson, E. N., Henderson, S. C., Maiti, A., ... Gewirtz, D. A. (2012). Dual functions of autophagy in the response of breast tumor cells to radiation. *Autophagy, 8*(5), 739–753. http://dx.doi.org/10.4161/auto.19313.

Budanov, A. V., & Karin, M. (2008). p53 target genes sestrin1 and sestrin2 connect genotoxic stress and mTOR signaling. *Cell, 134*(3), 451–460. http://dx.doi.org/10.1016/j.cell.2008.06.028.

Burman, C., & Ktistakis, N. T. (2010). Regulation of autophagy by phosphatidylinositol 3-phosphate. *FEBS Letters*, *584*(7), 1302–1312. http://dx.doi.org/10.1016/j.febslet.2010.01.011.

Chakradeo, S., Sharma, K., Alhaddad, A., Bakhshwin, D., Le, N., Harada, H., … Gewirtz, D. A. (2015). Yet another function of p53—The switch that determines whether radiation-induced autophagy will be cytoprotective or nonprotective: Implications for autophagy inhibition as a therapeutic strategy. *Molecular Pharmacology*, *87*(5), 803–814. http://dx.doi.org/10.1124/mol.114.095273.

Chen, N., Eritja, N., Lock, R., & Debnath, J. (2013). Autophagy restricts proliferation driven by oncogenic phosphatidylinositol 3-kinase in three-dimensional culture. *Oncogene*, *32*(20), 2543–2554. http://dx.doi.org/10.1038/onc.2012.277.

Choi, A. M. K., Ryter, S. W., & Levine, B. (2013). Autophagy in human health and disease. *New England Journal of Medicine*, *368*(7), 651–662. http://dx.doi.org/10.1056/NEJMra1205406.

Choudhury, S., Kolukula, V. K., Preet, A., Albanese, C., & Avantaggiati, M. L. (2013). Dissecting the pathways that destabilize mutant p53: The proteasome or autophagy? *Cell Cycle*, *12*(7), 1022–1029. http://dx.doi.org/10.4161/cc.24128.

Chourasia, A. H., Boland, M. L., & Macleod, K. F. (2015). Mitophagy and cancer. *Cancer & Metabolism*, *3*, 4. http://dx.doi.org/10.1186/s40170-015-0130-8.

Cianfanelli, V., Fuoco, C., Lorente, M., Salazar, M., Quondamatteo, F., Gherardini, P. F., … Cecconi, F. (2015). AMBRA1 links autophagy to cell proliferation and tumorigenesis by promoting c-Myc dephosphorylation and degradation. *Nature Cell Biology*, *17*(1), 20–30. http://dx.doi.org/10.1038/ncb3072. http://www.nature.com/ncb/journal/v17/n1/abs/ncb3072.html. supplementary-information.

Clarke, M. F., Dick, J. E., Dirks, P. B., Eaves, C. J., Jamieson, C. H. M., Jones, D. L., … Wahl, G. M. (2006). Cancer stem cells—Perspectives on current status and future directions: AACR Workshop on cancer stem cells. *Cancer Research*, *66*(19), 9339–9344. http://dx.doi.org/10.1158/0008-5472.can-06-3126.

Collado, M., & Serrano, M. (2010). Senescence in tumours: Evidence from mice and humans. *Nature Reviews. Cancer*, *10*(1), 51–57. Retrieved from, http://dx.doi.org/10.1038/nrc2772.

Coppé, J.-P., Desprez, P.-Y., Krtolica, A., & Campisi, J. (2010). The senescence-associated secretory phenotype: The dark side of tumor suppression. *Annual Review of Pathology*, *5*, 99–118. http://dx.doi.org/10.1146/annurev-pathol-121808-102144.

Courtois-Cox, S., Jones, S. L., & Cichowski, K. (2008). Many roads lead to oncogene-induced senescence. *Oncogene*, *27*(20), 2801–2809. Retrieved from, http://dx.doi.org/10.1038/sj.onc.1210950.

Coussens, L. M., & Werb, Z. (2002). Inflammation and cancer. *Nature*, *420*(6917), 860–867. Retrieved from, http://dx.doi.org/10.1038/nature01322.

Crazzolara, R., Cisterne, A., Thien, M., Hewson, J., Baraz, R., Bradstock, K. F., & Bendall, L. J. (2009). Potentiating effects of RAD001 (Everolimus) on vincristine therapy in childhood acute lymphoblastic leukemia. *Blood*, *113*(14), 3297–3306. http://dx.doi.org/10.1182/blood-2008-02-137752.

Crighton, D., Wilkinson, S., O'Prey, J., Syed, N., Smith, P., Harrison, P. R., … Ryan, K. M. (2006). DRAM, a p53-induced modulator of autophagy, is critical for apoptosis. *Cell*, *126*(1), 121–134. http://dx.doi.org/10.1016/j.cell.2006.05.034.

Cuervo, A. M., & Wong, E. (2014). Chaperone-mediated autophagy: Roles in disease and aging. *Cell Research*, *24*(1), 92–104. http://dx.doi.org/10.1038/cr.2013.153.

Degenhardt, K., Mathew, R., Beaudoin, B., Bray, K., Anderson, D., Chen, G., … White, E. (2006). Autophagy promotes tumor cell survival and restricts necrosis, inflammation, and tumorigenesis. *Cancer Cell*, *10*(1), 51–64. http://dx.doi.org/10.1016/j.ccr.2006.06.001.

Deosaran, E., Larsen, K. B., Hua, R., Sargent, G., Wang, Y., Kim, S., ... Kim, P. K. (2013). NBR1 acts as an autophagy receptor for peroxisomes. *Journal of Cell Science, 126*(4), 939–952. http://dx.doi.org/10.1242/jcs.114819.

Deretic, V., Saitoh, T., & Akira, S. (2013). Autophagy in infection, inflammation and immunity. *Nature Reviews. Immunology, 13*(10), 722–737. http://dx.doi.org/10.1038/nri3532.

DeSelm, Carl J., Miller, Brian C., Zou, W., Beatty, Wandy L., van Meel, E., Takahata, Y., ... Virgin, H. W. (2011). Autophagy proteins regulate the secretory component of osteoclastic bone resorption. *Developmental Cell, 21*(5), 966–974. http://dx.doi.org/10.1016/j.devcel.2011.08.016.

Di Vizio, D., Morello, M., Sotgia, F., Pestell, R. G., Freeman, M. R., & Lisanti, M. P. (2009). An absence of stromal caveolin-1 is associated with advanced prostate cancer, metastatic disease and epithelial Akt activation. *Cell cycle (Georgetown, TX), 8*(15), 2420–2424. Retrieved from, http://www.ncbi.nlm.nih.gov/pmc/articles/PMC2927821/.

Ding, Z.-B., Hui, B., Shi, Y.-H., Zhou, J., Peng, Y.-F., Gu, C.-Y., ... Fan, J. (2011). Autophagy activation in hepatocellular carcinoma contributes to the tolerance of oxaliplatin via reactive oxygen species modulation. *Clinical Cancer Research, 17*(19), 6229–6238. http://dx.doi.org/10.1158/1078-0432.ccr-11-0816.

Dou, Z., Xu, C., Donahue, G., Shimi, T., Pan, J. A., Zhu, J., ... Berger, S. L. (2015). Autophagy mediates degradation of nuclear lamina. *Nature, 527*(7576), 105–109. http://dx.doi.org/10.1038/nature15548.

Duffy, A., Le, J., Sausville, E., & Emadi, A. (2015). Autophagy modulation: A target for cancer treatment development. *Cancer Chemotherapy and Pharmacology, 75*(3), 439–447. http://dx.doi.org/10.1007/s00280-014-2637-z.

Dupont, N., Jiang, S., Pilli, M., Ornatowski, W., Bhattacharya, D., & Deretic, V. (2011). Autophagy-based unconventional secretory pathway for extracellular delivery of IL-1β. *The EMBO Journal, 30*(23), 4701–4711. http://dx.doi.org/10.1038/emboj.2011.398.

Duran, A., Amanchy, R., Linares, Juan F., Joshi, J., Abu-Baker, S., Porollo, A., ... Diaz-Meco, Maria T. (2011). p62 is a key regulator of nutrient sensing in the mTORC1 pathway. *Molecular Cell, 44*(1), 134–146. http://dx.doi.org/10.1016/j.molcel.2011.06.038.

Duran, J. M., Anjard, C., Stefan, C., Loomis, W. F., & Malhotra, V. (2010). Unconventional secretion of Acb1 is mediated by autophagosomes. *The Journal of Cell Biology, 188*(4), 527–536. http://dx.doi.org/10.1083/jcb.200911154.

Duran, A., Linares, J. F., Galvez, A. S., Wikenheiser, K., Flores, J. M., Diaz-Meco, M. T., & Moscat, J. (2008). The signaling adaptor p62 is an important NF-κB mediator in tumorigenesis. *Cancer Cell, 13*(4), 343–354. http://dx.doi.org/10.1016/j.ccr.2008.02.001.

Eng, C. H., Wang, Z., Tkach, D., Toral-Barza, L., Ugwonali, S., Liu, S., ... Nyfeler, B. (2016). Macroautophagy is dispensable for growth of KRAS mutant tumors and chloroquine efficacy. *Proceedings of the National Academy of Sciences of the United States of America, 113*(1), 182–187. http://dx.doi.org/10.1073/pnas.1515617113.

Ertmer, A., Huber, V., Gilch, S., Yoshimori, T., Erfle, V., Duyster, J., ... Schätzl, H. M. (2007). The anticancer drug imatinib induces cellular autophagy. *Leukemia, 21*(5), 936–942. http://dx.doi.org/10.1038/sj.leu.2404606.

Fader, C. M., Sánchez, D. G., Mestre, M. B., & Colombo, M. I. (2009). TI-VAMP/VAMP7 and VAMP3/cellubrevin: Two v-SNARE proteins involved in specific steps of the autophagy/multivesicular body pathways. *Biochimica et Biophysica Acta (BBA), 1793*(12), 1901–1916.

Fass, E., Shvets, E., Degani, I., Hirschberg, K., & Elazar, Z. (2006). Microtubules support production of starvation-induced autophagosomes but not their targeting and fusion with lysosomes. *Journal of Biological Chemistry, 281*(47), 36303–36316. http://dx.doi.org/10.1074/jbc.M607031200.

Fei, P., Wang, W., Kim, S. H., Wang, S., Burns, T. F., Sax, J. K., ... El-Deiry, W. S. (2004). Bnip3L is induced by p53 under hypoxia, and its knockdown promotes tumor growth. *Cancer Cell, 6*(6), 597–609. http://dx.doi.org/10.1016/j.ccr.2004.10.012.

Feng, Z., Hu, W., de Stanchina, E., Teresky, A. K., Jin, S., Lowe, S., & Levine, A. J. (2007). The regulation of AMPK beta1, TSC2, and PTEN expression by p53: Stress, cell and tissue specificity, and the role of these gene products in modulating the IGF-1-AKT-mTOR pathways. *Cancer Research, 67*(7), 3043–3053. http://dx.doi.org/10.1158/0008-5472.CAN-06-4149.

Filimonenko, M., Stuffers, S., Raiborg, C., Yamamoto, A., Malerød, L., Fisher, E. M. C., ... Simonsen, A. (2007). Functional multivesicular bodies are required for autophagic clearance of protein aggregates associated with neurodegenerative disease. *The Journal of Cell Biology, 179*(3), 485–500. http://dx.doi.org/10.1083/jcb.200702115.

Fimia, G. M., Stoykova, A., Romagnoli, A., Giunta, L., Di Bartolomeo, S., Nardacci, R., ... Cecconi, F. (2007). Ambra1 regulates autophagy and development of the nervous system. *Nature, 447*(7148), 1121–1125. http://www.nature.com/nature/journal/v447/n7148/suppinfo/nature05925_S1.html.

Fujii, S., Mitsunaga, S., Yamazaki, M., Hasebe, T., Ishii, G., Kojima, M., ... Ochiai, A. (2008). Autophagy is activated in pancreatic cancer cells and correlates with poor patient outcome. *Cancer Science, 99*(9), 1813–1819. http://dx.doi.org/10.1111/j.1349-7006.2008.00893.x.

Fujita, N., Itoh, T., Omori, H., Fukuda, M., Noda, T., & Yoshimori, T. (2008). The Atg16L complex specifies the site of LC3 lipidation for membrane biogenesis in autophagy. *Molecular Biology of the Cell, 19*(5), 2092–2100. http://dx.doi.org/10.1091/mbc.E07-12-1257.

Fujiwara, M., Marusawa, H., Wang, H. Q., Iwai, A., Ikeuchi, K., Imai, Y., ... Chiba, T. (2008). Parkin as a tumor suppressor gene for hepatocellular carcinoma. *Oncogene, 27*(46), 6002–6011. http://www.nature.com/onc/journal/v27/n46/suppinfo/onc2008199s1.html.

Fukuda, T., Oda, K., Wada-Hiraike, O., Sone, K., Inaba, K., Ikeda, Y., ... Fujii, T. (2015). The anti-malarial chloroquine suppresses proliferation and overcomes cisplatin resistance of endometrial cancer cells via autophagy inhibition. *Gynecologic Oncology, 137*(3), 538–545. http://dx.doi.org/10.1016/j.ygyno.2015.03.053.

Füllgrabe, J., Klionsky, D. J., & Joseph, B. (2014). The return of the nucleus: Transcriptional and epigenetic control of autophagy. *Nature Reviews. Molecular Cell Biology, 15*(1), 65–74. http://dx.doi.org/10.1038/nrm3716.

Füllgrabe, J., Lynch-Day, M. A., Heldring, N., Li, W., Struijk, R. B., Ma, Q., ... Joseph, B. (2013). The histone H4 lysine 16 acetyltransferase hMOF regulates the outcome of autophagy. *Nature, 500*(7463), 468–471. http://dx.doi.org/10.1038/nature12313. http://www.nature.com/nature/journal/v500/n7463/abs/nature12313.html. supplementary-information.

Fung, C., Lock, R., Gao, S., Salas, E., & Debnath, J. (2008). Induction of autophagy during extracellular matrix detachment promotes cell survival. *Molecular Biology of the Cell, 19*(3), 797–806. http://dx.doi.org/10.1091/mbc.E07-10-1092.

Galluzzi, L., Pietrocola, F., Bravo-San Pedro, J. M., Amaravadi, R. K., Baehrecke, E. H., Cecconi, F., ... Kroemer, G. (2015). Autophagy in malignant transformation and cancer progression. *The EMBO Journal, 34*(7), 856–880. http://dx.doi.org/10.15252/embj.201490784.

Gee, H. Y., Noh, S. H., Tang, B. L., Kim, K. H., & Lee, M. G. (2011). Rescue of ΔF508-CFTR trafficking via a GRASP-dependent unconventional secretion pathway. *Cell, 146*(5), 746–760. http://dx.doi.org/10.1016/j.cell.2011.07.021.

Goldsmith, J., Levine, B., & Debnath, J. (2014). Chapter Two—Autophagy and cancer metabolism. In G. Lorenzo & K. Guido (Eds.), *Methods in enzymology: Vol. 542* (pp. 25–57): Cambridge, MA: Academic Press.

Gong, C., Bauvy, C., Tonelli, G., Yue, W., Delomenie, C., Nicolas, V., … Mehrpour, M. (2013). Beclin 1 and autophagy are required for the tumorigenicity of breast cancer stem-like/progenitor cells. *Oncogene, 32*(18), 2261–2272. http://dx.doi.org/10.1038/onc.2012.252.

Goussetis, D. J., Gounaris, E., Wu, E. J., Vakana, E., Sharma, B., Bogyo, M., … Platanias, L. C. (2012). Autophagic degradation of the BCR-ABL oncoprotein and generation of antileukemic responses by arsenic trioxide. *Blood, 120*(17), 3555–3562. http://dx.doi.org/10.1182/blood-2012-01-402578.

Guan, J. L., Simon, A. K., Prescott, M., Menendez, J. A., Liu, F., Wang, F., … Zhang, J. (2013). Autophagy in stem cells. *Autophagy, 9*(6), 830–849. http://dx.doi.org/10.4161/auto.24132.

Guo, J. Y., Chen, H.-Y., Mathew, R., Fan, J., Strohecker, A. M., Karsli-Uzunbas, G., … White, E. (2011). Activated Ras requires autophagy to maintain oxidative metabolism and tumorigenesis. *Genes & Development, 25*(5), 460–470. http://dx.doi.org/10.1101/gad.2016311.

Guo, J. Y., Karsli-Uzunbas, G., Mathew, R., Aisner, S. C., Kamphorst, J. J., Strohecker, A. M., … White, E. (2013). Autophagy suppresses progression of K-ras-induced lung tumors to oncocytomas and maintains lipid homeostasis. *Genes & Development, 27*(13), 1447–1461. http://dx.doi.org/10.1101/gad.219642.113.

Gupta, A., Roy, S., Lazar, A. J. F., Wang, W.-L., McAuliffe, J. C., Reynoso, D., … Rubin, B. P. (2010). Autophagy inhibition and antimalarials promote cell death in gastrointestinal stromal tumor (GIST). *Proceedings of the National Academy of Sciences of the United States of America, 107*(32), 14333–14338. http://dx.doi.org/10.1073/pnas.1000248107.

Gutierrez, M. G., Master, S. S., Singh, S. B., Taylor, G. A., Colombo, M. I., & Deretic, V. (2004). Autophagy is a defense mechanism inhibiting BCG and mycobacterium tuberculosis survival in infected macrophages. *Cell, 119*(6), 753–766. http://dx.doi.org/10.1016/j.cell.2004.11.038.

Gutierrez, M. G., Munafó, D. B., Berón, W., & Colombo, M. I. (2004). Rab7 is required for the normal progression of the autophagic pathway in mammalian cells. *Journal of Cell Science, 117*(13), 2687–2697. http://dx.doi.org/10.1242/jcs.01114.

Gwinn, D. M., Shackelford, D. B., Egan, D. F., Mihaylova, M. M., Mery, A., Vasquez, D. S., … Shaw, R. J. (2008). AMPK phosphorylation of raptor mediates a metabolic checkpoint. *Molecular Cell, 30*(2), 214–226. http://dx.doi.org/10.1016/j.molcel.2008.03.003.

Han, W., Pan, H., Chen, Y., Sun, J., Wang, Y., Li, J., … Jin, H. (2011). EGFR tyrosine kinase inhibitors activate autophagy as a cytoprotective response in human lung cancer cells. *PLoS One, 6*(6), e18691. http://dx.doi.org/10.1371/journal.pone.0018691.

Hanada, T., Noda, N. N., Satomi, Y., Ichimura, Y., Fujioka, Y., Takao, T., … Ohsumi, Y. (2007). The Atg12-Atg5 conjugate has a novel E3-like activity for protein lipidation in autophagy. *Journal of Biological Chemistry, 282*(52), 37298–37302. http://dx.doi.org/10.1074/jbc.C700195200.

Harris, J. (2011). Autophagy and cytokines. *Cytokine, 56*(2), 140–144. http://dx.doi.org/10.1016/j.cyto.2011.08.022.

Harris, J., De Haro, S. A., Master, S. S., Keane, J., Roberts, E. A., Delgado, M., & Deretic, V. (2007). T helper 2 cytokines inhibit autophagic control of intracellular Mycobacterium tuberculosis. *Immunity, 27*(3), 505–517. http://dx.doi.org/10.1016/j.immuni.2007.07.022.

Hart, L. S., Cunningham, J. T., Datta, T., Dey, S., Tameire, F., Lehman, S. L., … Koumenis, C. (2012). ER stress–mediated autophagy promotes Myc-dependent transformation and tumor growth. *The Journal of Clinical Investigation, 122*(12), 4621–4634. http://dx.doi.org/10.1172/JCI62973.

He, C., & Klionsky, D. J. (2009). Regulation mechanisms and signaling pathways of autophagy. *Annual Review of Genetics, 43*(1), 67–93. http://dx.doi.org/10.1146/annurev-genet-102808-114910.

Höckel, M., & Vaupel, P. (2001). Tumor hypoxia: Definitions and current clinical, biologic, and molecular aspects. *Journal of the National Cancer Institute, 93*(4), 266–276. http://dx.doi.org/10.1093/jnci/93.4.266.

Horikawa, I., Fujita, K., Jenkins, L. M. M., Hiyoshi, Y., Mondal, A. M., Vojtesek, B., ... Harris, C. C. (2014). Autophagic degradation of the inhibitory p53 isoform Δ133p53α as a regulatory mechanism for p53-mediated senescence. *Nature Communications, 5.* http://dx.doi.org/10.1038/ncomms5706.

Hosokawa, N., Hara, T., Kaizuka, T., Kishi, C., Takamura, A., Miura, Y., ... Mizushima, N. (2009). Nutrient-dependent mTORC1 association with the ULK1-Atg13–FIP200 complex required for autophagy. *Molecular Biology of the Cell, 20*(7), 1981–1991. http://dx.doi.org/10.1091/mbc.E08-12-1248.

Howell, J. J., & Manning, B. D. (2011). mTOR couples cellular nutrient sensing to organismal metabolic homeostasis. *Trends in Endocrinology & Metabolism, 22*(3), 94–102. http://dx.doi.org/10.1016/j.tem.2010.12.003.

Høyer-Hansen, M., Bastholm, L., Szyniarowski, P., Campanella, M., Szabadkai, G., Farkas, T., ... Jäättelä, M. (2007). Control of macroautophagy by calcium, calmodulin-dependent kinase kinase-β, and Bcl-2. *Molecular Cell, 25*(2), 193–205. http://dx.doi.org/10.1016/j.molcel.2006.12.009.

Høyer-Hansen, M., & Jäättelä, M. (2007). Connecting endoplasmic reticulum stress to autophagy by unfolded protein response and calcium. *Cell Death and Differentiation, 14*(9), 1576–1582. Retrieved from, http://dx.doi.org/10.1038/sj.cdd.4402200.

Hu, Y.-L., DeLay, M., Jahangiri, A., Molinaro, A. M., Rose, S. D., Carbonell, W. S., & Aghi, M. K. (2012). Hypoxia-induced autophagy promotes tumor cell survival and adaptation to antiangiogenic treatment in glioblastoma. *Cancer Research, 72*(7), 1773–1783. http://dx.doi.org/10.1158/0008-5472.can-11-3831.

Huang, Y., Guerrero-Preston, R., & Ratovitski, E. A. (2012). Phospho-DeltaNp63alpha-dependent regulation of autophagic signaling through transcription and micro-RNA modulation. *Cell Cycle, 11*(6), 1247–1259. http://dx.doi.org/10.4161/cc.11.6.19670.

Inami, Y., Waguri, S., Sakamoto, A., Kouno, T., Nakada, K., Hino, O., ... Komatsu, M. (2011). Persistent activation of Nrf2 through p62 in hepatocellular carcinoma cells. *The Journal of Cell Biology, 193*(2), 275–284. http://dx.doi.org/10.1083/jcb.201102031.

Inoki, K., Zhu, T., & Guan, K.-L. (2003). TSC2 mediates cellular energy response to control cell growth and survival. *Cell, 115*(5), 577–590. http://dx.doi.org/10.1016/S0092-8674(03)00929-2.

Inoue, D., Suzuki, T., Mitsuishi, Y., Miki, Y., Suzuki, S., Sugawara, S., ... Yamamoto, M. (2012). Accumulation of p62/SQSTM1 is associated with poor prognosis in patients with lung adenocarcinoma. *Cancer Science, 103*(4), 760–766. http://dx.doi.org/10.1111/j.1349-7006.2012.02216.x.

Itakura, E., Kishi, C., Inoue, K., & Mizushima, N. (2008). Beclin 1 forms two distinct phosphatidylinositol 3-kinase complexes with mammalian Atg14 and UVRAG. *Molecular Biology of the Cell, 19*(12), 5360–5372. http://dx.doi.org/10.1091/mbc.E08-01-0080.

Itakura, E., Kishi-Itakura, C., & Mizushima, N. (2012). The hairpin-type tail-anchored SNARE syntaxin 17 targets to autophagosomes for fusion with endosomes/lysosomes. *Cell, 151*(6), 1256–1269. http://dx.doi.org/10.1016/j.cell.2012.11.001.

Itakura, E., & Mizushima, N. (2010). Characterization of autophagosome formation site by a hierarchical analysis of mammalian Atg proteins. *Autophagy, 6*(6), 764–776. http://dx.doi.org/10.4161/auto.6.6.12709.

Ito, H., Daido, S., Kanzawa, T., Kondo, S., & Kondo, Y. (2005). Radiation-induced autophagy is associated with LC3 and its inhibition sensitizes malignant glioma cells. *International Journal of Oncology, 26*(5), 1401–1410. Retrieved from, http://www.ncbi. nlm.nih.gov/pubmed/15809734.

Jäger, S., Bucci, C., Tanida, I., Ueno, T., Kominami, E., Saftig, P., & Eskelinen, E.-L. (2004). Role for Rab7 in maturation of late autophagic vacuoles. *Journal of Cell Science, 117*(20), 4837–4848. http://dx.doi.org/10.1242/jcs.01370.

Jahreiss, L., Menzies, F. M., & Rubinsztein, D. C. (2008). The itinerary of autophagosomes: From peripheral formation to kiss-and-run fusion with lysosomes. *Traffic, 9*(4), 574–587. http://dx.doi.org/10.1111/j.1600-0854.2008.00701.x.

Jin, S. (2006). Autophagy, mitochondrial quality control, and oncogenesis. *Autophagy, 2*(2), 80–84. http://dx.doi.org/10.4161/auto.2.2.2460.

Jones, R. G., & Thompson, C. B. (2009). Tumor suppressors and cell metabolism: A recipe for cancer growth. *Genes & Development, 23*(5), 537–548. http://dx.doi.org/10.1101/gad,1756509.

Jounai, N., Takeshita, F., Kobiyama, K., Sawano, A., Miyawaki, A., Xin, K.-Q., ... Okuda, K. (2007). The Atg5–Atg12 conjugate associates with innate antiviral immune responses. *Proceedings of the National Academy of Sciences of the United States of America, 104*(35), 14050–14055. http://dx.doi.org/10.1073/pnas.0704014104.

Jung, C. H., Jun, C. B., Ro, S.-H., Kim, Y.-M., Otto, N. M., Cao, J., ... Kim, D.-H. (2009). ULK-Atg13-FIP200 complexes mediate mTOR signaling to the autophagy machinery. *Molecular Biology of the Cell, 20*(7), 1992–2003. http://dx.doi.org/10.1091/mbc.E08-12-1249.

Kanematsu, S., Uehara, N., Miki, H., Yoshizawa, K., Kawanaka, A., Yuri, T., & Tsubura, A. (2010). Autophagy inhibition enhances sulforaphane-induced apoptosis in human breast cancer cells. *Anticancer Research, 30*(9), 3381–3390. Retrieved from, http://www.ncbi. nlm.nih.gov/pubmed/20944112.

Kang, M. R., Kim, M. S., Oh, J. E., Kim, Y. R., Song, S. Y., Kim, S. S., ... Lee, S. H. (2009). Frameshift mutations of autophagy-related genes ATG2B, ATG5, ATG9B and ATG12 in gastric and colorectal cancers with microsatellite instability. *The Journal of Pathology, 217*(5), 702–706. http://dx.doi.org/10.1002/path.2509.

Kanzawa, T., Germano, I. M., Komata, T., Ito, H., Kondo, Y., & Kondo, S. (2004). Role of autophagy in temozolomide-induced cytotoxicity for malignant glioma cells. *Cell Death and Differentiation, 11*(4), 448–457. http://dx.doi.org/10.1038/sj.cdd.4401359.

Karantza-Wadsworth, V., Patel, S., Kravchuk, O., Chen, G., Mathew, R., Jin, S., & White, E. (2007). Autophagy mitigates metabolic stress and genome damage in mammary tumorigenesis. *Genes & Development, 21*(13), 1621–1635. http://dx.doi.org/10.1101/gad.1565707.

Kenific, C. M., & Debnath, J. (2015). Cellular and metabolic functions for autophagy in cancer cells. *Trends in Cell Biology, 25*(1), 37–45. http://dx.doi.org/10.1016/j.tcb.2014.09.001.

Kenific, C. M., Thorburn, A., & Debnath, J. (2010). Autophagy and metastasis: Another double-edged sword. *Current Opinion in Cell Biology, 22*(2), 241–245. http://dx.doi.org/10.1016/j.ceb.2009.10.008.

Kenzelmann Broz, D., Spano Mello, S., Bieging, K. T., Jiang, D., Dusek, R. L., Brady, C. A., ... Attardi, L. D. (2013). Global genomic profiling reveals an extensive p53-regulated autophagy program contributing to key p53 responses. *Genes & Development, 27*(9), 1016–1031. http://dx.doi.org/10.1101/gad.212282.112.

Kim, P. K., Hailey, D. W., Mullen, R. T., & Lippincott-Schwartz, J. (2008). Ubiquitin signals autophagic degradation of cytosolic proteins and peroxisomes. *Proceedings of the National Academy of Sciences of the United States of America, 105*(52), 20567–20574. http://dx.doi.org/10.1073/pnas.0810611105.

Kim, J., Kim, Y. C., Fang, C., Russell, R. C., Kim, J. H., Fan, W., … Guan, K.-L. (2013). Differential regulation of distinct Vps34 complexes by AMPK in nutrient stress and autophagy. *Cell*, *152*(1), 290–303. http://dx.doi.org/10.1016/j.cell.2012.12.016.

Kim, J., Kundu, M., Viollet, B., & Guan, K.-L. (2011). AMPK and mTOR regulate autophagy through direct phosphorylation of Ulk1. *Nature Cell Biology*, *13*(2), 132–141. http://www.nature.com/ncb/journal/v13/n2/abs/ncb2152.html supplementary-information.

Kimura, S., Noda, T., & Yoshimori, T. (2008). Dynein-dependent movement of autophagosomes mediates efficient encounters with lysosomes. *Cell Structure and Function*, *33*(1), 109–122. http://dx.doi.org/10.1247/csf.08005.

Kirisako, T., Ichimura, Y., Okada, H., Kabeya, Y., Mizushima, N., Yoshimori, T., … Ohsumi, Y. (2000). The reversible modification regulates the membrane-binding state of Apg8/Aut7 essential for autophagy and the cytoplasm to vacuole targeting pathway. *The Journal of Cell Biology*, *151*(2), 263–276. http://dx.doi.org/10.1083/jcb.151.2.263.

Kiyono, K., Suzuki, H. I., Matsuyama, H., Morishita, Y., Komuro, A., Kano, M. R., … Miyazono, K. (2009). Autophagy is activated by TGF-β and potentiates TGF-β–mediated growth inhibition in human hepatocellular carcinoma cells. *Cancer Research*, *69*(23), 8844–8852. http://dx.doi.org/10.1158/0008-5472.can-08-4401.

Klionsky, D. J. (2007). Autophagy: From phenomenology to molecular understanding in less than a decade. *Nature Reviews. Molecular Cell Biology*, *8*(11), 931–937. http://www.nature.com/nrm/journal/v8/n11/suppinfo/nrm2245_S1.html.

Ko, A., Kanehisa, A., Martins, I., Senovilla, L., Chargari, C., Dugue, D., … Deutsch, E. (2014). Autophagy inhibition radiosensitizes in vitro, yet reduces radioresponses in vivo due to deficient immunogenic signalling. *Cell Death and Differentiation*, *21*(1), 92–99. http://dx.doi.org/10.1038/cdd.2013.124.

Köchl, R., Hu, X. W., Chan, E. Y. W., & Tooze, S. A. (2006). Microtubules facilitate autophagosome formation and fusion of autophagosomes with endosomes. *Traffic*, *7*(2), 129–145. http://dx.doi.org/10.1111/j.1600-0854.2005.00368.x.

Komatsu, M., & Ichimura, Y. (2010). Physiological significance of selective degradation of p62 by autophagy. *FEBS Letters*, *584*(7), 1374–1378. http://dx.doi.org/10.1016/j.febslet.2010.02.017.

Komatsu, M., Kurokawa, H., Waguri, S., Taguchi, K., Kobayashi, A., Ichimura, Y., … Yamamoto, M. (2010). The selective autophagy substrate p62 activates the stress responsive transcription factor Nrf2 through inactivation of Keap1. *Nature Cell Biology*, *12*(3), 213–223. http://www.nature.com/ncb/journal/v12/n3/suppinfo/ncb2021_S1.html.

Komatsu, M., Waguri, S., Koike, M., Sou, Y.-S., Ueno, T., Hara, T., … Tanaka, K. (2007). Homeostatic levels of p62 control cytoplasmic inclusion body formation in autophagy-deficient mice. *Cell*, *131*(6), 1149–1163. http://dx.doi.org/10.1016/j.cell.2007.10.035.

Kouroku, Y., Fujita, E., Tanida, I., Ueno, T., Isoai, A., Kumagai, H., … Momoi, T. (2007). ER stress (PERK/eIF2[alpha] phosphorylation) mediates the polyglutamine-induced LC3 conversion, an essential step for autophagy formation. *Cell Death and Differentiation*, *14*(2), 230–239. http://www.nature.com/cdd/journal/v14/n2/suppinfo/4401984 s1.html.

Kraya, A. A., Piao, S., Xu, X., Zhang, G., Herlyn, M., Gimotty, P., … Speicher, D. W. (2015). Identification of secreted proteins that reflect autophagy dynamics within tumor cells. *Autophagy*, *11*(1), 60–74. http://dx.doi.org/10.4161/15548627.2014.984273.

Kroemer, G., Mariño, G., & Levine, B. (2010). Autophagy and the integrated stress response. *Molecular Cell*, *40*(2), 280–293. http://dx.doi.org/10.1016/j.molcel.2010.09.023.

Kumar, D., Gupta, D., Shankar, S., & Srivastava, R. K. (2015). Biomolecular characterization of exosomes released from cancer stem cells: Possible implications for biomarker and treatment of cancer. *Oncotarget*, *6*, 3280–3291.

Laddha, S. V., Ganesan, S., Chan, C. S., & White, E. (2014). Mutational landscape of the essential autophagy gene BECN1 in human cancers. *Molecular Cancer Research*, *12*(4), 485–490. http://dx.doi.org/10.1158/1541-7786.mcr-13-0614.

Lamb, C. A., Yoshimori, T., & Tooze, S. A. (2013). The autophagosome: Origins unknown, biogenesis complex. *Nature Reviews. Molecular Cell Biology*, *14*(12), 759–774. http://dx. doi.org/10.1038/nrm3696.

Lau, A., Wang, X.-J., Zhao, F., Villeneuve, N. F., Wu, T., Jiang, T., … Zhang, D. D. (2010). A noncanonical mechanism of Nrf2 activation by autophagy deficiency: Direct interaction between Keap1 and p62. *Molecular and Cellular Biology*, *30*(13), 3275–3285. http://dx.doi.org/10.1128/mcb.00248-10.

Lazarou, M., Sliter, D. A., Kane, L. A., Sarraf, S. A., Wang, C., Burman, J. L., … Youle, R. J. (2015). The ubiquitin kinase PINK1 recruits autophagy receptors to induce mitophagy. *Nature*, *524*(7565), 309–314. http://dx.doi.org/10.1038/nature14893. http://www.nature. com/nature/journal/v524/n7565/abs/nature14893.html. supplementary-information.

Lee, J.-A., Beigneux, A., Ahmad, S. T., Young, S. G., & Gao, F.-B. (2007). ESCRT-III dysfunction causes autophagosome accumulation and neurodegeneration. *Current Biology*, *17*(18), 1561–1567. http://dx.doi.org/10.1016/j.cub.2007.07.029.

Lee, J. Y., Koga, H., Kawaguchi, Y., Tang, W., Wong, E., Gao, Y. S., … Yao, T. P. (2010). HDAC6 controls autophagosome maturation essential for ubiquitin-selective quality-control autophagy. *The EMBO Journal*, *29*(5), 969–980. Retrieved from, http://emboj.embopress.org/content/29/5/969.abstract.

Lee, J. M., Wagner, M., Xiao, R., Kim, K. H., Feng, D., Lazar, M. A., & Moore, D. D. (2014). Nutrient-sensing nuclear receptors coordinate autophagy. *Nature*, *516*(7529), 112–115. http://dx.doi.org/10.1038/nature13961. http://www.nature.com/nature/journal/v516/n7529/abs/nature13961.html. supplementary-information.

Levine, B., & Kroemer, G. (2008). Autophagy in the pathogenesis of disease. *Cell*, *132*(1), 27–42. http://dx.doi.org/10.1016/j.cell.2007.12.018.

Levine, B., & Yuan, J. (2005). Autophagy in cell death: An innocent convict? *The Journal of Clinical Investigation*, *115*(10), 2679–2688. http://dx.doi.org/10.1172/JCI26390.

Levy, J. M. M., Thompson, J. C., Griesinger, A. M., Amani, V., Donson, A. M., Birks, D. K., … Thorburn, A. (2014). Autophagy inhibition improves chemosensitivity in BRAFV600E brain tumors. *Cancer Discovery*, *4*(7), 773–780. http://dx.doi.org/10.1158/2159-8290.cd-14-0049.

Li, M., Hou, Y., Wang, J., Chen, X., Shao, Z.-M., & Yin, X.-M. (2011). Kinetics comparisons of mammalian Atg4 homologues indicate selective preferences toward diverse Atg8 substrates. *Journal of Biological Chemistry*, *286*(9), 7327–7338. http://dx.doi.org/10.1074/jbc.M110.199059.

Li, W.-W., Li, J., & Bao, J. K. (2012). Microautophagy: Lesser-known self-eating. *Cellular and Molecular Life Sciences*, *69*(7), 1125–1136. http://dx.doi.org/10.1007/s00018-011-0865-5.

Li, N., Wu, X., Holzer, R. G., Lee, J.-H., Todoric, J., Park, E.-J., … Karin, M. (2013). Loss of acinar cell IKKα triggers spontaneous pancreatitis in mice. *The Journal of Clinical Investigation*, *123*(5), 2231–2243. http://dx.doi.org/10.1172/JCI64498.

Liang, C., Feng, P., Ku, B., Dotan, I., Canaani, D., Oh, B.-H., & Jung, J. U. (2006). Autophagic and tumour suppressor activity of a novel Beclin1-binding protein UVRAG. *Nature Cell Biology*, *8*(7), 688–698. http://www.nature.com/ncb/journal/v8/n7/suppinfo/ncb1426_S1.html.

Liang, X. H., Jackson, S., Seaman, M., Brown, K., Kempkes, B., Hibshoosh, H., & Levine, B. (1999). Induction of autophagy and inhibition of tumorigenesis by beclin 1. *Nature*, *402*(6762), 672–676. Retrieved from, http://dx.doi.org/10.1038/45257.

Liang, C., Lee, J.-S., Inn, K.-S., Gack, M. U., Li, Q., Roberts, E. A., & Jung, J. U. (2008). Beclin1-binding UVRAG targets the class C Vps complex to coordinate autophagosome maturation and endocytic trafficking. *Nature Cell Biology, 10*(7), 776–787. http://www.nature.com/ncb/journal/v10/n7/suppinfo/ncb1740_S1.html.

Liu, L., Feng, D., Chen, G., Chen, M., Zheng, Q., Song, P., … Chen, Q. (2012). Mitochondrial outer-membrane protein FUNDC1 mediates hypoxia-induced mitophagy in mammalian cells. *Nature Cell Biology, 14*(2), 177–185. http://www.nature.com/ncb/journal/v14/n2/abs/ncb2422.html supplementary-information.

Liu, H., He, Z., von Rütte, T., Yousefi, S., Hunger, R. E., & Simon, H.-U. (2013). Down-regulation of autophagy-related protein 5 (ATG5) contributes to the pathogenesis of early-stage cutaneous melanoma. *Science Translational Medicine, 5*(202), 202ra123. http://dx.doi.org/10.1126/scitranslmed.3005864.

Liu, Y., & Levine, B. (2015). Autosis and autophagic cell death: The dark side of autophagy. *Cell Death and Differentiation, 22*(3), 367–376. http://dx.doi.org/10.1038/cdd.2014.143.

Liu, D., & Xu, Y. (2010). p53, oxidative stress, and aging. *Antioxidants & Redox Signaling, 15*(6), 1669–1678. http://dx.doi.org/10.1089/ars.2010.3644.

Lock, R., Kenific, C. M., Leidal, A. M., Salas, E., & Debnath, J. (2014). Autophagy-dependent production of secreted factors facilitates oncogenic RAS-driven invasion. *Cancer Discovery, 4*(4), 466–479. http://dx.doi.org/10.1158/2159-8290.cd-13-0841.

Lock, R., Roy, S., Kenific, C. M., Su, J. S., Salas, E., Ronen, S. M., & Debnath, J. (2011). Autophagy facilitates glycolysis during Ras-mediated oncogenic transformation. *Molecular Biology of the Cell, 22*(2), 165–178. http://dx.doi.org/10.1091/mbc.E10-06-0500.

Lopez-Castejon, G., & Brough, D. (2011). Understanding the mechanism of IL-1β secretion. *Cytokine and Growth Factor Reviews, 22*(4), 189–195. http://dx.doi.org/10.1016/j.cytogfr.2011.10.001.

Lu, Z., Luo, R. Z., Lu, Y., Zhang, X., Yu, Q., Khare, S., … Bast, R. C., Jr. (2008). The tumor suppressor gene ARHI regulates autophagy and tumor dormancy in human ovarian cancer cells. *The Journal of Clinical Investigation, 118*(12), 3917–3929. http://dx.doi.org/10.1172/JCI35512.

Ma, Y., Galluzzi, L., Zitvogel, L., & Kroemer, G. (2013). Autophagy and cellular immune responses. *Immunity, 39*(2), 211–227. http://dx.doi.org/10.1016/j.immuni.2013.07.017.

Maes, H., Kuchnio, A., Peric, A., Moens, S., Nys, K., De Bock, K., … Carmeliet, P. (2014). Tumor vessel normalization by chloroquine independent of autophagy. *Cancer Cell, 26*(2), 190–206. http://dx.doi.org/10.1016/j.ccr.2014.06.025.

Maes, H., Rubio, N., Garg, A. D., & Agostinis, P. (2013). Autophagy: Shaping the tumor microenvironment and therapeutic response. *Trends in Molecular Medicine, 19*(7), 428–446. http://dx.doi.org/10.1016/j.molmed.2013.04.005.

Mahalingam, D., Mita, M., Sarantopoulos, J., Wood, L., Amaravadi, R. K., Davis, L. E., … Carew, J. S. (2014). Combined autophagy and HDAC inhibition: A phase I safety, tolerability, pharmacokinetic, and pharmacodynamic analysis of hydroxychloroquine in combination with the HDAC inhibitor vorinostat in patients with advanced solid tumors. *Autophagy, 10*(8), 1403–1414. http://dx.doi.org/10.4161/auto.29231.

Manjithaya, R., Anjard, C., Loomis, W. F., & Subramani, S. (2010). Unconventional secretion of Pichia pastoris Acb1 is dependent on GRASP protein, peroxisomal functions, and autophagosome formation. *The Journal of Cell Biology, 188*(4), 537–546. http://dx.doi.org/10.1083/jcb.200911149.

Mar, F. A., Debnath, J., & Stohr, B. A. (2015). Autophagy-independent senescence and genome instability driven by targeted telomere dysfunction. *Autophagy, 11*(3), 527–537. http://dx.doi.org/10.1080/15548627.2015.1017189.

Martinez-Outschoorn, U. E., Balliet, R. M., Rivadeneira, D. B., Chiavarina, B., Pavlides, S., Wang, C., … Lisanti, M. P. (2010). Oxidative stress in cancer associated fibroblasts drives tumor-stroma co-evolution: A new paradigm for understanding tumor metabolism, the field effect and genomic instability in cancer cells. *Cell Cycle*, *9*(16), 3256–3276. http://dx.doi.org/10.4161/cc.9.16.12553.

Martinez-Outschoorn, U., Sotgia, F., & Lisanti, M. P. (2014). Tumor microenvironment and metabolic synergy in breast cancers: Critical importance of mitochondrial fuels and function. *Seminars in Oncology*, *41*(2), 195–216. http://dx.doi.org/10.1053/j.seminoncol.2014.03.002.

Martinez-Outschoorn, U. E., Trimmer, C., Lin, Z., Whitaker-Menezes, D., Chiavarina, B., Zhou, J., … Sotgia, F. (2010). Autophagy in cancer associated fibroblasts promotes tumor cell survival: Role of hypoxia, HIF1 induction and NFκB activation in the tumor stromal microenvironment. *Cell Cycle*, *9*(17), 3515–3533. http://dx.doi.org/10.4161/cc.9.17.12928.

Mathew, R., Karp, C. M., Beaudoin, B., Vuong, N., Chen, G., Chen, H.-Y., … White, E. (2009). Autophagy suppresses tumorigenesis through elimination of p62. *Cell*, *137*(6), 1062–1075. http://dx.doi.org/10.1016/j.cell.2009.03.048.

Mathew, R., Kongara, S., Beaudoin, B., Karp, C. M., Bray, K., Degenhardt, K., … White, E. (2007). Autophagy suppresses tumor progression by limiting chromosomal instability. *Genes & Development*, *21*(11), 1367–1381. http://dx.doi.org/10.1101/gad.1545107.

Matsunaga, K., Saitoh, T., Tabata, K., Omori, H., Satoh, T., Kurotori, N., … Yoshimori, T. (2009). Two Beclin 1-binding proteins, Atg14L and Rubicon, reciprocally regulate autophagy at different stages. *Nature Cell Biology*, *11*(4), 385–396. http://www.nature.com/ncb/journal/v11/n4/suppinfo/ncb1846_S1.html.

Maycotte, P., Aryal, S., Cummings, C. T., Thorburn, J., Morgan, M. J., & Thorburn, A. (2012). Chloroquine sensitizes breast cancer cells to chemotherapy independent of autophagy. *Autophagy*, *8*(2), 200–212. http://dx.doi.org/10.4161/auto.8.2.18554.

Maycotte, P., Jones, K. L., Goodall, M. L., Thorburn, J., & Thorburn, A. (2015). Autophagy supports breast cancer stem cell maintenance by regulating IL6 secretion. *Molecular Cancer Research*, *13*(4), 651–658. http://dx.doi.org/10.1158/1541-7786.mcr-14-0487.

Mazure, N. M., & Pouysségur, J. (2010). Hypoxia-induced autophagy: Cell death or cell survival? *Current Opinion in Cell Biology*, *22*(2), 177–180. http://dx.doi.org/10.1016/j.ceb.2009.11.015.

Michaud, M., Martins, I., Sukkurwala, A. Q., Adjemian, S., Ma, Y., Pellegatti, P., … Kroemer, G. (2011). Autophagy-dependent anticancer immune responses induced by chemotherapeutic agents in mice. *Science*, *334*(6062), 1573–1577. http://dx.doi.org/10.1126/science.1208347.

Mirzoeva, O., Hann, B., Hom, Y., Debnath, J., Aftab, D., Shokat, K., & Korn, W. M. (2011). Autophagy suppression promotes apoptotic cell death in response to inhibition of the PI3K—mTOR pathway in pancreatic adenocarcinoma. *Journal of Molecular Medicine*, *89*(9), 877–889. http://dx.doi.org/10.1007/s00109-011-0774-y.

Mizushima, N. (2007). Autophagy: Process and function. *Genes & Development*, *21*(22), 2861–2873. http://dx.doi.org/10.1101/gad.1599207.

Mizushima, N. (2010). The role of the Atg1/ULK1 complex in autophagy regulation. *Current Opinion in Cell Biology*, *22*(2), 132–139. http://dx.doi.org/10.1016/j.ceb.2009.12.004.

Monastyrska, I., Rieter, E., Klionsky, D. J., & Reggiori, F. (2009). Multiple roles of the cytoskeleton in autophagy. *Biological Reviews*, *84*(3), 431–448. http://dx.doi.org/10.1111/j.1469-185X.2009.00082.x.

Mortensen, M., Soilleux, E. J., Djordjevic, G., Tripp, R., Lutteropp, M., Sadighi-Akha, E., … Simon, A. K. (2011). The autophagy protein Atg7 is essential for hematopoietic stem cell maintenance. *The Journal of Experimental Medicine*, *208*(3), 455–467. http://dx.doi.org/10.1084/jem.20101145.

Moscat, J., & Diaz-Meco, M. T. (2009). p62 at the crossroads of autophagy, apoptosis, and cancer. *Cell*, *137*(6), 1001–1004. http://dx.doi.org/10.1016/j.cell.2009.05.023.

Mostowy, S., Sancho-Shimizu, V., Hamon, M. A., Simeone, R., Brosch, R., Johansen, T., & Cossart, P. (2011). p62 and NDP52 proteins target intracytosolic Shigella and Listeria to different autophagy pathways. *Journal of Biological Chemistry*, *286*(30), 26987–26995. http://dx.doi.org/10.1074/jbc.M111.223610.

Muñoz-Gámez, J. A., Rodríguez-Vargas, J. M., Quiles-Pérez, R., Aguilar-Quesada, R., Martín-Oliva, D., de Murcia, G., ... Oliver, F. J. (2009). PARP-1 is involved in autophagy induced by DNA damage. *Autophagy*, *5*(1), 61–74. http://dx.doi.org/10.4161/auto.5.1.7272.

Murrow, L., & Debnath, J. (2013). Autophagy as a stress-response and quality-control mechanism: Implications for cell injury and human disease. *Annual Review of Pathology: Mechanisms of Disease*, *8*(1), 105–137. http://dx.doi.org/10.1146/annurev-pathol-020712-163918.

Murrow, L., Malhotra, R., & Debnath, J. (2015). ATG12–ATG3 interacts with Alix to promote basal autophagic flux and late endosome function. *Nature Cell Biology*, *17*(3), 300–310. http://dx.doi.org/10.1038/ncb3112. http://www.nature.com/ncb/journal/v17/n3/abs/ncb3112.html supplementary-information.

Nair, U., Yen, W.-L., Mari, M., Cao, Y., Xie, Z., Baba, M., ... Klionsky, D. J. (2012). A role for Atg8–PE deconjugation in autophagosome biogenesis. *Autophagy*, *8*(5), 780–793. http://dx.doi.org/10.4161/auto.19385.

Nakahira, K., Haspel, J. A., Rathinam, V. A. K., Lee, S.-J., Dolinay, T., Lam, H. C., ... Choi, A. M. K. (2011). Autophagy proteins regulate innate immune responses by inhibiting the release of mitochondrial DNA mediated by the NALP3 inflammasome. *Nature Immunology*, *12*(3), 222–230. http://www.nature.com/ni/journal/v12/n3/abs/ni.1980.html supplementary-information.

Nakatogawa, H. (2013). Two ubiquitin-like conjugation systems that mediate membrane formation during autophagy. *Essays in Biochemistry*, *55*, 39–50. http://dx.doi.org/10.1042/bse0550039.

Nakatogawa, H., Suzuki, K., Kamada, Y., & Ohsumi, Y. (2009). Dynamics and diversity in autophagy mechanisms: Lessons from yeast. *Nature Reviews. Molecular Cell Biology*, *10*(7), 458–467. Retrieved from, http://dx.doi.org/10.1038/nrm2708.

Narita, M., Young, A. R. J., Arakawa, S., Samarajiwa, S. A., Nakashima, T., Yoshida, S., ... Narita, M. (2011). Spatial coupling of mTOR and autophagy augments secretory phenotypes. *Science*, *332*(6032), 966–970. http://dx.doi.org/10.1126/science.1205407.

Narita, M., Young, A. R. J., & Narita, M. (2009). Autophagy facilitates oncogene-induced senescence. *Autophagy*, *5*(7), 1046–1047. http://dx.doi.org/10.4161/auto.5.7.9444.

Nguyen, H. G., Yang, J. C., Kung, H. J., Shi, X. B., Tilki, D., Lara, P. N., ... Evans, C. P. (2014). Targeting autophagy overcomes Enzalutamide resistance in castration-resistant prostate cancer cells and improves therapeutic response in a xenograft model. *Oncogene*, *33*(36), 4521–4530. http://dx.doi.org/10.1038/onc.2014.25.

Nickel, W., & Rabouille, C. (2009). Mechanisms of regulated unconventional protein secretion. *Nature Reviews. Molecular Cell Biology*, *10*(2), 148–155. Retrieved from, http://dx.doi.org/10.1038/nrm2617.

Nixon, R. A. (2013). The role of autophagy in neurodegenerative disease. *Nature Medicine*, *19*(8), 983–997. http://dx.doi.org/10.1038/nm.3232.

Nobukuni, T., Joaquin, M., Roccio, M., Dann, S. G., Kim, S. Y., Gulati, P., ... Thomas, G. (2005). Amino acids mediate mTOR/raptor signaling through activation of class 3 phosphatidylinositol 3OH-kinase. *Proceedings of the National Academy of Sciences of the United States of America*, *102*(40), 14238–14243. http://dx.doi.org/10.1073/pnas.0506925102.

Noman, M. Z., Janji, B., Kaminska, B., Van Moer, K., Pierson, S., Przanowski, P., ... Chouaib, S. (2011). Blocking hypoxia-induced autophagy in tumors restores cytotoxic T-cell activity and promotes regression. *Cancer Research*, *71*(18), 5976–5986. http://dx.doi.org/10.1158/0008-5472.can-11-1094.

Ogata, M., Hino, S. I., Saito, A., Morikawa, K., Kondo, S., Kanemoto, S., ... Imaizumi, K. (2006). Autophagy is activated for cell survival after endoplasmic reticulum stress. *Molecular and Cellular Biology*, *26*(24), 9220–9231. http://dx.doi.org/10.1128/mcb.01453-06.

Paglin, S., Hollister, T., Delohery, T., Hackett, N., McMahill, M., Sphicas, E., ... Yahalom, J. (2001). A novel response of cancer cells to radiation involves autophagy and formation of acidic vesicles. *Cancer Research*, *61*(2), 439–444. Retrieved from, http://www.ncbi.nlm.nih.gov/pubmed/11212227.

Paillas, S., Causse, A., Marzi, L., de Medina, P., Poirot, M., Denis, V., ... Gongora, C. (2012). MAPK14/p38α confers irinotecan resistance to TP53-defective cells by inducing survival autophagy. *Autophagy*, *8*(7), 1098–1112. http://dx.doi.org/10.4161/auto.20268.

Paltridge, J. L., Belle, L., & Khew-Goodall, Y. (2013). The secretome in cancer progression. *Biochimica et Biophysica Acta*, *1834*(11), 2233–2241. http://dx.doi.org/10.1016/j.bbapap.2013.03.014.

Palumbo, S., Pirtoli, L., Tini, P., Cevenini, G., Calderaro, F., Toscano, M., ... Comincini, S. (2012). Different involvement of autophagy in human malignant glioma cell lines undergoing irradiation and temozolomide combined treatments. *Journal of Cellular Biochemistry*, *113*(7), 2308–2318. http://dx.doi.org/10.1002/jcb.24102.

Papandreou, I., Lim, A. L., Laderoute, K., & Denko, N. C. (2008). Hypoxia signals autophagy in tumor cells via AMPK activity, independent of HIF-1, BNIP3, and BNIP3L. *Cell Death and Differentiation*, *15*(10), 1572–1581. http://www.nature.com/cdd/journal/v15/n10/suppinfo/cdd200884s1.html.

Park, H.-J., Lee, S. J., Kim, S.-H., Han, J., Bae, J., Kim, S. J., ... Chun, T. (2011). IL-10 inhibits the starvation induced autophagy in macrophages via class I phosphatidylinositol 3-kinase (PI3K) pathway. *Molecular Immunology*, *48*(4), 720–727. http://dx.doi.org/10.1016/j.molimm.2010.10.020.

Parkhitko, A., Myachina, F., Morrison, T. A., Hindi, K. M., Auricchio, N., Karbowniczek, M., ... Henske, E. P. (2011). Tumorigenesis in tuberous sclerosis complex is autophagy and p62/sequestosome 1 (SQSTM1)-dependent. *Proceedings of the National Academy of Sciences of the United States of America*, *108*(30), 12455–12460. http://dx.doi.org/10.1073/pnas.1104361108.

Parzych, K. R., & Klionsky, D. J. (2014). An overview of autophagy: Morphology, mechanism, and regulation. *Antioxidants & Redox Signaling*, *20*(3), 460–473. http://dx.doi.org/10.1089/ars.2013.5371.

Pattingre, S., Bauvy, C., & Codogno, P. (2003). Amino acids interfere with the ERK1/2-dependent control of macroautophagy by controlling the activation of Raf-1 in human colon cancer HT-29 cells. *Journal of Biological Chemistry*, *278*(19), 16667–16674. http://dx.doi.org/10.1074/jbc.M210998200.

Pattingre, S., Tassa, A., Qu, X., Garuti, R., Liang, X. H., Mizushima, N., ... Levine, B. (2005). Bcl-2 antiapoptotic proteins inhibit Beclin 1-dependent autophagy. *Cell*, *122*(6), 927–939. http://dx.doi.org/10.1016/j.cell.2005.07.002.

Paul, S., Kashyap, Anuj K., Jia, W., He, Y.-W., & Schaefer, B. C. (2012). Selective autophagy of the adaptor protein Bcl10 modulates T cell receptor activation of NF-κB. *Immunity*, *36*(6), 947–958. http://dx.doi.org/10.1016/j.immuni.2012.04.008.

Pavlides, S., Vera, I., Gandara, R., Sneddon, S., Pestell, R. G., Mercier, I., ... Lisanti, M. P. (2012). Warburg meets autophagy: Cancer-associated fibroblasts accelerate tumor growth and metastasis via oxidative stress, mitophagy, and aerobic glycolysis. *Antioxidants & Redox Signaling*, *16*(11), 1264–1284. http://dx.doi.org/10.1089/ars.2011.4243.

Perera, R. M., Stoykova, S., Nicolay, B. N., Ross, K. N., Fitamant, J., Boukhali, M., … Bardeesy, N. (2015). Transcriptional control of autophagy-lysosome function drives pancreatic cancer metabolism. *Nature, 524*(7565), 361–365. http://dx.doi.org/10.1038/nature14587. http://www.nature.com/nature/journal/v524/n7565/abs/nature14587.html. supplementary-information.

Pérez-Mancera, P. A., Young, A. R. J., & Narita, M. (2014). Inside and out: The activities of senescence in cancer. *Nature Reviews. Cancer, 14*(8), 547–558. http://dx.doi.org/10.1038/nrc3773.

Pietras, K., & Östman, A. (2010). Hallmarks of cancer: Interactions with the tumor stroma. *Experimental Cell Research, 316*(8), 1324–1331.

Pilli, M., Arko-Mensah, J., Ponpuak, M., Roberts, E., Master, S., Mandell, M. A., … Deretic, V. (2012). TBK-1 promotes autophagy-mediated antimicrobial defense by controlling autophagosome maturation. *Immunity, 37*(2), 223–234. http://dx.doi.org/10.1016/j.immuni.2012.04.015.

Polager, S., Ofir, M., & Ginsberg, D. (2008). E2F1 regulates autophagy and the transcription of autophagy genes. *Oncogene, 27*(35), 4860–4864.

Ponpuak, M., Mandell, M. A., Kimura, T., Chauhan, S., Cleyrat, C., & Deretic, V. (2015). Secretory autophagy. *Current Opinion in Cell Biology, 35*, 106–116. http://dx.doi.org/10.1016/j.ceb.2015.04.016.

Puissant, A., Fenouille, N., & Auberger, P. (2012). When autophagy meets cancer through p62/SQSTM1. *American Journal of Cancer Research, 2*(4), 397–413. Retrieved from, http://www.ncbi.nlm.nih.gov/pmc/articles/PMC3410580/.

Qu, X., Yu, J., Bhagat, G., Furuya, N., Hibshoosh, H., Troxel, A., … Levine, B. (2003). Promotion of tumorigenesis by heterozygous disruption of the beclin 1 autophagy gene. *The Journal of Clinical Investigation, 112*(12), 1809–1820. http://dx.doi.org/10.1172/JCI20039.

Quail, D. F., & Joyce, J. A. (2013). Microenvironmental regulation of tumor progression and metastasis. *Nature Medicine, 19*(11), 1423–1437. http://dx.doi.org/10.1038/nm.3394.

Rabinowitz, J. D., & White, E. (2010). Autophagy and metabolism. *Science, 330*(6009), 1344–1348. http://dx.doi.org/10.1126/science.1193497.

Rabouille, C., Malhotra, V., & Nickel, W. (2012). Diversity in unconventional protein secretion. *Journal of Cell Science, 125*(22), 5251–5255. http://dx.doi.org/10.1242/jcs.103630.

Rahim, R., & Strobl, J. S. (2009). Hydroxychloroquine, chloroquine, and all-trans retinoic acid regulate growth, survival, and histone acetylation in breast cancer cells. *Anti-Cancer Drugs, 20*(8), 736–745. http://dx.doi.org/10.1097/CAD.0b013e32832f4e50.

Rangwala, R., Chang, Y. C., Hu, J., Algazy, K. M., Evans, T. L., Fecher, L. A., … Amaravadi, R. K. (2014). Combined MTOR and autophagy inhibition: Phase I trial of hydroxychloroquine and temsirolimus in patients with advanced solid tumors and melanoma. *Autophagy, 10*(8), 1391–1402. http://dx.doi.org/10.4161/auto.29119.

Rangwala, R., Leone, R., Chang, Y. C., Fecher, L. A., Schuchter, L. M., Kramer, A., … Amaravadi, R. K. (2014). Phase I trial of hydroxychloroquine with dose-intense temozolomide in patients with advanced solid tumors and melanoma. *Autophagy, 10*(8), 1369–1379. http://dx.doi.org/10.4161/auto.29118.

Rao, S., Tortola, L., Perlot, T., Wirnsberger, G., Novatchkova, M., Nitsch, R., … Penninger, J. M. (2014). A dual role for autophagy in a murine model of lung cancer. *Nature Communications, 5*. http://dx.doi.org/10.1038/ncomms4056.

Rautou, P.-E., Mansouri, A., Lebrec, D., Durand, F., Valla, D., & Moreau, R. (2010). Autophagy in liver diseases. *Journal of Hepatology, 53*(6), 1123–1134. http://dx.doi.org/10.1016/j.jhep.2010.07.006.

Reggiori, F., & Klionsky, D. J. (2002). Autophagy in the eukaryotic cell. *Eukaryotic Cell, 1*(1), 11–21. http://dx.doi.org/10.1128/ec.01.1.11-21.2002.

Rieber, M., & Strasberg Rieber, M. (2008). Sensitization to radiation-induced DNA damage accelerates loss of bcl-2 and increases apoptosis and autophagy. *Cancer Biology & Therapy*, 7(10), 1561–1566. http://dx.doi.org/10.4161/cbt.7.10.6540.

Roca, H., Varsos, Z. S., Sud, S., Craig, M. J., Ying, C., & Pienta, K. J. (2009). CCL2 and interleukin-6 promote survival of human CD11b + peripheral blood mononuclear cells and induce M2-type macrophage polarization. *Journal of Biological Chemistry*, 284(49), 34342–34354. http://dx.doi.org/10.1074/jbc.M109.042671.

Rosenfeld, M. R., Ye, X., Supko, J. G., Desideri, S., Grossman, S. A., Brem, S., … Amaravadi, R. K. (2014). A phase I/II trial of hydroxychloroquine in conjunction with radiation therapy and concurrent and adjuvant temozolomide in patients with newly diagnosed glioblastoma multiforme. *Autophagy*, 10(8), 1359–1368. http://dx. doi.org/10.4161/auto.28984.

Rosenfeldt, M. T., O'Prey, J., Morton, J. P., Nixon, C., MacKay, G., Mrowinska, A., … Ryan, K. M. (2013). p53 status determines the role of autophagy in pancreatic tumour development. *Nature*, 504(7479), 296–300. http://dx.doi.org/10.1038/nature12865.

Rosich, L., Xargay-Torrent, S., López-Guerra, M., Campo, E., Colomer, D., & Roué, G. (2012). Counteracting autophagy overcomes resistance to everolimus in mantle cell lymphoma. *Clinical Cancer Research*, 18(19), 5278–5289. http://dx.doi.org/10.1158/1078-0432.ccr-12-0351.

Rubinsztein, D. C., Mariño, G., & Kroemer, G. (2011). Autophagy and aging. *Cell*, 146(5), 682–695. http://dx.doi.org/10.1016/j.cell.2011.07.030.

Russell, R. C., Yuan, H.-X., & Guan, K.-L. (2014). Autophagy regulation by nutrient signaling. *Cell Research*, 24(1), 42–57. http://dx.doi.org/10.1038/cr.2013.166.

Rusten, T. E., Vaccari, T., Lindmo, K., Rodahl, L. M. W., Nezis, I. P., Sem-Jacobsen, C., … Stenmark, H. (2007). ESCRTs and Fab1 regulate distinct steps of autophagy. *Current Biology*, 17(20), 1817–1825. http://dx.doi.org/10.1016/j.cub.2007.09.032.

Sakaguchi, M. (1997). Eukaryotic protein secretion. *Current Opinion in Biotechnology*, 8(5), 595–601. http://dx.doi.org/10.1016/S0958-1669(97)80035-3.

Salas, E., Roy, S., Marsh, T., Rubin, B., & Debnath, J. (2015). Oxidative pentose phosphate pathway inhibition is a key determinant of antimalarial induced cancer cell death. *Oncogene*. http://dx.doi.org/10.1038/onc.2015.348.

Sancak, Y., Peterson, T. R., Shaul, Y. D., Lindquist, R. A., Thoreen, C. C., Bar-Peled, L., & Sabatini, D. M. (2008). The Rag GTPases bind raptor and mediate amino acid signaling to mTORC1. *Science*, 320(5882), 1496–1501. http://dx.doi.org/10.1126/science.1157535.

Scherz-Shouval, R., Shvets, E., Fass, E., Shorer, H., Gil, L., & Elazar, Z. (2007). Reactive oxygen species are essential for autophagy and specifically regulate the activity of Atg4. *The EMBO Journal*, 26(7), 1749–1760. http://dx.doi.org/10.1038/sj.emboj.7601623.

Schoenlein, P. V., Periyasamy-Thandavan, S., Samaddar, J. S., Jackson, W. H., & Barrett, J. T. (2009). Autophagy facilitates the progression of ERα-positive breast cancer cells to antiestrogen resistance. *Autophagy*, 5(3), 400–403. http://dx.doi.org/10.4161/auto.5.3.7784.

Schreiber, R. D., Old, L. J., & Smyth, M. J. (2011). Cancer immunoediting: Integrating immunity's roles in cancer suppression and promotion. *Science*, 331(6024), 1565–1570. http://dx.doi.org/10.1126/science.1203486.

Settembre, C., Di Malta, C., Polito, V. A., Arencibia, M. G., Vetrini, F., Erdin, S., … Ballabio, A. (2011). TFEB links autophagy to lysosomal biogenesis. *Science*, 332(6036), 1429–1433. http://dx.doi.org/10.1126/science.1204592.

Shao, Y., Gao, Z., Marks, P. A., & Jiang, X. (2004). Apoptotic and autophagic cell death induced by histone deacetylase inhibitors. *Proceedings of the National Academy of Sciences of the United States of America*, 101(52), 18030–18035. http://dx.doi.org/10.1073/pnas.0408345102.

Shen, H.-M., & Liu, Z.-G. (2006). JNK signaling pathway is a key modulator in cell death mediated by reactive oxygen and nitrogen species. *Free Radical Biology and Medicine, 40*(6), 928–939. http://dx.doi.org/10.1016/j.freeradbiomed.2005.10.056.

Shi, C.-S., & Kehrl, J. H. (2008). MyD88 and Trif target Beclin 1 to trigger autophagy in macrophages. *Journal of Biological Chemistry, 283*(48), 33175–33182. http://dx.doi.org/10.1074/jbc.M804478200.

Shi, C.-S., Shenderov, K., Huang, N.-N., Kabat, J., Abu-Asab, M., Fitzgerald, K. A., … Kehrl, J. H. (2012). Activation of autophagy by inflammatory signals limits IL-1[beta] production by targeting ubiquitinated inflammasomes for destruction. *Nature Immunology, 13*(3), 255–263. http://www.nature.com/ni/journal/v13/n3/abs/ni.2215.html. supplementary-information.

Shpilka, T., Mizushima, N., & Elazar, Z. (2012). Ubiquitin-like proteins and autophagy at a glance. *Journal of Cell Science, 125*(10), 2343–2348. http://dx.doi.org/10.1242/jcs.093757.

Sosa, M., Bragado, P., Debnath, J., & Aguirre-Ghiso, J. (2013). Regulation of tumor cell dormancy by tissue microenvironments and autophagy. In H. Enderling, N. Almog, & L. Hlatky (Eds.), *Systems biology of tumor dormancy: Vol. 734* (pp. 73–89). New York: Springer.

Strohecker, A. M., Guo, J. Y., Karsli-Uzunbas, G., Price, S. M., Chen, G. J., Mathew, R., … White, E. (2013). Autophagy sustains mitochondrial glutamine metabolism and growth of BrafV600E–driven lung tumors. *Cancer Discovery, 3*(11), 1272–1285. http://dx.doi.org/10.1158/2159-8290.cd-13-0397.

Sun, Q., Fan, W., Chen, K., Ding, X., Chen, S., & Zhong, Q. (2008). Identification of Barkor as a mammalian autophagy-specific factor for Beclin 1 and class III phosphatidylinositol 3-kinase. *Proceedings of the National Academy of Sciences of the United States of America, 105*(49), 19211–19216. http://dx.doi.org/10.1073/pnas.0810452105.

Suzuki, K., Kirisako, T., Kamada, Y., Mizushima, N., Noda, T., & Ohsumi, Y. (2001). The pre-autophagosomal structure organized by concerted functions of APG genes is essential for autophagosome formation. *The EMBO Journal, 20*(21), 5971–5981. http://dx.doi.org/10.1093/emboj/20.21.5971.

Takahashi, Y., Coppola, D., Matsushita, N., Cualing, H. D., Sun, M., Sato, Y., … Wang, H.-G. (2007). Bif-1 interacts with Beclin 1 through UVRAG and regulates autophagy and tumorigenesis. *Nature Cell Biology, 9*(10), 1142–1151. http://www.nature.com/ncb/journal/v9/n10/suppinfo/ncb1634_S1.html.

Takahashi, Y., Hori, T., Cooper, T. K., Liao, J., Desai, N., Serfass, J. M., … Wang, H.-G. (2013). Bif-1 haploinsufficiency promotes chromosomal instability and accelerates Myc-driven lymphomagenesis via suppression of mitophagy. *Blood, 121*(9), 1622–1632. http://dx.doi.org/10.1182/blood-2012-10-459826.

Takamura, A., Komatsu, M., Hara, T., Sakamoto, A., Kishi, C., Waguri, S., … Mizushima, N. (2011). Autophagy-deficient mice develop multiple liver tumors. *Genes & Development, 25*(8), 795–800. http://dx.doi.org/10.1101/gad.2016211.

Takeuchi, H., Kondo, Y., Fujiwara, K., Kanzawa, T., Aoki, H., Mills, G. B., & Kondo, S. (2005). Synergistic augmentation of rapamycin-induced autophagy in malignant glioma cells by phosphatidylinositol 3-kinase/protein kinase B inhibitors. *Cancer Research, 65*(8), 3336–3346. http://dx.doi.org/10.1158/0008-5472.CAN-04-3640.

Tang, D., Kang, R., Livesey, K. M., Cheh, C.-W., Farkas, A., Loughran, P., … Lotze, M. T. (2010). Endogenous HMGB1 regulates autophagy. *The Journal of Cell Biology, 190*(5), 881–892. http://dx.doi.org/10.1083/jcb.200911078.

Tang, D., & Lotze, M. (2013). Autophagy and the tumor microenvironment. In H.-G. Wang (Ed.), *Autophagy and cancer: Vol. 8* (pp. 167–189). New York: Springer.

Tanida, I., Ueno, T., & Kominami, E. (2004). LC3 conjugation system in mammalian autophagy. *The International Journal of Biochemistry & Cell Biology, 36*(12), 2503–2518. http://dx.doi.org/10.1016/j.biocel.2004.05.009.

Tasdemir, E., Maiuri, M. C., Galluzzi, L., Vitale, I., Djavaheri-Mergny, M., D'Amelio, M., … Kroemer, G. (2008). Regulation of autophagy by cytoplasmic p53. *Nature Cell Biology*, *10*(6), 676–687. http://dx.doi.org/10.1038/ncb1730.

Torisu, T., Torisu, K., Lee, I. H., Liu, J., Malide, D., Combs, C. A., … Finkel, T. (2013). Autophagy regulates endothelial cell processing, maturation and secretion of von Willebrand factor. *Nature Medicine*, *19*(10), 1281–1287. http://dx.doi.org/10.1038/nm.3288. http://www.nature.com/nm/journal/v19/n10/abs/nm.3288.html. supplementary-information.

Vader, P., Breakefield, X. O., & Wood, M. J. A. (2014). Extracellular vesicles: Emerging targets for cancer therapy. *Trends in Molecular Medicine*, *20*(7), 385–393. http://dx.doi.org/10.1016/j.molmed.2014.03.002.

Van Grol, J., Subauste, C., Andrade, R. M., Fujinaga, K., Nelson, J., & Subauste, C. S. (2010). HIV-1 Inhibits autophagy in bystander macrophage/monocytic cells through Src-Akt and STAT3. *PLoS One*, *5*(7), e11733. http://dx.doi.org/10.1371/journal.pone.0011733.

Vander Heiden, M. G., Cantley, L. C., & Thompson, C. B. (2009). Understanding the Warburg effect: The metabolic requirements of cell proliferation. *Science*, *324*(5930), 1029–1033. http://dx.doi.org/10.1126/science.1160809.

Velikkakath, A. K. G., Nishimura, T., Oita, E., Ishihara, N., & Mizushima, N. (2012). Mammalian Atg2 proteins are essential for autophagosome formation and important for regulation of size and distribution of lipid droplets. *Molecular Biology of the Cell*, *23*(5), 896–909. http://dx.doi.org/10.1091/mbc.E11-09-0785.

Viale, A., Pettazzoni, P., Lyssiotis, C. A., Ying, H., Sanchez, N., Marchesini, M., … Draetta, G. F. (2014). Oncogene ablation-resistant pancreatic cancer cells depend on mitochondrial function. *Nature*, *514*(7524), 628–632. http://dx.doi.org/10.1038/nature13611.

Villarreal, L., Méndez, O., Salvans, C., Gregori, J., Baselga, J., & Villanueva, J. (2013). Unconventional secretion is a major contributor of cancer cell line secretomes. *Molecular & Cellular Proteomics*, *12*(5), 1046–1060. http://dx.doi.org/10.1074/mcp.M112.021618.

Vogl, D. T., Stadtmauer, E. A., Tan, K. S., Heitjan, D. F., Davis, L. E., Pontiggia, L., … Amaravadi, R. K. (2014). Combined autophagy and proteasome inhibition: A phase 1 trial of hydroxychloroquine and bortezomib in patients with relapsed/refractory myeloma. *Autophagy*, *10*(8), 1380–1390. http://dx.doi.org/10.4161/auto.29264.

Wang, R. C., Wei, Y., An, Z., Zou, Z., Xiao, G., Bhagat, G., … Levine, B. (2012). Akt-mediated regulation of autophagy and tumorigenesis through Beclin 1 phosphorylation. *Science*, *338*(6109), 956–959. http://dx.doi.org/10.1126/science.1225967.

Ward, P. S., & Thompson, C. B. (2012). Metabolic reprogramming: A cancer hallmark even Warburg did not anticipate. *Cancer Cell*, *21*(3), 297–308. http://dx.doi.org/10.1016/j.ccr.2012.02.014.

Waris, G., & Ahsan, H. (2006). Reactive oxygen species: Role in the development of cancer and various chronic conditions. *Journal of Carcinogenesis*, *5*(1), 14. http://dx.doi.org/10.1186/1477-3163-5-14.

Wei, Y., Pattingre, S., Sinha, S., Bassik, M., & Levine, B. (2008). JNK1-mediated phosphorylation of Bcl-2 regulates starvation-induced autophagy. *Molecular Cell*, *30*(6), 678–688. http://dx.doi.org/10.1016/j.molcel.2008.06.001.

Wei, H., Wang, C., Croce, C. M., & Guan, J.-L. (2014). p62/SQSTM1 synergizes with autophagy for tumor growth in vivo. *Genes & Development*, *28*(11), 1204–1216. http://dx.doi.org/10.1101/gad.237354.113.

Wei, H., Wei, S., Gan, B., Peng, X., Zou, W., & Guan, J.-L. (2011). Suppression of autophagy by FIP200 deletion inhibits mammary tumorigenesis. *Genes & Development*, *25*(14), 1510–1527. http://dx.doi.org/10.1101/gad.2051011.

Wei, Y., Zou, Z., Becker, N., Anderson, M., Sumpter, R., Xiao, G., … Levine, B. (2013). EGFR-mediated Beclin 1 phosphorylation in autophagy suppression, tumor progression, and tumor chemoresistance. *Cell, 154*(6), 1269–1284. http://dx.doi.org/10.1016/j.cell.2013.08.015.

Weidberg, H., Shvets, E., & Elazar, Z. (2011). Biogenesis and cargo selectivity of autophagosomes. *Annual Review of Biochemistry, 80*(1), 125–156. http://dx.doi.org/10.1146/annurev-biochem-052709-094552.

Weidberg, H., Shvets, E., Shpilka, T., Shimron, F., Shinder, V., & Elazar, Z. (2010). LC3 and GATE-16/GABARAP subfamilies are both essential yet act differently in autophagosome biogenesis. *The EMBO Journal, 29*(11), 1792–1802. http://dx.doi.org/10.1038/emboj.2010.74.

White, E. (2012). Deconvoluting the context-dependent role for autophagy in cancer. *Nature Reviews. Cancer, 12*(6), 401–410. Retrieved from, http://dx.doi.org/10.1038/nrc3262.

White, E. (2015). The role for autophagy in cancer. *The Journal of Clinical Investigation, 125*(1), 42–46. http://dx.doi.org/10.1172/JCI73941.

Wilkinson, S., O'Prey, J., Fricker, M., & Ryan, K. M. (2009). Hypoxia-selective macroautophagy and cell survival signaled by autocrine PDGFR activity. *Genes & Development, 23*(11), 1283–1288. http://dx.doi.org/10.1101/gad.521709.

Witkiewicz, A. K., Dasgupta, A., Sotgia, F., Mercier, I., Pestell, R. G., Sabel, M., … Lisanti, M. P. (2009). An absence of stromal caveolin-1 expression predicts early tumor recurrence and poor clinical outcome in human breast cancers. *The American Journal of Pathology, 174*(6), 2023–2034. http://dx.doi.org/10.2353/ajpath.2009.080873.

Wu, W. K., Coffelt, S. B., Cho, C. H., Wang, X. J., Lee, C. W., Chan, F. K., … Sung, J. J. (2012). The autophagic paradox in cancer therapy. *Oncogene, 31*(8), 939–953. http://dx.doi.org/10.1038/onc.2011.295.

Xie, X., White, E. P., & Mehnert, J. M. (2013). Coordinate autophagy and mTOR pathway inhibition enhances cell death in melanoma. *PLoS One, 8*(1), e55096. http://dx.doi.org/10.1371/journal.pone.0055096.

Yadav, R. K., Chae, S.-W., Kim, H.-R., & Chae, H. J. (2014). Endoplasmic reticulum stress and cancer. *Journal of Cancer Prevention, 19*(2), 75–88. http://dx.doi.org/10.15430/JCP.2014.19.2.75.

Yang, Z., & Klionsky, D. (2009). An overview of the molecular mechanism of autophagy. In B. Levine, T. Yoshimori, & V. Deretic (Eds.), *Autophagy in infection and immunity: Vol. 335.* (pp. 1–32). Berlin, Heidelberg: Springer.

Yang, Z., & Klionsky, D. J. (2010). Mammalian autophagy: Core molecular machinery and signaling regulation. *Current Opinion in Cell Biology, 22*(2), 124–131. http://dx.doi.org/10.1016/j.ceb.2009.11.014.

Yang, A., Rajeshkumar, N. V., Wang, X., Yabuuchi, S., Alexander, B. M., Chu, G. C., … Kimmelman, A. C. (2014). Autophagy is critical for pancreatic tumor growth and progression in tumors with p53 alterations. *Cancer Discovery, 4*(8), 905–913. http://dx.doi.org/10.1158/2159-8290.cd-14-0362.

Yang, S., Wang, X., Contino, G., Liesa, M., Sahin, E., Ying, H., … Kimmelman, A. C. (2011). Pancreatic cancers require autophagy for tumor growth. *Genes & Development, 25*(7), 717–729. http://dx.doi.org/10.1101/gad.2016111.

Yazbeck, V. Y., Buglio, D., Georgakis, G. V., Li, Y., Iwado, E., Romaguera, J. E., … Younes, A. (2008). Temsirolimus downregulates p21 without altering cyclin D1 expression and induces autophagy and synergizes with vorinostat in mantle cell lymphoma. *Experimental Hematology, 36*(4), 443–450. http://dx.doi.org/10.1016/j.exphem.2007.12.008.

Yeh, A. C., & Ramaswamy, S. (2015). Mechanisms of cancer cell dormancy—Another hall-mark of cancer? *Cancer Research, 75*, 5014–5022. http://dx.doi.org/10.1158/0008-5472. can-15-1370.

Yoshioka, A., Miyata, H., Doki, Y., Yamasaki, M., Sohma, I., Gotoh, K., … Monden, M. (2008). LC3, an autophagosome marker, is highly expressed in gastrointestinal cancers. *International Journal of Oncology, 33*(3), 461–468. Retrieved from, http://www.ncbi.nlm. nih.gov/pubmed/18695874.

Young, A. R. J., Narita, M., Ferreira, M., Kirschner, K., Sadaie, M., Darot, J. F. J., … Narita, M. (2009). Autophagy mediates the mitotic senescence transition. *Genes & Development, 23*(7), 798–803. http://dx.doi.org/10.1101/gad.519709.

Yue, Z., Jin, S., Yang, C., Levine, A. J., & Heintz, N. (2003). Beclin 1, an autophagy gene essential for early embryonic development, is a haploinsufficient tumor suppressor. *Proceedings of the National Academy of Sciences of the United States of America, 100*(25), 15077–15082. http://dx.doi.org/10.1073/pnas.2436255100.

Zhan, Z., Xie, X., Cao, H., Zhou, X., Zhang, X. D., Fan, H., & Liu, Z. (2014). Autophagy facilitates TLR4- and TLR3-triggered migration and invasion of lung cancer cells through the promotion of TRAF6 ubiquitination. *Autophagy, 10*(2), 257–268. http://dx.doi.org/10.4161/auto.27162.

Zhang, Y., Cheng, Y., Ren, X., Zhang, L., Yap, K. L., Wu, H., … Yang, J. M. (2012). NAC1 modulates sensitivity of ovarian cancer cells to cisplatin by altering the HMGB1-mediated autophagic response. *Oncogene, 31*(8), 1055–1064. http://www. nature.com/onc/journal/v31/n8/suppinfo/onc2011290s1.html.

Zhang, M., Kenny, S., Ge, L., Xu, K., & Schekman, R. (2015). Translocation of interleukin-1β into a vesicle intermediate in autophagy-mediated secretion. *eLife.* http://dx.doi.org/ 10.7554/eLife.11205.

Zhang, M., & Schekman, R. (2013). Unconventional secretion, unconventional solutions. *Science, 340*(6132), 559–561. http://dx.doi.org/10.1126/science.1234740.

Zhao, J., Brault, J. J., Schild, A., Cao, P., Sandri, M., Schiaffino, S., … Goldberg, A. L. (2007). FoxO3 coordinately activates protein degradation by the autophagic/lysosomal and proteasomal pathways in atrophying muscle cells. *Cell Metabolism, 6*(6), 472–483. http://dx.doi.org/10.1016/j.cmet.2007.11.004.

Zhao, Z., Han, F.-H., Yang, S.-B., Hua, L.-X., Wu, J.-H., & Zhan, W.-H. (2015). Loss of stromal caveolin-1 expression in colorectal cancer predicts poor survival. *World Journal of Gastroenterology, 21*(4), 1140–1147. http://dx.doi.org/10.3748/wjg.v21.i4.1140.

Zhong, Y., Wang, Q. J., Li, X., Yan, Y., Backer, J. M., Chait, B. T., … Yue, Z. (2009). Distinct regulation of autophagic activity by Atg14L and Rubicon associated with Beclin 1-phosphatidylinositol-3-kinase complex. *Nature Cell Biology, 11*(4), 468–476. http:// www.nature.com/ncb/journal/v11/n4/suppinfo/ncb1854_S1.html.

Zhou, R., Yazdi, A. S., Menu, P., & Tschopp, J. (2011). A role for mitochondria in NLRP3 inflammasome activation. *Nature, 469*(7329), 221–225. http://www.nature.com/ nature/journal/v469/n7329/abs/nature09663.html, supplementary-information.

Zou, Y., Ling, Y.-H., Sironi, J., Schwartz, E. L., Perez-Soler, R., & Piperdi, B. (2013). The autophagy inhibitor chloroquine overcomes the innate resistance of wild-type EGFR non-small-cell lung cancer cells to erlotinib. *Journal of Thoracic Oncology, 8*(6), 693–702. http://dx.doi.org/10.1097/JTO.0b013e31828c7210.

> CHAPTER TWO

Inhibitors of DNA Methylation, Histone Deacetylation, and Histone Demethylation: A Perfect Combination for Cancer Therapy

C.A. Zahnow[1], M. Topper, M. Stone, T. Murray-Stewart, H. Li, S.B. Baylin, R.A. Casero Jr.

The Sidney Kimmel Comprehensive Cancer Center, Johns Hopkins University, Baltimore, MD, United States
[1]Corresponding author: e-mail address: zahnoci@jhmi.edu

Contents

Abstract

Epigenetic silencing and inappropriate activation of gene expression are frequent events during the initiation and progression of cancer. These events involve a complex interplay between the hypermethylation of CpG dinucleotides within gene promoter and enhancer regions, the recruitment of transcriptional corepressors and the deacetylation and/or methylation of histone tails. These epigenetic regulators act in concert to block transcription or interfere with the maintenance of chromatin boundary regions. However, DNA/histone methylation and histone acetylation states are reversible, enzyme-mediated processes and as such, have emerged as promising targets for cancer therapy. This review will focus on the potential benefits and synergistic/additive effects of combining DNA-demethylating agents and histone deacetylase inhibitors or lysine-specific demethylase inhibitors together in epigenetic therapy for solid tumors and will highlight what is known regarding the mechanisms of action that contribute to the antitumor response.

1. INTRODUCTION

Epigenetics refers to functionally relevant changes in gene expression that are not the result of changes in the DNA sequence, but rather changes in histone modifications, DNA methylation, and chromatin structure (Allis, Jenuwein, Reinberg, & Caparros, 2015; Baylin & Jones, 2011; Herman & Baylin, 2003; Jones & Baylin, 2007). Epigenetic processes are mitotically heritable and critically important for gene silencing that is necessary during development and normal cellular functioning in eukaryotes (Allis et al., 2015). However, epigenetic processes can become dysregulated and contribute to the evolution of diseased states such as cancer (Baylin & Jones, 2011; Portela & Esteller, 2010). To date, the most intensely studied epigenetic changes observed in cancer are changes in DNA methylation that can result in both decreased gene body CpG methylation (Hansen et al., 2011) and increased methylation of CpG islands in the promoter regions of genes (Baylin & Jones, 2011; Jones & Baylin, 2002, 2007; Rodriguez-Paredes & Esteller, 2011) as well as deacetylation or methylation of histone tails, which regulate chromatin conformational states (Chi, Allis, & Wang, 2010; Jenuwein & Allis, 2001). Chromatin consists of DNA, histones, and nonhistone proteins, which constitute nucleosome structures. Chromatin can exist as heterochromatin, which is densely compacted and transcriptionally inactive, or euchromatin, wherein nucleosomes are less compacted and arranged more linearly resulting in more open and accessible regions for transcription (Li, Carey, & Workman, 2007; Tessarz & Kouzarides, 2014). The balance and interplay between DNA methylation, histone modification, and nucleosome positioning determines if a particular gene or genes within regions are transcriptionally expressed or silent (Allis et al., 2015; Guil & Esteller, 2009).

Numerous associations exist between DNA methylation and posttranslational histone modification. Histone deacetylases (HDACs, detailed in a later section) are often found to be overexpressed in cancer cells (Ellis, Atadja, & Johnstone, 2009), lead to histone hypoacetylation around the transcription start site of genes, and are associated with compact chromatin near silenced genes. It has been established that CpG island promoter DNA methylation can attract methylcytosine-binding proteins (MBD1, MBD2, MBD4 and MeCP1, MeCP2) and other associated proteins that mediate transcriptional repression during gene silencing and heterochromatin formation (Nan et al., 1998; Parry & Clarke, 2011). The MeCP1/2 proteins, in turn, recruit corepressor complexes to the DNA consisting of HDACs 1 and 2 and mSin3a (Nan et al., 1998). Methyl-binding proteins, MBD2 or MBD3, are mutually exclusive and have been shown to interact individually with the nucleosomal-remodeling complex (NuRD) (Zhang et al., 1999). Moreover, CHD4, a key component of the NuRD repressive remodeling complex, binds HDACs 1 and 2 and may be critical in maintaining the transcriptional repression of DNA hypermethylated genes (Cai et al., 2014). Lastly, polycomb group (PcG) proteins are required for stable long-term silencing of specific genes, and complexes containing PcG proteins, DNA methyltransferases (DNMTs), and SIRT1 have been linked to hypermethylated gene promoters during tumorigenesis (O'Hagan, Mohammad, & Baylin, 2008; O'Hagan et al., 2011). This growing body of evidence demonstrates that HDACs 1 and 2 and the Class III HDAC Sirtuin 1 (SIRT1) are linked to the initiation and/or maintenance of repression for DNA hypermethylated genes, and studies have demonstrated that the simultaneous targeting of both DNA methylation and histone deacetylation leads to additive or synergistic effects to reactivate aberrantly silenced genes (Allis et al., 2015; Arrowsmith, Bountra, Fish, Lee, & Schapira, 2012).

Moreover, links between DNA methylation and histone methylation have also been described (Ahuja, Easwaran, & Baylin, 2014). The histone methyltransferase SUV39H1/2 moves to centromeres during mitosis to methylate lysine 9 of histone H3 (H3K9) and plays a vital role in heterochromatin organization, chromosome segregation, and mitotic progression (Aagaard et al., 1999). This histone methyltransferase has been shown to interact with DNMT3a (Fuks, Hurd, Deplus, & Kouzarides, 2003) and MBD1 (Fujita et al., 2003). In *Arabidopsis* and *Neurospora*, H3K9 methylation seems to be a prerequisite for DNA methylation (Jackson, Lindroth, Cao, & Jacobsen, 2002). Lysine-specific demethylase, LSD1 (see later section), is also upregulated in cancer and selectively demethylates H3K4me1/2 (Lim et al., 2010), leading to transcriptional repression. Reduced H3K9me3 levels and increased H3ac and H3K4me3 modifications are associated with gene promoter regions in hypomethylated genes. As both DNA and histone methylation play a role in gene silencing, combination therapy using both DNMT and KDM (lysine demethylase) inhibitors may be a rational anticancer strategy.

2. DNMTs: THE ENZYMES RESPONSIBLE FOR DNA METHYLATION

There are three enzymatically active DNMTs in eukaryotic cells, DNMT1, 3a, and 3b (for review, see Denis, Ndlovu, & Fuks, 2011), and each are known to bind HDAC1 and HDAC2 (Bachman, Rountree, & Baylin, 2001; Fuks, Burgers, Brehm, Hughes-Davies, & Kouzarides, 2000; Ling et al., 2004; Robertson et al., 2000; Rountree, Bachman, & Baylin, 2000). These are the only enzymes known to catalyze the transfer of a methyl group from S-adenosylmethionine to cytosine (Goll & Bestor, 2005). DNMT1 is the predominant methyltransferase and is important for the maintenance of postreplicative DNA methylation. DNMT1 localizes to DNA replication foci during S phase and preferentially methylates hemimethylated CpG dinucleotides via its interaction with the SRA domain of ubiquitin-like containing PHD and RING finger domains 1 (UHFR1) (Avvakumov et al., 2008; Sharif et al., 2007). DNMT1 can also contribute to de novo methylation in human cancer cells (Jair et al., 2006), and its loss can lead to genomic instability (Chen, Pettersson, Beard, Jackson-Grusby, & Jaenisch, 1998; Li, Bestor, & Jaenisch, 1992). DNMT3a and 3b are known as de novo methyltransferases and play a role in the establishment of methylation patterns during development. Sequence preferences for DNMT3a and 3b have been suggested to be important for their de novo activity. It is not yet clear what determines their activity, but interactions with other factors may be important for locus-specific DNA methylation (Jurkowska, Jurkowski, & Jeltsch, 2011).

DNMT3L, a related protein that lacks methyltransferase activity, recognizes histone H3 tails that are unmethylated at lysine 4 (Ooi et al., 2007). DNMT3L is necessary for de novo methylation of imprinted loci in germ cells via stabilization of the active site loop of DNMT3a and increases in the binding of S-adenosylmethionine (Jia, Jurkowska, Zhang, Jeltsch, & Cheng, 2007; Ooi et al., 2007). DNMT2 is an RNA methyltransferase and catalyzes the methylation of tRNA^{Asp} at cytosine 38 and cytosine 48 (Goll et al., 2006; Schaefer, Hagemann, Hanna, & Lyko, 2009).

3. DNA-DEMETHYLATING AGENTS

The two best studied of the nucleoside analogue-based DNA-demethylating agents that are currently being used in clinical trials for solid tumors are azacytidine (AZA, 5-azacytidine, 5-AZA-CR, trade name Vidaza, Celgene), a derivative of the nucleoside cytidine, and decitabine (DAC, 5-deoxy azacytidine, 5-aza-2′-deoxycytidine-5′-triphosphate, 5-AZA-dC, 5-AZA-Cdr, trade name Dacogen, Eisai), the deoxyribose analogue of 5-azacytidine. Azacytidine and decitabine were synthesized as cytostatic agents in 1964 (Sorm, Piskala, Cihak, & Vesely, 1964) and azacytidine was later found to be a natural product of *Streptoverticillium ladakanus* (Bergy & Herr, 1966; Hanka, Evans, Mason, & Dietz, 1966). Early clinical trials found both compounds to be too toxic for use, but in the 1980s, it was discovered that azacytidine could induce differentiation in cultured mouse embryo cells and inhibit the methylation of newly synthesized DNA (Jones & Taylor, 1980; Taylor & Jones, 1982). Studies were also emerging from the Baylin laboratory and others in the 1980s and 1990s regarding the existence of promoter CpG island hypermethylation and the correlation with transcriptional repression. Moreover, work by Issa and colleagues suggested that pharmacologic inhibition of DNMT activity and resultant DNA methylation might be a promising new therapy to reactivate tumor suppressor gene expression (Baylin, 1997; Baylin, Herman, Graff, Vertino, & Issa, 1998; Baylin et al., 1991; Issa, Baylin, & Herman, 1997). Taken together, these studies prompted its re-evaluation in patients and led to the approval for clinical use of azacytidine in 2004 and decitabine in 2006 (Egger, Liang, Aparicio, & Jones, 2004). Both agents are FDA approved for use in myelodysplastic syndromes (MDSs) and chronic myelomonocytic leukemia, but not yet in solid tumors.

After cellular uptake, azacytidine and decitabine are phosphorylated sequentially by uridine-cytidine and diphosphate kinases, which convert them to the active triphosphate forms 5-Aza-CTP and 5-AZA-dCTP, respectively (Fig. 1). Decitabine is incorporated into DNA in place of cytidine. Ten to twenty percent of intracellular azacytidine can also incorporate into DNA after it is converted to decitabine via ribonucleotide reductase (Fig. 1; Stresemann & Lyko, 2008). The remaining 80% of azacytidine incorporates into RNA (Li, Olin, Buskirk, & Reineke, 1970) to affect nuclear and cytoplasmic RNA metabolism including ribosome biogenesis and protein synthesis (Cihak, 1974; see Section 4).

S phase is required for effective incorporation of decitabine into DNA. The incorporated decitabine, recognized as a natural cytosine by the

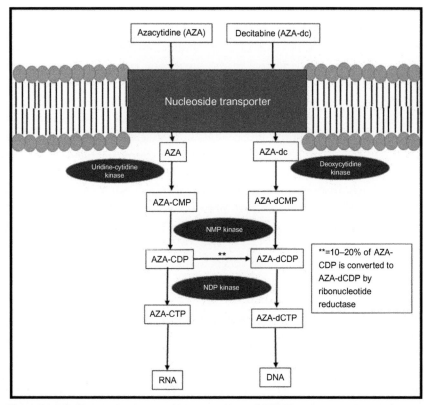

Fig. 1 Metabolism, activation, and incorporation of DNMT active cytosine analogues. (See the color plate.)

DNMTs, is methylated via nucleophilic attack and forms a strong covalent bond with the enzyme, known as covalent trapping, which leads to degradation of the DNMTs (Chen et al., 1991; Santi, Norment, & Garrett, 1984). As a consequence, in the presence of reduced DNMT levels, DNA methylation will be lost rather than maintained with each cellular division via the passive dilution of methylated cytosines; this is in contrast to active demethylation (Ghoshal et al., 2005; Kuo, Griffith, & Kreuzer, 2007). This covalent interaction can also function as a bulky decitabine-DNMT adduct to trigger a DNA damage signal (Juttermann, Li, & Jaenisch, 1994). Moreover, the DNA damage signal may arise from the nitrogen at the 5′ position of the heterocyclic ring in the demethylating agent, which can destabilize and destroy the ring, leading to DNA damage (Sampath, Rao, & Plunkett, 2003). Other studies have shown that decitabine can induce selective degradation of DNMT1 in the nucleus via activation of an ubiquitin-dependent proteasomal pathway (Ghoshal et al., 2005).

Although azacytidine can incorporate into RNA, evidence in studies using HCT-116 DNMT knockout cells shows that the mRNA expression profile between DNMT knockout cells and azacytidine- or decitabine-treated cells is similar (Li et al., 2014). This demonstrates the significance of the DNMTs as specific targets of nucleoside analogues and that both azacytidine and decitabine are capable of degrading DNMTs in a manner that yield similar changes in gene expression. Other DNMT inhibitors (DNMTi) include the following:

Guadecitabine (SGI-110, Astex) is a novel hypomethylating dinucleotide of decitabine and deoxyguanosine that is more resistant to degradation by cytidine deaminase. This nucleoside was developed to increase the stability and half-life of decitabine to improve bioavailability and uptake into cancer cells and is currently being tested in clinical trials for selected solid tumors, the results of which are not yet published for solid tumors, but have been for MDS/acute myeloid leukemia (AML) (Issa et al., 2015).

Hydralazine, also currently being used in clinical trials, is a small-molecule, non-nucleoside compound commonly used to treat hypertension (Segura-Pacheco et al., 2003). It is a weak inhibitor of DNMTs and is able to reactivate the expression of several tumor suppressor genes in solid tumors (Candelaria et al., 2007). Clinical trials have shown that hydralazine is better able to reactivate silenced genes in the presence of the HDAC inhibitor valproic acid.

Zebularine (1-(β-D-ribofuranosyl)-2(1H)-pyrimidinone) is a cytidine lacking the 4-amino group of the pyrimidine ring (Champion et al., 2010).

Synthesized in 1961, it was found to be an inhibitor of cytidine deaminase with antitumor properties (Kim, Marquez, Mao, Haines, & McCormack, 1986) and serves as a DNMTi (Zhou et al., 2002) leading to DNA demethylation (Stresemann & Lyko, 2008) and reactivation of tumor suppressor genes (Billam, Sobolewski, & Davidson, 2010). Zebularine is considered less toxic than azacytidine and decitabine, which allows it to be administered continuously for long periods of time to prevent the recurrence of methylation (Yoo et al., 2008). However, the actions of zebularine are not well understood or without drawbacks, and this drug is being re-examined before further use in the clinic (Ren et al., 2011).

5-Fluoro-2′-deoxycytidine (FdCyd, NSC 48006) inhibits DNMT in a manner similar to AZA and DAC, by forming a covalent bond with DNMTs after incorporation into DNA. It was initially investigated, however, as a prodrug for the thymidylate synthase inhibitor, 5-fluoro-2′-dUMP (FdUMP) (Van Triest, Pinedo, Giaccone, & Peters, 2000). Although FdCyd is chemically stable in aqueous environments, it is deaminated by cytidine deaminase to generate FdUMP (Beumer et al., 2006). In a phase I clinical trial of mixed solid tumors FdCyd is being used in combination with the deamination inhibitor tetrahydrouridine to improve its stability as a demethylating agent (Newman et al., 2015).

The nucleoside inhibitors, azacytidine, decitabine, guadecitabine, and zebularine, are metabolized before being incorporated into DNA (Fig. 1). After incorporation, they function as suicide substrates for DNMT enzymes. Non-nucleoside inhibitors, EGCG and RG108, inhibit DNMTs by blocking the active site of the enzyme (EGCG, RG108) (Lyko & Brown, 2005). It is felt, however, that the non-nucleoside compounds induce limited epigenetic changes in cells (Chuang et al., 2005).

RG108 was developed by rational drug design to block the active sites of DNMTs with very little toxicity. Although antitumor effects in human prostate cancer cells (Graca et al., 2014) have been observed, the mechanism of action of this agent is unclear and additional studies of this compound are underway (Asgatay et al., 2014).

EGCG (−)-epigallocatechin-3-gallate, the main polyphenol compound in green tea, inhibits DNMT activity by blocking the active site of human DNMT1 (Fang et al., 2003).

SGI-1027 is a lipophilic, quinolone-based compound containing a decitabine moiety that acts as a DNMTi. This agent is not incorporated into

DNA and has shown reactivation of hypermethylated genes (Amato, 2007). For additional review on DNA-demethylating agents, see Ren et al. (2011).

4. AZACYTIDINE IN RNA METABOLISM

As mentioned previously, only about 10–20% of azacytidine is converted to 2-deoxy-5-azacytidine (decitabine) by ribonucleotide reductase in treated cells, which can be further incorporated into DNA, leading to hypomethylation (Stresemann & Lyko, 2008). Approximately 80–90% of azacytidine is incorporated into RNA (Li et al., 1970). RNA serves as a critical mediator between DNA and protein. Disruptions of RNA will eventually result in aberrant protein translation and may ultimately lead to cell death. Apart from the common belief that azacytidine functions through DNA hypomethylation, Aimiuwu et al. (2012) have reported that azacytidine can inhibit ribonucleotide reductase M2 (RRM2) mRNA expression by direct RNA incorporation and resultant decreases in RRM2 mRNA stability. As a result of ribonucleotide reductase inhibition, azacytidine can reduce the overall deoxyribonucleotide pool, and profoundly impair DNA synthesis and repair (Aimiuwu et al., 2012).

Although proper methylation of RNA is very important for its function, the reports on the effect of azacytidine on RNA methylation are relatively few and focused on tRNA. Similar to DNA methylation, cytosine-5-methylation (m^5C) is also detected in RNA (Motorin, Lyko, & Helm, 2010). There are six major families of m^5C RNA methyltransferases: (1) RsmB/Nol1/NSUN1, (2) RsmF/YebU/NSUN2, (3) RlmI, (4) Ynl022, (5) NSUN6, and (6) DNMT2 (Motorin et al., 2010). Only DNMT2 works on a single cytosine, while the other five families target two cytosines (Jurkowski et al., 2008; King & Redman, 2002). In a manner similar to DNMTs, all m^5C RNA transferases mediate methylation by forming covalent bonds with their target (Motorin et al., 2010). Incorporated azacytidine in RNA can deplete m^5C RNA methyltransferases by stabilizing the covalent bond (Lu, Chiang, Medina, & Randerath, 1976; Lu & Randerath, 1979; Schaefer et al., 2009). It has not been demonstrated that azacytidine degrades DNMT2, but RNA methylation at DNMT2 target sites has been shown to be inhibited by azacytidine (Schaefer et al., 2009). DNMT2 contains all the catalytic motifs of traditional DNMTs and shares conserved motifs with bacterial DNMT; however, it has neither DNMT activity nor CpG methylation regulation capability (Defossez, 2013; Hermann, Schmitt, & Jeltsch, 2003).

Although the exact biological function of tRNA demethylation remains unknown, the alterations mediated by azacytidine might have an impact on tRNA folding and stability, leading to mismatch and further impairment of protein synthesis. It has been observed that in vivo treatment with azacytidine inhibits mouse liver tRNA m^5C RNA methyltransferase function (Lu & Randerath, 1979). Moreover, tRNA^{Asp}, tRNA^{Gly}, and tRNA^{Val} have been reported as substrates for DNMT2 (Goll et al., 2006; Jurkowski et al., 2008; Khoddami & Cairns, 2013; Rai et al., 2007; Schaefer & Lyko, 2010), and azacytidine can inhibit the methylation (eg, C38) of tRNA^{Asp}, but decitabine cannot (Schaefer et al., 2009). Using azacytidine pull down and RNA sequencing, it was found that azacytidine can cause both mutation and transversion (C to G) at m^5C sites of DNMT2 and NSUN2 targets (tRNA: tRNA^{Asp}, tRNA^{Gly}, tRNA^{Val}, and tRNA^{Leu}) and noncoding RNAs, which can lead to the disruption of a wide range of RNA structures and consequent binding to ribonucleosomes (Khoddami & Cairns, 2013). Besides its effects on tRNA, azacytidine can also disrupt ribosomal RNA. In a study using radiolabeled azacytidine, treatment of Novikoff hepatoma cells resulted in approximately 37% of the cytidines in the 45S rRNA being replaced by azacytidine (Weiss & Pitot, 1975). The incorporated azacytidine alters the secondary structure of the 45S molecule and greatly reduces the conversion into 28S and 18S rRNA as well as maturation of the precursor 45S (Weiss & Pitot, 1975). rRNA is the most dominant form of RNA and a major component of ribosomal organization, which is responsible for protein translation. Indeed, decreased protein synthesis has been observed in azacytidine-treated cells, but not those treated with decitabine (Hollenbach et al., 2010).

Taken together, the ability of azacytidine to activate hypermethylated and silenced genes as well as its effects on tRNA and rRNA suggest more complex mechanisms of action for this drug than for decitabine. Although reports show that azacytidine can interfere with rRNA, mRNA, and tRNA synthesis, stability, and function, the precise mechanisms and biological outcomes are still not clear. Studies of the nondemethylating effects of azacytidine on noncoding RNA, such as lncRNA and miRNA, are also largely unknown. One might speculate that because azacytidine is effectively incorporated into RNA, the azacytidine-containing RNA might subsequently serve as an intracellular pool for the "slow-release" of azacytidine. A better understanding of the RNA mechanism of azacytidine action will improve clinical drug monitoring, combination therapy design, prognosis prediction, and may even uncover more significant potentials of epigenetic drugs for clinical applications.

5. HISTONE ACETYLATION

As stated earlier, dysregulation of epigenetic gene regulation is a hallmark of cancer. Aberrant silencing of important tumor suppressor or other growth regulatory genes by the combination of hypoacetylation and hypermethylation of promoter regions results in loss of normal growth control. As such, the histone acetylation state is a critical determinant in the transcriptional regulation of important growth regulatory genes, and thus HDACs are interesting drug targets that have the potential to reactivate aberrantly silenced genes in cancer.

Histone acetylation is an active process regulated by both the relative abundance and localization of histone acetyltransferases (HATs) and nuclear-localized HDACs (Ropero & Esteller, 2007). The posttranslational modification of acetylation is extremely dynamic with a half-life of less than 15 min for all modified histones; this necessitates continual maintenance of the mark (Barth & Imhof, 2010). Protein acetylation induces charge neutralization of histone lysine tails, inducing dissociation of the tails from the negatively charged DNA phosphodiester backbone. This removes steric hindrance for transcription factor association, thus creating a transcriptionally permissive state at a specified locus (Ropero & Esteller, 2007).

5.1 Histone Deacetylases

HDAC enzymes are classified based on cellular localization and cofactor dependence. The predominant function of this enzyme class is to act as an eraser of one of the marks in the histone code; specifically the removal of an acetyl moiety from lysines in histone tails. In addition, some of the HDACs do function as scaffolds and readers of the histone code. Thus far, 18 HDACs have been identified to date, with 11 HDACs comprising the classical zinc-dependent HDACs, and the remaining 7 being the Class III NAD-dependent Sirtuins (SIRT 1–7). The presence or lack of a nuclear localization signal is critical for determining the cellular distribution of the classical zinc-dependent deacetylases. These HDACs are subcategorized into three distinct classes: Class I, Class II, and Class IV (Falkenberg & Johnstone, 2014; Ropero & Esteller, 2007; Witt, Deubzer, Milde, & Oehme, 2009).

5.1.1 Class I HDACs

Class I HDACs are predominantly nuclear localized, consisting of HDACs 1, 2, 3, and 8 (Table 1). Class I HDACs have near ubiquitous expression across many disparate cell lineages (Falkenberg & Johnstone, 2014; Witt

Table 1 Zinc-Dependent HDAC Classes with Associated Isoforms

HDAC Class	HDAC Isoforms	Cellular Distribution	Nuclear Localization Signal Present	Size—Amino Acids
Class I	1	Nuclear	Yes	482
	2	Nuclear	No	488
	3	Nuclear and cytoplasmic	Yes	428
	8	Nuclear and cytoplasmic	Yes	377
Class IIa	4	Nuclear and cytoplasmic	Yes	1084
	5	Nuclear and cytoplasmic	Yes	1122
	7	Nuclear and cytoplasmic	Yes	855
	9	Nuclear and cytoplasmic	Yes	1011
Class IIb	6	Cytoplasmic	No	1215
	10	Cytoplasmic	No	669
Class IV	11	Cytoplasmic	No	347

et al., 2009). HDACs 1 and 2 are key in terms of histone acetylation regulation as these HDACs form the catalytic core of multiple corepressor complexes (Bantscheff et al., 2011). These complexes recognize methylated CpG DNA through the presence of methyl–binding domain proteins such as MeCP2 and MBD2 and facilitate the localization of these complexes to areas of CpG island methylation in the genome (Denslow & Wade, 2007; Ebert et al., 2013). HDAC3, another critical regulator of histone acetylation, can translocate between the nuclear and cytoplasmic compartment, with the primary site of action being the nuclear compartment. This particular HDAC isoform must associate with the NCoR complex to attain a catalytically permissive conformation, free of repressive chaperones (Codina et al., 2005; Guenther, Barak, & Lazar, 2001). HDAC8 has lower enzymatic functionality, relative to other Class I isoforms, but has been implicated in the acetylation of both histone and nonhistone substrates (Witt et al., 2009). Overexpression of Class I HDAC isoforms 1, 2, and 3 has been detected in a wide range of malignancies including prostate, gastric, and colon cancers. This overexpression is correlated with p21 downregulation resulting in dysregulation of the cell cycle (Glozak & Seto, 2007). Critical to the epigenetic therapy focus of this review is the link of HDACs 1 and 2 to the DNA methylation processes discussed earlier. These two proteins, as mentioned earlier and further later, bind to the DNMTs as well as to key complexes that interact with DNA methylation such as the MBDs, the SIN transcription repression complexes, and the NURD complex, among others (Ahuja et al., 2014; Cai et al., 2014; Deaton & Bird, 2011; Fuks et al., 2003; O'Hagan et al., 2008; Rountree et al., 2000).

5.1.2 Class II HDACs

Class II HDACs function more in terms of nonhistone substrate modification and display tissue specificity in terms of expression (Verdin, Dequiedt, & Kasler, 2003). Class II HDACs are further subsetted into two broad categories: Class IIa and Class IIb (Table 1). Both of these subclasses are zinc dependent and thus subcategorization is based more on enzyme activity and the presence of a nuclear localization signal (Falkenberg & Johnstone, 2014; Witt et al., 2009). Class IIa HDACs, HDACs 4, 5, 7, and 9, have low enzymatic activity and act more as readers of acetylated lysine tails and scaffolding than erasers (Bradner et al., 2010). Class IIa HDACs do contain a nuclear localization signal, allowing these enzymes to shuttle between the nuclear and cytoplasmic compartments. Class IIb HDACs, HDACs 6 and 10, actively deacetylate nonhistone substrates and act to augment protein stability and activation status. This class of enzymes lacks a nuclear localization signal and is strictly comprised of cytoplasmic deacetylases (Falkenberg & Johnstone, 2014; Verdin et al., 2003). HDAC6 is a critical regulator of the unfolded protein response: in this context, HDAC6 deacetylates HSP90 and HSP70, allowing for binding of ATP and target proteins (Rao, Nalluri, et al., 2010). The overexpression of HDAC6 has been demonstrated in a wide range of cancers including osteosarcoma, AML, and ovarian cancers (Aldana-Masangkay & Sakamoto, 2011; Glozak & Seto, 2007). Additionally, it was elucidated in a study by Lee et al. (2008) that HDAC6 is a critical determinant of anchorage-independent growth of RAS-transformed MEF cells, implicating a crucial role for this HDAC in RAS-mediated tumorigenesis.

5.1.3 Class IV HDAC

The Class IV HDAC, HDAC11 is a zinc-dependent HDAC whose function is largely unknown. Sharing significant homology with both Class I and Class II HDACs, HDAC11 does not possess a nuclear localization signal and is thought to act more as a cytoplasmic HDAC (Table 1) (Ropero & Esteller, 2007; Witt et al., 2009).

6. NUCLEAR REPRESSIVE COMPLEXES

6.1 Nucleosome Remodeling and Deacetylase Complex: A Link Between DNA Methylation, Histone Deacetylation, and Nucleosome Remodeling

As discussed in Section 1, the nucleosome remodeling and deacetylase complex or NuRD nuclear repressive complex provides a link between DNA methylation, histone deacetylation, and nucleosome remodeling. The interaction of this complex may have very special connections to the gene silencing associated with DNA methylation and HDACs and for strategies to target abnormalities involving these proteins in cancer (Cai et al., 2014). Table 2 provides a summary of the study by Bantscheff et al. (2011), which elucidated NuRD complex-associated chromatin modifiers. The NuRD complex contains the core enzymatic components of an HDAC1:HDAC2 dimer, which facilitates the deacetylase function of the complex (Bantscheff et al., 2011). Nucleosome remodeling is enabled by the presence of two Mi-2 proteins: CHD3 and CHD4. These SWI/SNF family ATPases compact nucleosome structure. Localization of the complex is permitted by the presence of methyl CpG island-binding proteins MBD2 and MBD3, with only MBD2 possessing the functionality of methylated DNA recognition (Denslow & Wade, 2007). The NuRD complex provides a direct mechanistic link between DNA methylation and alteration of chromatin structure at the level of histone modification and nucleosome remodeling (Wong, Guo, & Zhang, 2014). This model predicts NuRD complex recognition

Table 2 HDAC and LSD1-Associated Nuclear Repressive Complexes

| Epigenetic Modifier | Associated Nuclear Repressive Complex | | |
	NuRD	CoREST	NCoR
HDAC1	Y	Y	
HDAC2	Y	Y	
HDAC3		Y	Y
LSD1	Y	Y	

Y = presence in repressive complex.
Adapted from Bantscheff, M., Hopf, C., Savitski, M. M., Dittmann, A., Grandi, P., Michon, A. M., et al. (2011). Chemoproteomics profiling of HDAC inhibitors reveals selective targeting of HDAC complexes. *Nature Biotechnology, 29*(3), 255–265.

of 5-methylcytosines of the DNA through interaction of the complex at the level of MBD2 proteins; after this localization, deacetylation of histones and nucleosome remodeling will facilitate acquisition of the transcriptionally repressive state (Fig. 2). The NuRD complex, in conjunction with DNA methylation, has demonstrated the propensity to act as a repressive complex in colorectal cancer, facilitating the stable repression of tumor suppressor genes such as SFRPs 1, 2, and 5 in human colorectal cancer cell lines (Cai et al., 2014).

6.2 NCoR and SMRT Corepressor Complex

Nuclear receptor corepressor (NCoR) and silencing mediator for retinoid and thyroid receptor (SMRT) corepressor are critical transcriptional repressors of nuclear receptors (Wong et al., 2014). Together, this complex interacts with multiple deacetylases including HDACs 3, 4, 5, and 7. With regard to deacetylase activity, HDAC3 has the highest functionality in this repressor complex, owing to its higher intrinsic enzymatic capacity (Bradner et al., 2010). Prior to interaction with the repressor complex, HDAC3 is inactive enzymatically due to occlusion of the enzyme active site by two protein chaperones: Hsc70 and TRiC. The DAD domain of the NCoR–SMRT complex binds HDAC3 at the N-terminus, facilitating a conformational change at the C-terminus. This conformational change expels the protein chaperones from the active site, thus activating the HDAC3 enzyme (Codina et al., 2005; Perissi, Jepsen, Glass, & Rosenfeld, 2010; Yang, Tsai, Wen, Fejer, & Seto, 2002; Zhang, Kalkum, Chait, & Roeder, 2002). In promyelocytic leukemia (PML) specifically, it has been demonstrated that NCoR occupancy of the retinoic acid (RA) promoter reduces the transcriptional induction of RA responsive genes; these cancers are thus immune to the differentiation effects of RA. This provides direct evidence of aberrant transcriptional regulation by NCoR in driving PML carcinogenesis (Wong et al., 2014).

MeCP2, a CpG methylation recognition protein, provides a direct link between NCoR–SMRT complexes and DNA methylation. A study by Ebert et al. (2013) found the ablation of the interaction between NCoR and MeCP2 reduced the ability of the methyl-binding protein to repress transcription (Ebert et al., 2013). The presence of this CpG recognition protein is critical to recruit the NCoR–SMRT complex to methylated CpG regions to instill repressive chromatin architecture at methylated loci.

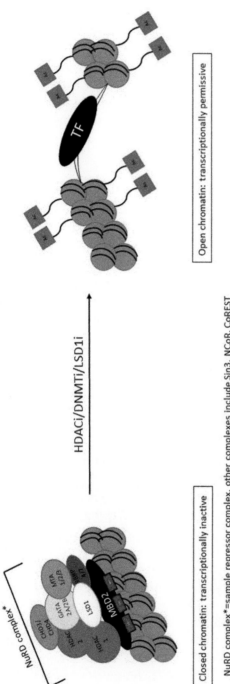

Fig. 2 Corepressor with associated chromatin modifier regulation of loci transcription. (See the color plate.)

6.3 Corepressor of RE1-Silencing Transcription Factor (CoREST) Repressor Complex

The CoREST complex is a functional deacetylase and demethylase complex whose activity is facilitated by the interaction of LSD1 (see Section 8.2) with an HDAC1:HDAC2 dimer (Table 2; Bantscheff et al., 2011). DNA binding and recognition by the CoREST complex is enabled by the SANT2 domain of CoREST (Boyer et al., 2002). In this model, the SANT2 domain binds the complex to the DNA, and the HDAC1:HDAC2 components of the complex create hypoacetylated nucleosomes upstream of LSD1. This facilitates substrate recognition by LSD1, which imparts demethylation of H3K4. Furthermore, the association of LSD1 (see later) with the CoREST complex protects the protein from degradative processes (Forneris, Binda, Adamo, Battaglioli, & Mattevi, 2007; Foster et al., 2010; Yang et al., 2006).

The downregulation of E-cadherin is considered an early step in tumorigenesis and a potent mediator of the epithelial-to-mesenchymal transition. In a study by Cowger, Zhao, Isovic, and Torchia (2007), a critical role for the CoREST complex was discovered in the facilitation of E-cadherin transcriptional repression, thus identifying a direct role for this complex in carcinogenesis.

H3K4 methylation provides a mechanistic link between the CoREST complex and DNA methylation. The presence of the H3K4me3 mark has been demonstrated to act as a block for DNMT3L association, while the lack of H3K4 methylation is permissive for the association of DNMT3a/b/l (Rose & Klose, 2014). In line with this, a study by Lu, Wajapeyee, Turker, and Glazer (2014) elucidated that after a transient exposure to DNMTi, knockdown of CoREST complex components prevents the remethylation of the MLH1 promoter. This demonstrates a differing but equally important role for the corepressor complex in regulating the epigenome, where the repressor complex actively enables the occurrence of DNA methylation through the deposition of repressive chromatin marks.

7. HDAC INHIBITORS: GENERAL MECHANISM OF ZINC CHELATORS

Current drug development strategies for targeting the classical HDACs center on the use of reversible inhibitors to chelate zinc away from the active site of the HDAC enzyme. This disrupts the ability of the enzyme to facilitate zinc-dependent substrate coordination and nucleophilic attack

Table 3 HDAC Inhibitors with Associated Classification

HDAC Inhibitor	Class	Clinical Trial Phase
Entinostat	Benzamide	III
Mocetinostat	Benzamide	II
Panobinostat	Hydroxamic acid	FDA approved
Belinostat	Hydroxamic acid	FDA approved
Givinostat	Hydroxamic acid	II
Vorinostat	Hydroxamic acid	FDA approved
Romidepsin	Cyclic peptide	FDA approved
Valproic acid	Aliphatic fatty acid	II
Butyrate	Aliphatic fatty acid	II

by water (Lombardi, Cole, Dowling, & Christianson, 2011). The general pharmacophore of an HDAC inhibitor follows the schematic of cap–linker–chelator. Inhibitor specificity is derived from the cap, while the inhibitory functionality is based on chelation of zinc away from the active site of the deacetylase (Bantscheff et al., 2011; Bradner et al., 2010; Falkenberg & Johnstone, 2014). The general classes of HDAC inhibitors are hydroxamic acids, benzamides, cyclic peptides, and aliphatic fatty acids. While the benzamides display Class I specificity in terms of inhibition, the other classes of inhibitors are broader spectrum. However, nuanced differences in isoform selectivity can be noted (Bradner et al., 2010; New, Olzscha, & La Thangue, 2012; Witt & Lindemann, 2009). Table 3 provides a brief summary of HDAC inhibitors with associated class and phase of clinical development.

7.1 Mechanisms of HDAC-Induced Anticancer Effects

HDAC inhibitors are pleiotropic drugs with a wide range of effects, both epigenetic- and nonepigenetic-based. HDAC inhibitors induce transcriptional changes in just 2–5% of genes, and these changes in isolation do not fully explain the drug response phenotype of cell cycle arrest and apoptosis. A well-known consequence of HDAC inhibition is the induction of p21 transcription; this cyclin-dependent kinase inhibitor has the potential to induce G1–S restriction point cell cycle arrest. p21 induction does correlate well with the often observed increase in G1 cell population after administration of high-dose HDAC inhibitors, and therefore has at least some phenotypic implications (Gui, Ngo, Xu, Richon, & Marks, 2004).

HDAC inhibitors also induce both caspase-dependent and caspase-independent cell death. Caspase 3-induced cell death is dependent on cytochrome c release, a hallmark of intrinsic apoptosis, while caspase-independent cell death is induced by autophagy (Shao, Gao, Marks, & Jiang, 2004). This cell death response has been demonstrated to be at least partly dependent on ROS production by HDAC inhibitors. In a study by Bhalla et al. (2009), a hydroxamic acid derivative HDAC inhibitor was able to induce a threefold increase in ROS with the apoptosis in this setting determined to be ROS dependent.

7.2 Hydroxamic Acid-Based Inhibitors: Vorinostat and Panobinostat

Vorinostat, or suberoylanilide hydroxamic acid (SAHA), is a hydroxamic acid-based HDAC inhibitor with FDA approval for the treatment of CTCL (Table 3; Mann, Johnson, Cohen, Justice, & Pazdur, 2007; Mann, Johnson, He, et al., 2007). Vorinostat displays a broad of spectrum of HDAC isoform inhibition, with K_i values measuring in the low nanomolar range for HDACs 1, 2, 3, and 6, a K_i of 480 nM for HDAC8 and a K_i of 3.6 μM for HDAC4; no measurable inhibition could be ascertained for the remaining HDACs (Bradner et al., 2010). Vorinostat is dosed at 400 mg daily for the treatment of CTCL patients who have failed two prior systemic therapies. A phase II trial in refractory CTCL patients noted a 31% response rate to vorinostat (Mann, Johnson, Cohen, et al., 2007; Mann, Johnson, He, et al., 2007). Panobinostat is a very potent, broad-spectrum hydroxamic acid HDAC inhibitor, displaying K_i values in the low nanomolar and picomolar range for HDACs 1, 2, 3, and 6. Relatively high potency was also noted for HDACs 4, 5, and 8, with K_i measurements of 550, 80, and 105 nM, respectively (Bradner et al., 2010). Panobinostat has been deployed clinically in combination with the proteasome inhibitor bortezomib, resulting in noted drug synergy. The mechanism of this synergy is based upon HDAC6-mediated deacetylation of HSP90 and the subsequent augmentation of the unfolded protein response (Rao, Nalluri, et al., 2010). The perturbation of this unfolded protein response is most acutely toxic in the immunoglobulin-secreting environment of multiple myeloma. In the PANORAMA trial, the combination of panobinostat + bortezomib + dexamethasone resulted in an increase of progression-free survival from 8.1 months in the bortezomib + dexamethasone group to 12 months in refractory mye-loma patients (Richardson et al., 2016; San-Miguel et al., 2013).

The FDA has granted accelerated approval to another hydroxamic acid derivative, belinostat (Table 3), for the treatment of relapsed or refractory peripheral T-cell lymphoma (PTCL), based on the results of a phase II trial (Lee et al., 2015). The FDA mandates that a phase III trial be conducted to explore belinostat in combination with cyclophosphamide, hydro-xydaunorubicin, oncovin, and prednisone (CHOP) vs CHOP alone as a part of this accelerated approval.

Thus far, HDAC inhibitors have demonstrated much promise for the treatment of hematological malignancies, but the results in solid malignan-cies have been disappointing to date.

7.3 Benzamide-Based HDAC Inhibitor: Entinostat

An exception to the lack of efficacy, to date, for HDAC inhibitors in solid tumors may be entinostat, which is gaining traction for the treatment of solid malignancies. Entinostat, or MS275, a benzamide-based HDAC inhibitor, has received breakthrough therapy status for advanced ER^+ breast cancer and has been deployed clinically for a wide range of malignancies (Table 3). As a benzamide-based inhibitor, entinostat displays selective inhi-bition of Class I HDACs with K_i's for HDACs 1 and 3 of 22 and 360 nM, respectively (Bradner et al., 2010). In a phase II clinical trial which compared the efficacy of 25 mg exemestane daily with placebo or 5 mg entinostat weekly in ER^+ breast cancer, the addition of entinostat led to a significant increase in progression-free survival and overall survival (Yardley et al., 2013).

7.4 Cyclic Tetrapeptide-Based Inhibitor: Romidepsin

Romidepsin, or FK228, is a cyclic tetrapeptide-based HDAC inhibitor with FDA approval for the treatment of CTCL and PTCL (Table 3). The FDA recommended dose and schedule is 14 mg/m^2 IV on days 1, 8, and 15 of a 28-day schedule. A phase II trial noted an overall response rate of 34%, with a durable response of 13–15 months in refractory CTCL patients (Jones et al., 2012; Kim, Thompson, Wenger, & O'Bryant, 2012). Romidepsin is a very potent HDAC inhibitor with biochemical K_i's in the picomolar range for all Class I HDACs. High potency was also noted against HDACs 4 and 6, with K_i's of 20.5 and 9.5 nM, respectively (Bradner et al., 2010).

7.5 Biomarkers of Response to HDAC Inhibition and Prognostic Indications

The search for prognostic indicators of HDAC inhibitor activity and patient response has been thus far rather difficult. The canonical and most deployed marker of HDAC inhibitor activity is augmentation of histone acetylation status; while potentially useful, it has been shown to not correlate with response to the therapeutic (Prince, Bishton, & Harrison, 2009). The induction of p21 has also been deployed as a marker of drug activity, due to its near ubiquitous induction in the presence of HDAC inhibition (Stimson & La Thangue, 2009). But similar to acetylation augmentation, p21 induction is not always correlated with response.

A potential prognostic indicator for response to HDAC inhibitors may lie in the detection of a dysregulated proteasome pathway. In a study by Fotheringham et al., a genome-wide loss-of-function screen in U2OS cells identified HR23B, a ubiquitin domain–containing protein, as a predictive biomarker for HDAC inhibitor response. Specifically, protein levels of HR23B were found to correlate directly with the sensitivity of cells to undergo HDAC inhibitor–induced apoptosis, in this setting. Additionally, in a later study by Kim et al., this same marker was found to drive sensitivity of CTCL to HDAC inhibitors in clinical samples with a positive predictive value of 71.7% noted between HR23B protein abundance, as discerned by immunostaining of CTCL biopsies, and sensitivity to SAHA (Fotheringham et al., 2009; Khan et al., 2010).

In summary, although the precise mechanisms by which HDAC inhibitors interfere with tumor growth have not yet been fully elucidated, encouraging clinical results in specific cancers with multiple classes of these inhibitors suggest a promising future for their use. Future studies must elucidate HDAC inhibitor sensitivity biomarkers to more accurately target patients for HDAC inhibitor–based therapies. Furthermore, the question of which HDACs should be inhibited and what schedule of drug should be used remains open and most likely will be mutational and lineage dependent.

8. HISTONE METHYLATION

8.1 Histone Methyltransferases

The histone lysine methyltransferases (KMTs) are epigenetic writers that mark lysines in histones and create substrates for the histone demethylases, including both the FAD-dependent demethylases LSD1 and LSD2, and the JmjC class of demethylases, KDM2–7, thus partnering with the KDMs to produce dynamic histone methylation states. McGrath and Trojer (2015) have recently reviewed the KMTs in detail; however, as several KMT inhibitors are entering clinical trials, some highlights of targeting KMTs are covered later.

KMTs, similar to the DNMTs, use S-adenosylmethionine as their methyl donor. The first KMT described was SUV39H1, a Su(var)3-9, enhancer of zeste, trithorax (SET) domain-containing KMT that targets H3K9, leading to the repressive H3K9me3 mark (Rea et al., 2000). Currently, two important KMTs are targets of small-molecule inhibitors in clinical trials. DOT1L targets H3K79 and can catalyze activating mono-, di-, and trimethylation marks (Lacoste, Utley, Hunter, Poirier, & Cote, 2002; McLean, Karemaker, & van Leeuwen, 2014), and EZH2, a polycomb protein family member, catalyzes the repressive H3K27me3 mark (Margueron & Reinberg, 2011).

DOT1L is responsible for several important cellular processes including, but not limited to, activation of gene expression. Importantly, DOT1L is critical in the development of mixed lineage leukemia (MLL)-rearranged leukemia (reviewed in McLean et al., 2014). DOT1L inhibitors have been developed through structure/activity approaches to target the catalytic domain of the enzyme with S-adenosylhomocysteine analogues (Basavapathruni et al., 2012; Yao et al., 2011). Of the several promising inhibitors, EPZ-5676 has entered phase I clinical trial for MLL–rearranged AML patients (NCT01684150). Additionally, recruitment is underway for a trial in pediatric patients with relapsed/refractory leukemias bearing the MLL rearrangement (NCT02141828).

As stated earlier, EZH2 and its homologue are members of the polycomb repressive complex 2 (PRC2) (Margueron & Reinberg, 2011). This complex is responsible for the methylation of H3K27, a transcriptionally repressive mark associated with chromatin condensation and transcriptional repression. It is also a mark that when found simultaneously in promoter regions with the activating marks H3K4me2/3, defines a chromatin state known as "bivalent chromatin." Such chromatin mediates a poised state of transcription, which can be activated or silenced during lineage commitment in embryogenesis (Baylin & Jones, 2011; Ohm et al., 2007).

The facts that EZH2 is frequently overexpressed in cancers and appears, in many cases, to be required for transformation and progression, have made it a rational target for antineoplastic drug development (Volkel, Dupret,

Le Bourhis, & Angrand, 2015). EZH2 overexpression is thought to play a role in many important solid tumors, including breast, lung, prostate, and ovarian cancers (Collett et al., 2006; Rao, Cai, et al., 2010; Sato et al., 2013; Varambally et al., 2002). Additionally, activating mutations have been described in follicular and B-cell lymphomas (Morin et al., 2010). Importantly, studies indicate that mutations in SWI–SNF complexes, which are negative regulators of EZH2, are critical to the phenotype of several cancers (Kim et al., 2015; Wilson et al., 2010); however, it is also interesting to note that some SWI/SNF-mutant cancers are primarily dependent on the non-catalytic role of EZH2, suggesting that inhibitors of EZH2 catalytic activity may not fully abrogate the oncogenic effects of EZH2 (Kim et al., 2015). Although most active compounds targeting EZH2 are thought to compete with S-adenosylmethionine, definitive crystal analysis has yet to prove this hypothesis.

There are currently four clinical trials recruiting for two different EZH2 inhibitors. EPZ-6438 is in three different trials at the phase I/II stage that include pediatric (NCT02601937) and adult (NCT02601950) patients with INI1-negative tumors or relapsed/refractory synovial sarcoma and in patients with B-cell lymphomas (phase I); advanced solid tumors (phase I); diffuse large B-cell lymphoma (phase II); and follicular lymphoma (phase II) (NCT01897571). Additionally, CPI-1205 is in a phase I trial for B-cell lymphoma.

Although the KTM inhibitors are in the early stages of clinical trial, the importance of both DOT1L and EZH2 in the cancer phenotype suggests great promise for these classes of inhibitors.

8.2 Histone Demethylation

In combination with DNA methylation, epigenetic regulation of gene expression results from posttranslational modifications of specific residues on the N-terminal tails of histone proteins. Once thought to be irreversible, the discovery and characterization of LSD1 (LSD1/KDM1A/AOF2/BHC110/KIAA0601) in 2004 (Shi et al., 2004) revealed that histone methylation is a dynamic process with direct implications on gene transcription. This N-methylation occurs primarily on specific lysine and arginine residues of histone proteins H3 and H4; however, evidence also exists for methylation of nonhistone proteins, including p53 (Chuikov et al., 2004). Unlike acetylation, the effect of histone methylation on transcription can be repressive or activating, depending on the position of the residue methylated and the extent of methylation. For example, the methylation of lysines 4 or 36 of histone H3 is typically associated with active transcription, while the methylation of lysines 9 or 27 on histone H3 contributes to repressed transcription. The overall combination of histone "marks," including methylation, acetylation, phosphorylation, and ubiquitination, as well as the presence of other regulatory factors and DNA methylation ultimately determine chromatin conformation and expression level of the associated gene. Interestingly, specific histone demethylation has also recently been suggested to be required for proper DNA replication origin firing.

Over the last decade, over 20 lysine demethylases (KDMs) have been discovered representing two distinct classes: the KDM1 subfamily containing the lysine-specific demethylase (LSD) enzymes (the focus of this section), and the KDM2–7 subfamilies consisting of the Jumonji C (JmjC) domain-containing enzymes, excellently reviewed by Klose and colleagues (Dimitrova, Turberfield, & Klose, 2015; Klose, Kallin, & Zhang, 2006). These classes differ with respect to their catalytic mechanisms and thus possess unique substrate specificities. The KDM1 subfamily members, LSD1 and LSD2 (KDM1B/AOF1; Karytinos et al., 2009), are flavin-dependent amine oxidases related to the monoamine and polyamine oxidases (Fitzpatrick, 2010; Forneris, Binda, Vanoni, Mattevi, & Battaglioli, 2005). As such, these enzymes rely on a lone electron pair within the lysine for catalysis and thereby can demethylate only mono- and dimethylated lysines. In contrast, the JmjC domain-containing KDMs are Fe(II) and 2-oxoglutarate-dependent dioxygenases capable of demethylating mono-, di-, or trimethylated lysines (Walport, Hopkinson, & Schofield, 2012). As a member of the CoREST complex (Humphrey et al., 2001), LSD1 catalyzes the specific demethylation of mono- and dimethylated lysine 4 on histone H3 (H3K4) (Forneris et al., 2007; Lee, Wynder, Cooch, & Shiekhattar, 2005; Shi et al., 2004), histone marks associated with active gene transcription. However, evidence suggests that this substrate specificity may be altered in the presence of certain interactions, such as that with the androgen receptor, which allows demethylation of the repressive marks H3K9me1 and H3K9me2 in the presence of LSD1 (Metzger et al., 2005). Additionally, LSD1 has been reported to demethylate modified lysine residues of several nonhistone proteins capable of regulating transcription, including p53 and DNA methyltransferase 1 (DNMT1) (Huang, Sengupta, et al., 2007; Wang et al., 2009); however, whether these proteins are truly substrates of LSD1 has been called into question, since the loss of LSD1 fails to alter the stability or function of either (Jin et al., 2013). Therefore, depending on the context, LSD1 may act as either a transcriptional repressor or facilitator of gene expression (Wang et al., 2007). Importantly, LSD1 is often dysregulated and/or oncogenic in both solid tumors and hematological malignancies, where aberrant histone modification patterns are associated with both cancer initiation and progression (Harris et al., 2012; Hayami et al., 2011; Kahl et al., 2006; Kauffman et al., 2011; Lim et al., 2010; Schulte et al., 2009; Shi, 2007). Furthermore, H3K4me2, the substrate of LSD1, is depleted at the promoters of genes silenced by DNA hypermethylation (McGarvey et al., 2006), suggesting the utility of inhibiting LSD1 activity with the goal of re-expressing silenced tumor suppressor genes as a means of chemotherapeutic intervention.

8.3 LSD1 Inhibitors

8.3.1 MAO Inhibitors and Derivatives

The amine oxidase catalytic domain of LSD1 is homologous to those of the monoamine oxidases (MAOs) A and B. Consequently, several well-studied MAO inhibitors, including phenelzine and tranylcypromine (TCP), an FDA-approved treatment for psychological disorders (Shih, Chen, & Ridd, 1999), have also been demonstrated to also inhibit LSD1 (Lee, Wynder, Schmidt, McCafferty, & Shiekhattar, 2006; Schmidt & McCafferty, 2007). A mechanism-based irreversible inhibitor, TCP forms a covalent adduct with the FAD cofactor within the active site of the enzyme (Schmidt & McCafferty, 2007; Yang, Culhane, Szewczuk, Gocke, et al., 2007; Yang, Culhane, Szewczuk, Jalili, et al., 2007). The use of TCP as an inhibitor of LSD1 has provided promising proof-of-principle data in mouse models and leukemia cell lines (Harris et al., 2012; Schenk et al., 2012), and TCP is currently undergoing phase I clinical trials in combination with all-*trans* retinoic acid (ATRA) in AML and MDS patients with the goal of resensitizing leukemic cells to the differentiation-inducing effects of ATRA (NCT02273102). However, nonspecific amine oxidase inhibitors such as TCP clearly have off-target effects, and second-generation TCP analogues and derivatives have since been developed with enhanced inhibitory efficacy and selectivity for LSD1 (reviewed in Hojfeldt, Agger, & Helin, 2013; Thinnes et al., 2014). ORY-1001, a selective and potent TCP-based LSD1 inhibitor developed by Oryzon Genomics (Maes et al., 2015), is currently undergoing a phase I/IIA clinical trial at centers in Spain, France, and the UK (EU Clinical Trial #2013-002447-29). According to the Oryzon website (www.oryzon.com), the initial multiple ascending dose stage has been completed in patients with relapsed/refractory acute leukemia, establishing a recommended dose for safety and tolerability. As of Nov. 2015, the extension arm of the study is ongoing, investigating preliminary efficacy in specific AML subpopulations, including MLL.

A second mechanism-based, cyclopropylamine-containing, irreversible LSD1 inhibitor, GSK2879552, has demonstrated antiproliferative activity in small cell lung cancer (SCLC) cells both in vitro and in vivo, as well as in AML cell lines (Mohammad et al., 2015). This study also identified a hypomethylated DNA biomarker signature capable of predicting sensitivity to the small-molecule inhibitor in SCLC patient-derived xenografts. GSK2879552 is currently enrolling relapsed or refractory SCLC and AML patients in phase I clinical trials (clinical trial identifiers NCT02034123 and NCT02177872, respectively).

Recently, Cole and colleagues have synthesized and examined a number of phenelzine analogues for LSD1 inhibitory activity, identifying some with nanomolar K_i's. Although quite promising, this series of compounds is still in the early stages of preclinical testing (Prusevich et al., 2014).

8.3.2 Polyamine Analogue-Based Inhibitors

In addition to the MAO enzymes, LSD1 has significant sequence and structural homology to the polyamine oxidases N^1-acetylpolyamine oxidase (PAOX) (Huang, Greene, et al., 2007; Vujcic, Liang, Diegelman, Kramer, & Porter, 2003; Wang et al., 2005) and spermine oxidase (Shi et al., 2004; Wang et al., 2001). The structures of known inhibitors of polyamine oxidation have therefore been used as the basis for polyamine analogue-based LSD1 inhibitors (Bianchi et al., 2006; Federico et al., 2001; Huang, Marton, Woster, & Casero, 2009; Sharma et al., 2012). Initially, a screen of (bis)guanidine and (bis)biguanide compounds identified compound **2d** (1,15-bis{N^5-[3,3-(diphenyl)propyl]-N^1-biguanido}-4,12-diazapentadecane) (verlindamycin) as a potent, noncompetitive inhibitor of LSD1. Treatment with **2d** increased H3K4me2, H3K4me1, and AcH3K9 abundance and decreased H3K9me2 abundance at the promoters of specific aberrantly silenced tumor suppressor genes in cell lines of colon cancer, breast cancer, and AML origin, thereby re-establishing gene expression (Huang, Stewart, et al., 2009; Murray-Stewart, Woster, & Casero, 2014; Zhu et al., 2012). Additionally, although not as effective as TCP, **2d** was capable of increasing the sensitivity of ATRA-resistant AML cells to differentiation therapy (Schenk et al., 2012). Further derivatization of these initial compounds into (bis)urea and (bis)thiourea compounds identified more effective inhibitors of LSD1 with increased potency (Nowotarski et al., 2015; Sharma et al., 2010). The most recently derived (bis) ureidopropyl- and (bis)thioureidopropyldiamine LSD1 inhibitors demonstrate antiproliferative effects in nonsmall cell lung carcinoma (NSCLC) and breast cancer cells and evoke histone modifications associated with the re-expression of specific aberrantly silenced tumor suppressor genes, including SFRP2, h-cadherin, p16, and GATA4, in NSCLC cells (Nowotarski et al., 2015). Meanwhile, studies investigating long-chain polyamine analogues known as oligoamines provided similar results in colon and breast cancer cell lines in vitro (Zhu et al., 2012) as well as in mouse xenografts of human colorectal cancer cells (Huang, Stewart, et al., 2009). In contrast to compound **2d**, the mechanism of inhibition by the oligoamine PG-11144 was found to be competitive (Huang, Stewart, et al., 2009).

In addition to the irreversible TCP-analogue inhibitors described earlier, several reversible, nonpolyamine-based inhibitors of LSD1 have also been identified and were recently reviewed by Mould, McGonagle, Wiseman, Williams, and Jordan (2015). For a list of LSD1 inhibitors in clinical trials and the preclinical pipeline, see Table 4.

8.4 Cross-Talk Between HDACs and LSD1

LSD1 is commonly found in association with the CoREST transcriptional repressor complex, where its interacting partners include HDACs 1 and 2 (Hakimi et al., 2002; Humphrey et al., 2001; You, Tong, Grozinger, & Schreiber, 2001), among others (for a review of LSD1-containing complexes, see Maes et al., 2015). Studies investigating the effects of HDAC inhibitors have demonstrated derepression of specific LSD1 target genes in HeLa cells (Shi et al., 2005) and increased levels of H3K4me2, the substrate of LSD1 in breast cancer cells (Huang, Vasilatos, Boric, Shaw, & Davidson, 2012). Conversely, pharmacologic or siRNA-mediated inhibition of LSD1 increases the abundance of AcH3K9, the substrate of HDACs (Huang et al., 2012). These studies indicated collaboration between LSD1 and HDACs in establishing transcriptionally repressive chromatin architecture and suggested the utility of combining epigenetic treatments targeting both LSD1 and HDAC inhibition as a means for re-expressing aberrantly silenced genes. In fact, studies in glioblastoma and breast cancer cell lines have demonstrated synergistic responses on cell proliferation in response to combined treatment with HDAC and LSD1 inhibitors (Huang et al., 2012; Singh et al., 2011). These studies also revealed cooperation in the induction of aberrantly silenced gene expression and the identification of

Table 4 LSD1 Inhibitors in Clinical Trials and the Preclinical Pipeline

LSD1 Inhibitor	Mode of Inhibition	Clinical Trial Phase	Notes
Tranylcypromine	Irreversible	FDA approved (antidepressant)	Increases concentration of norepinephrine and epinephrine in nervous system (www.accessdata.fda.gov/drugsatfda_docs/label/2010/012342s063lbl.pdf)
ORY-1001	Irreversible	Phase I	Tranylcypromine derivative
GSK-2879552	Irreversible	Phase I	Small cell lung cancer clinical trial, first solid malignancy for LSD1 clinical trial
GSK-354	Reversible	Preclinical	High potency
CBB-1007	Reversible	Preclinical	
2d/verlindamycin	Noncompetitive	Preclinical	(Bis)biguanide; synergistic with AZA in vivo
PG-11144	Competitive	Preclinical	Oligoamine; synergistic with AZA in vivo
(Bis)alkylthiourea derivatives of **2d**	ND	Preclinical	No published in vivo results
(Bis)aralkylthiourea analogues	Competitive	Preclinical	Most potent inhibitors to date; no published in vivo results

a unique subset of genes upregulated by the combination treatment (Huang et al., 2012). Further studies investigating HDAC/LSD1 cross-talk using shRNA strategies in the triple-negative breast cancer (TNBC) subtype provided evidence that LSD1 activity mediates the mRNA expression levels of multiple HDAC isozymes; furthermore, of the individual HDAC isotypes, downregulation of HDAC5 caused the greatest induction of H3K4me2 abundance (Vasilatos et al., 2013). Interestingly, cotreatment with HDAC and LSD1 inhibitors enhanced growth inhibition and apoptosis only in the TNBC subtype, and knockdown of LSD1 enhanced the re-expression of aberrantly silenced genes when exposed to the HDAC inhibitor vorinostat (Vasilatos et al., 2013). Finally, a recent proteomics study quantified histone lysine acetylation and methylation levels following the treatment of HEK293 and K562 cells with the HDAC inhibitors vorinostat, entinostat, or mocetinostat (Lillico, Sobral, Stesco, & Lakowski, 2016). Although with some variability, each of these inhibitors induced alterations in lysine methylation levels in addition to chromatin hyperacetylation. This study also provided insight into the downregulation of specific KDMs by the various HDAC inhibitors: for example, entinostat specifically reduced LSD1 expression, while vorinostat downregulated certain other members of the KDM family.

In summary, LSD1 inhibitors have demonstrated promising results in preclinical models. Although it is too early to speculate as to their clinical effectiveness in multiple tumor settings, the information gained to date holds considerable promise.

9. EXPERIMENTAL EVIDENCE AND MECHANISMS BY WHICH DNMT AND HDAC INHIBITORS CAN SYNERGIZE TO REACTIVATE GENE EXPRESSION: CELL CULTURE STUDIES

As indicated earlier, the silencing of genes in cancer is controlled by a complex interplay between DNA methylation, the acetylation and methylation status of histones, and chromatin conformation. Thus, an effective anticancer therapy might contain a combination of demethylating agents, HDAC inhibitors or other chromatin modifying drugs (Ahuja et al., 2014). Both DNA-demethylating agents and HDAC inhibitors have shown clinical efficacy as single agents (Table 5), but although numerous trials have tested combination therapy, to date, no clinical trials have been designed in solid tumors to test the efficacy of combination therapy versus the DNMTi and HDACi as single agents. For a list of clinical trials using a DNMTi alone and in combination with other epigenetic agents or therapeutics, see Table 5 and reviews by Juo et al. (2015), Nervi, De Marinis, and Codacci-Pisanelli (2015), and Pasini, Delmonte, Tesei, Calistri, and Giordano (2015).

Experimental preclinical evidence suggests that epigenetic therapies used in combination can lead to synergistic effects on apoptosis, antiproliferative effects, the reactivation of silenced genes and of course, at higher doses, cytotoxicity. Studies focusing on combination treatment with both a DNA-demethylating agent and an HDACi can be divided into those using high-dose epigenetic agents, which usually lead to cytotoxic effects and apoptosis, or those using drug combinations at lower doses, which lead to less cytotoxic

Table 5 Clinical Trials of DNMT Inhibitors in Combination with Other Epigenetic or Therapeutic Agents

Treatment	References	Cancer Type (# of Patients), Phase	Clinical Results
Demethylating agent: monotherapy			
Decitabine	Abele et al. (1987)	CRC, head and neck, melanoma, RCC (101), II	One partial response (PR)
Decitabine	Clavel et al. (1992)	Noseminomatous testicular cancer	No responses
Decitabine	Momparler et al. (1997)	Metastatic NSCLC (15), I/II	Stable disease (SD) for at least 6 months, prolonged survival up to 15 months in three patients
Decitabine	Schrump et al. (2006)	NSCLC (20), I	SD in two patients up to 12 months
Demethylating agent and HDACi or other epigenetic agent and chemotherapeutic agent			
Azacytidine and phenylbutyrate	Lin et al. (2009)	Mixed tumors (27), I	No responses
Azacytidine and entinostat	Juergens et al. (2011)	Refractory, advanced NSCLC (45), I/II	1 complete response (CR) (14 months), 1 PR (8 months), SD in 10 patients (≥12 weeks and <18 months), sensitization to subsequent chemo in 4/19 patients, sensitization to immune therapy 5/6 patients
Azacytidine and valproate	Braiteh et al. (2008)	Mixed tumors (55)	SD of 4–12 months observed in 14 patients
Decitabine and vorinostat	Stathis et al. (2011)	Advanced solid tumors, non–Hodgkin's lymphoma (43), I	SD observed in 11 patients ≥4 cycles

Decitabine and valproic acid	Chu et al. (2013)	NSCLC (8), I	SD observed in one patient
Decitabine, panobinostat, and temozolomide	Xia et al. (2014)	Resistant melanoma I	No DLTs were observed, MTD was not reached
5-Fluoro-2′-deoxycytidine, and tetrahydrouridine	Newman et al. (2015)	Advanced solid tumors, I	One refractory breast cancer patient experienced a PR with >90% decrease in tumor size, lasting over a year
Hydralazine/valproate and chemotherapy	Candelaria et al. (2007)	Refractory solid tumors (32), II	A clinical benefit was observed in 12 (80%) patients: four PR and eight SD
Hydralazine, valproate cisplatin, and topotecan	Coronel et al. (2011)	Advanced cervical cancer (36), III	Four PRs for CT + HV and one in CT + placebo. The median progression-free survival (PFS) was 6 months for CT + placebo and 10 months for CT + HV. A significant advantage in PFS for epigenetic therapy over the current standard chemo combination in cervical cancer
Hydralazine, valproate doxorubicin, and cyclophosphamide	Arce et al. (2006)	Neoadjuvant breast (16), II	Five (31%) patients had clinical CRs and eight (50%) had PRs for an ORR of 81%. No patient progressed. One of 15 operated patients (6.6%) had pathological CR and 70% had residual disease <3 cm
Azacytidine and entinostat	Connolly (unpublished)	Advanced HER2 negative breast cancer	Completed, awaiting analysis
Azacytidine and entinostat	Azad (unpublished)	Colorectal cancer	Completed, awaiting analysis
Azacytidine, entinostat and nivolumab	Brahmer (unpublished)	NSCLC	Ongoing

Continued

Table 5 Clinical Trials of DNMT Inhibitors in Combination with Other Epigenetic or Therapeutic Agents—cont'd

Treatment	References	Cancer Type (# of Patients), Phase	Clinical Results
Demethylating agent and conventional anticancer drug			
Azacytidine and erlotinib	Bauman et al. (2012)	Mixed tumors (30), I	PRs in lung and ovarian cancer patients with SD noted in 2 lung and 11 ovarian patients
Azacytidine and carboplatin	Fu et al. (2011)	Ovarian cancer, platinum resistant (30), Ib–IIa	1 CR, 3 PRs, objective response rate (ORR) was 13.8%, with 10 cases of SD
Azacytidine, docetaxel, and prednisone	Singal et al. (2015)	Metastatic, castrate-resistant prostate cancer (22), I/II	PSA response in 10 of 19 evaluable patients and objective response was observed in 3 of 10 patients
Decitabine and carboplatin	Appleton et al. (2007)	Mixed tumors (33), I	No responses
Decitabine and carboplatin	Matei et al. (2012)	Ovarian cancer (17)	35% ORR and PFS of 10.2 months, with nine patients (53%) free of progression at 6 months
Decitabine and carboplatin	Fang et al. (2010)	Recurrent ovarian cancer (10), I	One CR was observed and three additional patients had SD for ≥ 6 months
Decitabine and temozolomide	Tawbi et al. (2013)	Refractory melanoma (35), I/II	2 CR, 4 PR, 14 SD, 18% ORR, and 61% clinical benefit rate (CR + PR + SD). The median overall survival (OS) was 12.4 months; the 1-year OS rate was 56%
Decitabine and cisplatin	Schwartsmann et al. (2000)	Solid tumors and inoperable NSCLC (35), I/II	3 PR which lasted for 4, 16, and 36 weeks. Median survival of patients was 15 weeks
Decitabine and cisplatin	Pohlmann et al. (2002)	Squamous cell carcinoma of cervix (25), II	8 (38.1%) achieved PR, SD was documented in five cases (23.8%)

effects and more changes in gene expression. The latter may be more relevant to patients because the clinical toxicities for higher doses may be hard to tolerate and these may be due to the many off-target effects of higher doses. In this regard, high doses of HDAC or LSD1 inhibitors may have actions in both the nuclear and cytoplasmic compartments, leading to changes in acetylation or methylation of nonhistone proteins that may also be important in regulating tumorigenesis, but are not associated with an epigenetic mechanism, thereby complicating our understanding of the mode of action of these epigenetic drugs. Consequently, many of the effects described in the following studies may be clinically off target because of high doses used for both the DNMT and HDAC inhibitors. Moreover, drug scheduling must be given considerable thought in combination therapy, because HDACi can cause cell cycle arrest and may limit the amount of a DNMTi that can be incorporated into nondividing DNA.

One of the first studies to address combination therapy was that of Cameron, Bachman, Myohanen, Herman, and Baylin (1999), who demonstrated, in colorectal cancer cells, that demethylating agents, given only prior to but not concordantly, or after, HDAC inhibitors can work together in an additive and/or synergistic manner to re-express some hypermethylated genes. Densely methylated DNA is associated with transcriptionally repressive chromatin and underacetylated histones (Antequera, Macleod, & Bird, 1989; Eden, Hashimshony, Keshet, Cedar, & Thorne, 1998). Using this information, the authors found that silenced, hypermethylated genes that could not be reactivated using the HDAC inhibitor trichostatin A (TSA) as a single agent, were robustly reactivated if the genes were partially demethylated first with a demethylating agent, such as decitabine (100 nM), followed by treatment with TSA (300 nM). Their results showed that the epigenetic treatments did not alter the chromatin structure associated with the hypermethylated promoter and suggested that dense DNA methylation is the dominant factor in the maintenance of silencing at CpG island promoters.

p53-independent apoptotic cell death was induced in a study using both depsipeptide (0.05–5 µM) and TSA (0.5–10 µM) to treat human lung cancer cell lines H23 and H719. PARP cleavage was demonstrated by flow analysis and Western blotting (Zhu, Lakshmanan, Beal, & Otterson, 2001). The HDAC inhibitor-induced apoptosis is greatly enhanced with the addition of DAC (1 µM) and may be related to increased acetylation of histones H3 and H4. The authors suspect that increased DNA demethylation and histone acetylation results in a decondensation of chromatin allowing easier access of endogenous proapoptotic endonucleases or that gene expression related to apoptotic pathways has increased. Similarly, a study in 2002 by Boivin, Momparler, Hurtubise, and Momparler (2002) in human lung carcinoma cells, demonstrated that combination therapy using DAC and phenylbutyrate led to a greater inhibition of DNA synthesis and loss of clonogenicity in A549 and Calu-6 lung carcinoma lines than with the single agents tested alone.

The next several studies show a synergistic response to both DNA-demethylating agents and HDAC inhibitors, but the authors believe the response to be methylation-independent and primarily due to DNA damage. Chai et al. (2008) observed synergy using decitabine and an HDACi in H719 and A549 human lung cancer cells. They found evidence of DNA damage and apoptosis in a dose-dependent manner, as decitabine induces DSB at 5 µM and SSB at 1 µM. Cell proliferation was inhibited by decitabine (1 µM) and the HDACi depsipeptide (0.1 µM). This inhibition was not observed in cells that had a knockdown of DNMT1/DNMT3a/DNMT3b, suggesting that the synergistic effects were methylation independent. The authors showed that there was an association between decitabine-induced DNA damage and the amount of $[^3H]$-decitabine incorporation into DNA. Over time, the incorporation of $[^3H]$-decitabine decreased, suggesting that it could be removed by a DNA repair mechanism. The addition of an HDACi did not play a role in the incorporation of $[^3H]$-decitabine into DNA but did slow the removal of $[^3H]$-decitabine, which prevented DNA repair and led to an inhibition of proliferation. It has been suggested that HDACi may somehow interfere with the repair process of nucleoside analogue-induced DNA damage and suppress expression or activity of enzymes that are involved in this repair process.

Luszczek, Cheriyath, Mekhail, and Borden (2010) demonstrated that decitabine (up to 1 µM) alone inhibited growth in two out of nine SCLC lines, while combination therapy with decitabine and the HDAC inhibitor LBH589 (up to 12.8 µM) reduced the proliferation of four out of nine SCLC lines (H526, H82, H146, and DMS114) and decitabine and the HDAC inhibitor MGCD0103 (up to 1.228 mM) reduced the proliferation of five lines (H526, H82, H146, DMS114, and H1048). Loss of viability of sensitive SCLC cells did not correlate with the degree of DNMT1 or HDAC inhibition on plastic, which suggested to the authors that non-epigenetic mechanisms might contribute to the synergy observed using the combination therapy. They found that combination treatment increased DNA damage, as assayed by comet assay, and γH2AX staining in sensitive cells but not resistant cells. Our laboratories have also observed that DNMT1 is effectively degraded with decitabine or azacytidine treatment, but that an antitumorigenic response does not always correlate with the degree of DNMT depletion. The loss of DNMT1 may serve as a biomarker for uptake of decitabine or azacytidine but not always as a marker for an anti-tumorigenic response.

Interestingly, Luszczek observed in the resistant cells an increase in expression of genes related to interferon expression, with IFI27 as the most highly expressed gene in the H196 resistant cell line. Their data suggested that a decitabine-induced elevation in interferon-related gene expression correlated with resistance to DNA damage. We have also reported that deci-tabine (100 nM) or azacytidine (500 nM) can induce expression of genes for interferon signaling (Li et al., 2014; Wrangle et al., 2013), and that this response can be mediated by the re-expression of methylated endogenous retroviruses that stimulate double-stranded RNA (dsRNA) sensors to stim-ulate an antiviral, interferon-mediated response (Chiappinelli et al., 2015; Roulois et al., 2015).

Lastly, synergy was observed using both DNMT and HDAC inhibitors to activate the methylated estrogen receptor (ER) promoter in ER-negative, MDA-MB-231 human breast cancer cells (Sharma et al., 2005). Cells were treated with exceedingly high, cytotoxic doses of decitabine (2.5 µM) for 96 h and TSA (100 ng/mL) for 12 h. At these doses, this combination facil-itates the release of a repressor complex containing various MBD proteins (MeCP2, MBD1, and MBD2), DNMTs (DNMT1 and DNMT3b), and HDAC1 from the ER promoter, with concomitant enrichment of acetyl-H4, acetyl-H3, and H3K4me2 and diminished methylation at H3K9, lead-ing to re-expression of ER.

10. EXPERIMENTAL EVIDENCE AND MECHANISMS BY WHICH DNMT AND HDAC OR LSD1 INHIBITORS CAN SYNERGIZE TO REACTIVATE GENE EXPRESSION: ANIMAL STUDIES

10.1 Chemosensitivity, Apoptotic Pathways, Inhibition of Tumor Growth

In many in vivo models of solid tumors, a demethylating agent combined with an HDAC inhibitor has been shown to reduce tumor burden more effectively than either epigenetic drug alone. This is often coupled with the observation of an enhanced upregulation of important genes with the combination therapy, whether those genes are important tumor suppressors or are involved in cell death pathways or processes leading to differentiation. The genes that are upregulated may have important implications for the sensitizing effect of combination epigenetic therapy. For example, epigenetically induced re-expression of silenced genes in chemoresistant tumors can resensitize those tumors to the initial chemotherapy to which they developed resistance, as discussed later.

In the following study by Steele, the addition of the HDAC inhibitor belinostat to a decitabine treatment regimen re-expressed genes in the xenografted tumors and increased their sensitivity to cisplatin. Immunodeficient mice engrafted with the cisplatin-resistant human ovarian cancer cell line (HEY) A2780/cp70 demonstrated in vivo re-expression of genes implicated in cisplatin sensitivity (MAGE-A1 and MLH1) in xenografted tumors after a high dose (5 mg/kg) of decitabine treatment, while belinostat (40 mg/kg) alone did not affect expression of those genes, as measured by immunohistochemical staining of the tumor cells (Steele, Finn, Brown, & Plumb, 2009). In combination, however, re-expression was enhanced compared to either decitabine or belinostat alone. While decitabine as a single agent did decrease methylation at the MAGE-A1 promoter region, there was no further decrease in methylation with belinostat treatment, indicating that different HDACi's may have separate mechanisms for increasing gene expression. The authors hypothesize that the HDAC inhibitor allows transcription factors to more easily access the DNA as a result of chromatin remodeling. Overall, the addition of the HDAC inhibitor belinostat to decitabine enhanced gene re-expression in xenografted tumors, and increased their sensitivity to cisplatin (6 mg/kg) (Steele et al., 2009).

The sensitization of resistant tumors to chemotherapy may be very dependent on the tumor type as well as the administration schedule of epigenetic agents and chemotherapeutics. In a study by Vendetti using cell lines and tissue derived from NSCLC patients, no differences in tumor chemosensitivity following epigenetic treatment with azacytidine (s.c. 0.5 mg/kg) and entinostat (i.p. 1 mg/kg) were observed with cisplatin; however, some tumor lines exhibited differential responses to irinotecan, especially those serially transplanted and treated for longer periods of time (Vendetti et al., 2015).

In addition to potentially sensitizing tumors to other agents, epigenetic therapies in combination can have potent antitumor effects themselves. For example, in a mouse model of ovarian cancer, decitabine and SAHA inhibited the growth of ovarian cancer cell lines and xenografts while inducing expression of imprinted tumor suppressor genes, apoptosis, G2/M arrest, and autophagy (Chen et al., 2011). The HEY was injected intraperitoneally into nude mice and treated with decitabine at 0.8 mg/kg/3 × per week and/ or SAHA at the high dose of 12.5 mg/kg/5 × per week for 21 days. The combination-treated xenografts showed re-expression of the tumor suppressor genes ARHI and PEG3, inhibited tumor growth, and increased autophagy. SAHA alone did not improve the survival of the mice but decitabine alone did, and there was a significant additive improvement of survival in the combination group. The inhibition of tumor growth may be caused in part by autophagy of the tumor cells, because there was an increase in the number of autophagosomes detected in the decitabine-treated groups, with the group treated with decitabine and SAHA having the greatest number of autophagosomes (Chen et al., 2011).

Another study, using again a very high dose of SAHA (50 mg/kg) and decitabine (1 mg/kg) in a mouse model xenografted with Huh7 hepatoma cells saw reduced tumor volume with single agents, but the only significant reduction was in the combination-treated group. Furthermore, histological analysis of normal liver tissue did not show any pathological changes with combination therapy, suggesting that the mice tolerated the drug well (Venturelli et al., 2007).

To test the effect of combination epigenetic therapy on tumor reduction and gene expression in vivo, the Belinsky laboratory used an interesting orthotopic lung cancer model in which human lung cancer lines are transplanted into the lung via orotracheal intubation into immunocompromised Rowett nude rats. Much of their research has focused on the Calu-6 cell line established from an anaplastic adenocarcinoma, containing mutant K-ras and p53 (Belinsky et al., 2003). They found that treatment with a moderately high dose of azacytidine (2 mg/kg), reduced tumor burden by 31% but combination therapy with both azacytidine and entinostat (1 mg/kg) reduced burden by 60%. Results were replicated using A549 and H1975 cells, in which tumor burden was reduced 40% and 53%, respectively, in the combination arm. In Calu-6 cells, pro-apoptotic genes (Bad, Bak, Bok, Bik) and p21 were increased in the combination group (Belinsky et al., 2003). This same model was used to test guadecitabine (SGI-110) at 20 mg/kg, s.c., twice weekly and entinostat 1 mg/kg, i.p., weekly for antitumorigenic properties (Tellez et al., 2014). SGI-110 alone was able to reduce tumors by 35%, and the combination with entinostat showed a reduction of 56%. There was toxicity observed, however, with the mice losing up to 18% of their body weight after 4 weeks of treatment. SGI-110 led to demethylation of promoter regions on a genome-wide level, but the number of genes demethylated was not significantly different between the

SGI-110 group and the SGI-110 plus entinostat group. There were overall greater changes in expression for tumors treated with the combination (Tellez et al., 2014). Unfortunately, in neither study was entinostat tested as a single agent. Overall, however, the combination of a demethylating agent and an HDAC inhibitor increased the expression level of pro-apoptotic genes in tumors and decreased tumor growth.

The in vivo therapeutic effect of LSD1-inhibiting polyamine analogues alone, and in combination with DNMTi, have been tested for their ability to inhibit LSD1 activity and tumor growth in a xenograft model of colon cancer (Huang, Greene, et al., 2007; Huang, Stewart, et al., 2009). HCT-116 colorectal tumor xenografts in athymic nude mice were treated with increasing doses of the decamine, PG-11144, or the biquanide polyamine analogue **2d** alone, or in combination with azacytidine. Treatment with either polyamine increased H3K4me2 in tumors and PG-11144 or azacytidine alone showed significant inhibition of the growth of established HCT-116 xenografts, but treatment with **2d** alone did not. However, a significant anti-tumor effect was observed for both polyamine analogues when combined with the DNMTi azacytidine (Huang, Greene, et al., 2007; Huang, Stewart, et al., 2009).

A majority of epigenetic studies published focus on mouse tumor xenograft models engrafted with human cancer cell lines. However, one study used genetically engineered, *Patched* (*Ptch*) heterozygous mice, which develop medulloblastoma and rhabdomyosarcoma resembling human tumor counterparts (Ecke et al., 2009). *Ptch* is a member of the hedgehog-signaling pathway and epigenetic silencing as well as mutational inactivation of *Ptch* has been identified in a variety of tumors (Evangelista, Tian, & de Sauvage, 2006). In vivo, combination treatment with 0.1 mg/kg per day decitabine and 100 mg/kg per day valproic acid prevented tumor incidence, while single agent therapy was less effective. Combination therapy led to a reduction in DNMT1 activity, and reactivated wild-type *Ptch* expression via decreased DNA promoter methylation and induction of histone hyper-acetylation (Ecke et al., 2009). Epigenetic therapy was not effective in advanced stage tumors, suggesting that these agents may be more effective in early-stage disease.

10.2 Activation of Tumor Immune Response, Depletion of MDSCs, Tregs

A series of preclinical, syngeneic animal experiments highlighted later demonstrate the promising interactions between epigenetic therapy and the activation of a tumor immune response. Epigenetic therapy can increase tumor immunoreactivity via four mechanisms: (1) cytotoxic death of the cancer cell releases tumor-associated antigens that will attract and activate T cells. (2) DNMTi demethylate and activate genes in the tumor cell involved in an immune response, such as cancer testis antigens, chemokines and cytokines, inflammatory processes, and interferon signaling (Li et al., 2014). (3) Demethylating agents can activate a dsRNA sensing, viral defense response, involving activation of endogenous retroviral transcripts and cellular sensors of these to stimulate interferon signaling in the cancer cell (Chiappinelli et al., 2015; Roulois et al., 2015). (4) Epigenetic agents can regulate immune cells and in particular are known to decrease populations of MDSCs and Tregs (Kim et al., 2014; Shen & Pili, 2012).

In a study of mesothelioma cells by Leclercq et al., epigenetic therapy increased tumor-specific antigens and tumor lymphocyte infiltration. Malignant pleural mesothelioma is a cancer that develops in the mesothelial cells of the pleura, a thin membrane of lubricating cells that lines the lungs and chest wall. To evaluate the efficacy of epigenetic therapy as an antitumor agent for this aggressive tumor, AK7 murine mesothelioma tumors were established in syngeneic mice and treated with high doses of decitabine (4 mg/kg) and valproic acid (5 mM) in the drinking water (Leclercq et al., 2011). Combination therapy produced the greatest decrease in tumor growth, promoted lymphocyte infiltration, and induced a specific antitumor response in the $CD8^+$ T cells of the mice, which primarily targeted treatment-induced antigens (Leclercq et al., 2011). Moreover, $CD8^+$ T cells were only found in tumors that had been treated with DAC and valproic acid. Overall, the results suggest that the combination of a hypomethylating agent and an HDAC inhibitor may be a promising therapy to induce cell death by increasing the immunogenicity of the tumor through the induced expression of tumor-associated antigens.

In a metastatic model of colon cancer, treatment with decitabine and vorinostat increased expression of the death receptor Fas in tumor cells, sensitizing them to Fas-ligand-mediated apoptosis and decreasing their metastatic potential (Yang et al., 2012). Fas-mediated apoptosis is dependent on the binding of the Fas ligand (FasL) to the receptor, and cancer cells can downregulate the receptor to become apoptosis resistant. This downregulation is an obstacle to Fas-based cytotoxic lymphocyte (CTL) immunotherapy. The authors investigated the effects of DAC and vorinostat in vivo on the colon carcinoma CT26 experimental lung metastasis model. Decitabine (0.1 mg/kg) and vorinostat (20 mg/kg) upregulate Fas in

CT26 cells in vitro, and the cells become sensitive to FasL-induced apopto-sis. In vivo, both agents had an antimetastatic effect individually, but there was a much greater effect with the combination treatment (Yang et al., 2012). The source of the FasL in the lung tissue was found to be both CD8[+] T cells (of which 24.8% expressed FasL) and non-CD8[+] T cells (of which 12.7% expressed FasL). Next, cells were transplanted into wild-type and FasL-deficient (Fas[gld]) mice. While in the untreated groups, there was no difference in the metastatic rates in the two types of mice; deci-tabine and vorinostat treatment was significantly more effective at suppressing the tumors in wild-type mice compared to FasL-deficient mice. This suggests that decitabine and vorinostat could sensitize colon cancers to FasL-mediated immunotherapy. Therefore, tumor-specific CTL adoptive immunotherapy was given to the mice that had either received decitabine and vorinostat or not. The most significant tumor reduction occurred with combinatorial epigenetic therapy followed by CTL immunotherapy, which enhanced tumor rejection efficacy in established lung metastases. Overall, the combination of decitabine and vorinostat was able to upregulate Fas-mediated apoptosis molecules in vitro and sensitize metastatic colon cancer to CTL adoptive immuno-therapy in vivo (Yang et al., 2012).

In addition to T-cell therapies, epigenetic therapy can also sensitize tumors to immune checkpoint blockade. In a study using two different syn-geneic models, the authors injected CT26, a modestly immunogenic colo-rectal carcinoma cell line, and 4T1, a poorly immunogenic breast cancer cell line into balb/c mice and treated the mice with azacytidine (0.8 mg/kg), a relatively high dose of entinostat (20 mg/kg), anti-CTLA-4 (10 mg/kg), and anti-PD-1 (10 mg/kg) together and with each epigenetic agent individ-ually (Kim et al., 2014). Tumors were unresponsive to anti-CTLA-4 and anti-PD1 treatment; however, combination treatment with all four drugs eradicated tumors in more than 80% of tumor-bearing mice. Entinostat led to a significant decrease in the number of FoxP3[+] T regulatory cells in the tumor and the number of circulating granulocytic myeloid-derived suppressor cells (gMDSCs). This study demonstrated that epigenetic therapy not only acts to re-express genes in cancer cells but can also affect immune cells such as MDSCs. Moreover, HDAC inhibitors such as entinostat may be more effective on immune populations of cells and at depleting MDSCs than are DNMTi. Other studies have also demonstrated that entinostat, at lower doses of 5 mg/kg, can reduce FoxP3 levels and block Treg suppressive func-tion in renal and prostate cancer models (Shen & Pili, 2012).

In the syngeneic BR5FVB1-Akt ovarian cancer mouse model, treatment with decitabine increased the expression of chemokines in tumor cells in vitro and then led to an increased number of activated NK and $CD8^+$ T cells in the ascites fluid and longer survival of the mice in vivo. Furthermore, decitabine improved the efficacy of anti-CTLA-4 immunotherapy, prolonging the CTL activity (Wang et al., 2015).

In another example of sensitization to anti-CTLA-4 immune checkpoint therapy, work by Chan, in mice with syngeneic B16-F10 melanoma tumors treated with AZA and anti-CTLA-4 showed significantly improved tumor growth inhibition as compared to the mice that received PBS, AZA alone (which had no effect as a single agent), or anti-CTLA-4 alone (Chiappinelli et al., 2015).

Finally, inhibition of DNMT1 and EZH2 in ovarian cancer increases tumor expression of T helper 1 (T_H1)-type chemokines CXCL9 and CXCL10 (Peng et al., 2015). The change in the tumor leads to increased tumor-infiltrating T effector cells, inhibits tumor growth, and increases the sensitivity of the tumor to adaptive T-cell transfusion therapy or PD-L1 blockade. The former study was done using a humanized mouse model in which human tumor and immune cells were transplanted into NSG mice, which were then treated with GSK126 (a selective EZH2 inhibitor) and decitabine, which improved the efficacy of the T-cell therapy but had no effect alone. The sensitization to PD-L1 blockade was studied in the syngeneic ID8 ovarian cancer model. The mice were treated with decitabine and/or DZNep (an inhibitor of all S-adenosyl-methionine-dependent enzymes, including EZH2). The combination of epigenetic therapy reduced tumor growth and increased T-cell infiltration and tumor T_H1 chemokine expression compared to the single agents. When anti-PD-L1 therapy was added to the combination epigenetic therapy, it enhanced both the anti-tumorigenic and immunogenic effects. As a whole, these studies suggest that epigenetic therapy can reprogram tumors in order to make them more immunogenic, leading to increased immune cell recruitment and sensitization to immune therapy.

11. SUMMARY

The earlier studies show that DNA methylation, posttranslational histone modification and chromatin structure are inextricably linked in the control of gene expression and suggests that dysregulation of these epigenetic processes is a fertile target for therapeutic intervention in cancer.

Several inhibitors of key enzymes responsible for epigenetic regulation have demonstrated impressive preclinical results, especially when used in combination, and some are now in early to mid-phase clinical trials. Azacytidine and decitabine are two examples of DNMTi that display additive or synergistic antitumorigenic effects when used in combination with an HDACi or KDMi in preclinical studies. However, these observations have not yet been validated in the clinic. Both DNA-demethylating agents and HDAC inhibitors have shown clinical efficacy as single agents, but although numerous trials have tested combination therapy, to date, no clinical trials have been designed in solid tumors to test the efficacy of combination therapy versus the DNMTi, HDACi, or KDMi as single agents. To move the combinations of these agents effectively into patients will require a better understanding of how to dose and schedule these epigenetic drugs, and to determine how they interact with each other and with other therapies. For example, sequential or simultaneous scheduling of the epigenetic agents in combination therapy is a critical parameter to define. This is because azacytidine or decitabine must incorporate into actively dividing DNA to be effective, and HDACi or KDMi are capable of inhibiting cell cycle progression. Dose of inhibitors is also important as high doses yield cytotoxic, off-target effects that limit their clinical usefulness. Maximum tolerated dose (MTD) is not an effective endpoint for most epigenetic drugs. Lastly, epigenetic therapy may be most successful when paired with chemo- or targeted therapy, such as checkpoint inhibitors, kinase inhibitors, or antiestrogens, because of the epigenetically induced re-expression of genes necessary for immune signaling and attraction, kinase signaling, and differentiated cellular states. In summary, experimental evidence overwhelmingly demonstrates that inhibitors of HDACs and lysine demethylases are more effective when paired with DNA-demethylating agents, but the final arbiter will be the cancer patients receiving this therapy.

REFERENCES

Aagaard, L., Laible, G., Selenko, P., Schmid, M., Dorn, R., Schotta, G., et al. (1999). Functional mammalian homologues of the *Drosophila* PEV-modifier Su(var)3-9 encode centromere-associated proteins which complex with the heterochromatin component M31. *The EMBO Journal, 18*(7), 1923–1938.

Abele, R., Clavel, M., Dodion, P., Bruntsch, U., Gundersen, S., Smyth, J., et al. (1987). The EORTC Early Clinical Trials Cooperative Group experience with 5-aza-2'-deoxycytidine (NSC 127716) in patients with colo-rectal, head and neck, renal carcinomas and malignant melanomas. *European Journal of Cancer and Clinical Oncology, 23*(12), 1921–1924.

Ahuja, N., Easwaran, H., & Baylin, S. B. (2014). Harnessing the potential of epigenetic therapy to target solid tumors. *The Journal of Clinical Investigation, 124*(1), 56–63.

Aimiuwu, J., Wang, H., Chen, P., Xie, Z., Wang, J., Liu, S., et al. (2012). RNA-dependent inhibition of ribonucleotide reductase is a major pathway for 5-azacytidine activity in acute myeloid leukemia. *Blood, 119*(22), 5229–5238.

Aldana-Masangkay, G. I., & Sakamoto, K. M. (2011). The role of HDAC6 in cancer. *Journal of Biomedicine & Biotechnology, 2011*, 875824.

Allis, C., Jenuwein, T., Reinberg, D., & Caparros, M. (2015). *Epigenetics. Vol. 2* (2nd ed.). New York: Cold Spring Harbor Laboratories Press.

Amato, R. J. (2007). Inhibition of DNA methylation by antisense oligonucleotide MG98 as cancer therapy. *Clinical Genitourinary Cancer, 5*(7), 422–426.

Antequera, F., Macleod, D., & Bird, A. P. (1989). Specific protection of methylated CpGs in mammalian nuclei. *Cell, 58*(3), 509–517.

Appleton, K., Mackay, H. J., Judson, I., Plumb, J. A., McCormick, C., Strathdee, G., et al. (2007). Phase I and pharmacodynamic trial of the DNA methyltransferase inhibitor decitabine and carboplatin in solid tumors. *Journal of Clinical Oncology, 25*(29), 4603–4609.

Arce, C., Perez-Plasencia, C., Gonzalez-Fierro, A., de la Cruz-Hernandez, E., Revilla-Vazquez, A., Chavez-Blanco, A., et al. (2006). A proof-of-principle study of epigenetic therapy added to neoadjuvant doxorubicin cyclophosphamide for locally advanced breast cancer. *PLoS One, 1*, e98.

Arrowsmith, C. H., Bountra, C., Fish, P. V., Lee, K., & Schapira, M. (2012). Epigenetic protein families: A new frontier for drug discovery. *Nature Reviews Drug Discovery, 11*(5), 384–400.

Asgatay, S., Champion, C., Marloie, G., Drujon, T., Senamaud-Beaufort, C., Ceccaldi, A., et al. (2014). Synthesis and evaluation of analogues of N-phthaloyl-l-tryptophan (RG108) as inhibitors of DNA methyltransferase 1. *Journal of Medicinal Chemistry, 57*(2), 421–434.

Avvakumov, G. V., Walker, J. R., Xue, S., Li, Y., Duan, S., Bronner, C., et al. (2008). Structural basis for recognition of hemi-methylated DNA by the SRA domain of human UHRF1. *Nature, 455*(7214), 822–825.

Bachman, K. E., Rountree, M. R., & Baylin, S. B. (2001). Dnmt3a and Dnmt3b are transcriptional repressors that exhibit unique localization properties to heterochromatin. *The Journal of Biological Chemistry, 276*(34), 32282–32287.

Bantscheff, M., Hopf, C., Savitski, M. M., Dittmann, A., Grandi, P., Michon, A. M., et al. (2011). Chemoproteomics profiling of HDAC inhibitors reveals selective targeting of HDAC complexes. *Nature Biotechnology, 29*(3), 255–265.

Barth, T., & Imhof, A. (2010). Fast signals and slow marks: The dynamics of histone modifications. *Trends in Biochemical Sciences, 35*(11), 618–626.

Basavapathruni, A., Jin, L., Daigle, S. R., Majer, C. R., Therkelsen, C. A., Wigle, T. J., et al. (2012). Conformational adaptation drives potent, selective and durable inhibition of the human protein methyltransferase DOT1L. *Chemical Biology & Drug Design, 80*(6), 971–980.

Bauman, J., Verschraegen, C., Belinsky, S., Muller, C., Rutledge, T., Fekrazad, M., et al. (2012). A phase I study of 5-azacytidine and erlotinib in advanced solid tumor malignancies. *Cancer Chemotherapy and Pharmacology, 69*(2), 547–554.

Baylin, S. B. (1997). Tying it all together: Epigenetics, genetics, cell cycle, and cancer. *Science, 277*(5334), 1948–1949.

Baylin, S. B., Herman, J. G., Graff, J. R., Vertino, P. M., & Issa, J. P. (1998). Alterations in DNA methylation: A fundamental aspect of neoplasia. *Advances in Cancer Research, 72*, 141–196.

Baylin, S. B., & Jones, P. A. (2011). A decade of exploring the cancer epigenome—Biological and translational implications. *Nature Reviews. Cancer, 11*(10), 726–734.

Baylin, S. B., Makos, M., Wu, J. J., Yen, R. W., de Bustros, A., Vertino, P., et al. (1991). Abnormal patterns of DNA methylation in human neoplasia: Potential consequences for tumor progression. *Cancer Cells, 3*(10), 383–390.

Belinsky, S. A., Klinge, D. M., Stidley, C. A., Issa, J. P., Herman, J. G., March, T. H., et al. (2003). Inhibition of DNA methylation and histone deacetylation prevents murine lung cancer. *Cancer Research, 63*(21), 7089–7093.

Bergy, M. E., & Herr, R. R. (1966). Microbiological production of 5-azacytidine. II. Isolation and chemical structure. *Antimicrobial Agents and Chemotherapy, 6*, 625–630.

Beumer, J. H., Eiseman, J. L., Parise, R. A., Joseph, E., Holleran, J. L., Covey, J. M., et al. (2006). Pharmacokinetics, metabolism, and oral bioavailability of the DNA methyltransferase inhibitor 5-fluoro-2′-deoxycytidine in mice. *Clinical Cancer Research, 12*(24), 7483–7491.

Bhalla, S., Balasubramanian, S., David, K., Sirisawad, M., Buggy, J., Mauro, L., et al. (2009). PCI-24781 induces caspase and reactive oxygen species-dependent apoptosis through NF-kappaB mechanisms and is synergistic with bortezomib in lymphoma cells. *Clinical Cancer Research, 15*(10), 3354–3365.

Bianchi, M., Polticelli, F., Ascenzi, P., Botta, M., Federico, R., Mariottini, P., et al. (2006). Inhibition of polyamine and spermine oxidases by polyamine analogues. *The FEBS Journal, 273*(6), 1115–1123.

Billam, M., Sobolewski, M. D., & Davidson, N. E. (2010). Effects of a novel DNA methyltransferase inhibitor zebularine on human breast cancer cells. *Breast Cancer Research and Treatment, 120*(3), 581–592.

Boivin, A. J., Momparler, L. F., Hurtubise, A., & Momparler, R. L. (2002). Antineoplastic action of 5-aza-2′-deoxycytidine and phenylbutyrate on human lung carcinoma cells. *Anti-Cancer Drugs, 13*(8), 869–874.

Boyer, L. A., Langer, M. R., Crowley, K. A., Tan, S., Denu, J. M., & Peterson, C. L. (2002). Essential role for the SANT domain in the functioning of multiple chromatin remodeling enzymes. *Molecular Cell, 10*(4), 935–942.

Bradner, J. E., West, N., Grachan, M. L., Greenberg, E. F., Haggarty, S. J., Warnow, T., et al. (2010). Chemical phylogenetics of histone deacetylases. *Nature Chemical Biology, 6*(3), 238–243.

Braiteh, F., Soriano, A. O., Garcia-Manero, G., Hong, D., Johnson, M. M., Silva Lde, P., et al. (2008). Phase I study of epigenetic modulation with 5-azacytidine and valproic acid in patients with advanced cancers. *Clinical Cancer Research, 14*(19), 6296–6301.

Cai, Y., Geutjes, E. J., de Lint, K., Roepman, P., Bruurs, L., Yu, L. R., et al. (2014). The NuRD complex cooperates with DNMTs to maintain silencing of key colorectal tumor suppressor genes. *Oncogene, 33*(17), 2157–2168.

Cameron, E. E., Bachman, K. E., Myohanen, S., Herman, J. G., & Baylin, S. B. (1999). Synergy of demethylation and histone deacetylase inhibition in the re-expression of genes silenced in cancer. *Nature Genetics, 21*(1), 103–107.

Candelaria, M., Gallardo-Rincon, D., Arce, C., Cetina, L., Aguilar-Ponce, J. L., Arrieta, O., et al. (2007). A phase II study of epigenetic therapy with hydralazine and magnesium valproate to overcome chemotherapy resistance in refractory solid tumors. *Annals of Oncology, 18*(9), 1529–1538.

Chai, G., Li, L., Zhou, W., Wu, L., Zhao, Y., Wang, D., et al. (2008). HDAC inhibitors act with 5-aza-2′-deoxycytidine to inhibit cell proliferation by suppressing removal of incorporated abases in lung cancer cells. *PLoS ONE, 3*(6), e2445.

Champion, C., Guianvarc'h, D., Senamaud-Beaufort, C., Jurkowska, R. Z., Jeltsch, A., Ponger, L., et al. (2010). Mechanistic insights on the inhibition of c5 DNA methyltransferases by zebularine. *PLoS ONE, 5*(8), e12388.

Chen, M. Y., Liao, W. S., Lu, Z., Bornmann, W. G., Hennessey, V., Washington, M. N., et al. (2011). Decitabine and suberoylanilide hydroxamic acid (SAHA) inhibit growth of ovarian cancer cell lines and xenografts while inducing expression of imprinted tumor suppressor genes, apoptosis, G2/M arrest, and autophagy. *Cancer, 117*(19), 4424–4438.

Chen, L., MacMillan, A. M., Chang, W., Ezaz-Nikpay, K., Lane, W. S., & Verdine, G. L. (1991). Direct identification of the active-site nucleophile in a DNA (cytosine-5)-methyltransferase. *Biochemistry, 30*(46), 11018–11025.

Chen, R. Z., Pettersson, U., Beard, C., Jackson-Grusby, L., & Jaenisch, R. (1998). DNA hypomethylation leads to elevated mutation rates. *Nature, 395*(6697), 89–93.

Chi, P., Allis, C. D., & Wang, G. G. (2010). Covalent histone modifications—Miswritten, misinterpreted and mis-erased in human cancers. *Nature Reviews. Cancer, 10*(7), 457–469.

Chiappinelli, K. B., Strissel, P. L., Desrichard, A., Li, H., Henke, C., Akman, B., et al. (2015). Inhibiting DNA methylation causes an interferon response in cancer via dsRNA including endogenous retroviruses. *Cell, 162*(5), 974–986.

Chu, B. F., Karpenko, M. J., Liu, Z., Aimiuwu, J., Villalona-Calero, M. A., Chan, K. K., et al. (2013). Phase I study of 5-aza-2'-deoxycytidine in combination with valproic acid in non-small-cell lung cancer. *Cancer Chemotherapy and Pharmacology, 71*(1), 115–121.

Chuang, J. C., Yoo, C. B., Kwan, J. M., Li, T. W., Liang, G., Yang, A. S., et al. (2005). Comparison of biological effects of non-nucleoside DNA methylation inhibitors versus 5-aza-2'-deoxycytidine. *Molecular Cancer Therapeutics, 4*(10), 1515–1520.

Chuikov, S., Kurash, J. K., Wilson, J. R., Xiao, B., Justin, N., Ivanov, G. S., et al. (2004). Regulation of p53 activity through lysine methylation. *Nature, 432*(7015), 353–360.

Cihak, A. (1974). Biological effects of 5-azacytidine in eukaryotes. *Oncology, 30*(5), 405–422.

Clavel, M., Monfardini, S., Fossa, S., Smyth, J., Renard, J., & Kaye, S. B. (1992). 5-Aza-2'-deoxycytidine (NSC 127716) in non-seminomatous testicular cancer. Phase II from the EORTC Early Clinical Trials Cooperative Group and Genito-Urinary Group. *Annals of Oncology, 3*(5), 399–400.

Codina, A., Love, J. D., Li, Y., Lazar, M. A., Neuhaus, D., & Schwabe, J. W. (2005). Structural insights into the interaction and activation of histone deacetylase 3 by nuclear receptor corepressors. *Proceedings of the National Academy of Sciences of the United States of America, 102*(17), 6009–6014.

Collett, K., Eide, G. E., Arnes, J., Stefansson, I. M., Eide, J., Braaten, A., et al. (2006). Expression of enhancer of zeste homologue 2 is significantly associated with increased tumor cell proliferation and is a marker of aggressive breast cancer. *Clinical Cancer Research, 12*(4), 1168–1174.

Coronel, J., Cetina, L., Pacheco, I., Trejo-Becerril, C., Gonzalez-Fierro, A., de la Cruz-Hernandez, E., et al. (2011). A double-blind, placebo-controlled, randomized phase III trial of chemotherapy plus epigenetic therapy with hydralazine valproate for advanced cervical cancer. Preliminary results. *Medical Oncology, 28*(Suppl. 1), S540–S546.

Cowger, J. J., Zhao, Q., Isovic, M., & Torchia, J. (2007). Biochemical characterization of the zinc-finger protein 217 transcriptional repressor complex: Identification of a ZNF217 consensus recognition sequence. *Oncogene, 26*(23), 3378–3386.

Deaton, A. M., & Bird, A. (2011). CpG islands and the regulation of transcription. *Genes and Development, 25*(10), 1010–1022.

Defossez, P. A. (2013). Ceci n'est pas une DNMT: Recently discovered functions of DNMT2 and their relation to methyltransferase activity (comment on DOI 10.1002/bies.201300088). *Bioessays, 35*(12), 1024.

Denis, H., Ndlovu, M. N., & Fuks, F. (2011). Regulation of mammalian DNA methyltransferases: A route to new mechanisms. *EMBO Reports, 12*(7), 647–656.

Denslow, S. A., & Wade, P. A. (2007). The human Mi-2/NuRD complex and gene regulation. *Oncogene, 26*(37), 5433–5438.

Dimitrova, E., Turberfield, A. H., & Klose, R. J. (2015). Histone demethylases in chromatin biology and beyond. *EMBO Reports, 16*(12), 1620–1639.

Ebert, D. H., Gabel, H. W., Robinson, N. D., Kastan, N. R., Hu, L. S., Cohen, S., et al. (2013). Activity-dependent phosphorylation of MeCP2 threonine 308 regulates interaction with NCoR. *Nature, 499*(7458), 341–345.

Ecke, I., Petry, F., Rosenberger, A., Tauber, S., Monkemeyer, S., Hess, I., et al. (2009). Antitumor effects of a combined 5-aza-2′deoxycytidine and valproic acid treatment on rhabdomyosarcoma and medulloblastoma in Ptch mutant mice. *Cancer Research, 69*(3), 887–895.

Eden, S., Hashimshony, T., Keshet, I., Cedar, H., & Thorne, A. W. (1998). DNA methylation models histone acetylation. *Nature, 394*(6696), 842.

Egger, G., Liang, G., Aparicio, A., & Jones, P. A. (2004). Epigenetics in human disease and prospects for epigenetic therapy. *Nature, 429*(6990), 457–463.

Ellis, L., Atadja, P. W., & Johnstone, R. W. (2009). Epigenetics in cancer: Targeting chromatin modifications. *Molecular Cancer Therapeutics, 8*(6), 1409–1420.

Evangelista, M., Tian, H., & de Sauvage, F. J. (2006). The hedgehog signaling pathway in cancer. *Clinical Cancer Research, 12*(20 Pt. 1), 5924–5928.

Falkenberg, K. J., & Johnstone, R. W. (2014). Histone deacetylases and their inhibitors in cancer, neurological diseases and immune disorders. *Nature Reviews. Drug Discovery, 13*(9), 673–691.

Fang, F., Balch, C., Schilder, J., Breen, T., Zhang, S., Shen, C., et al. (2010). A phase 1 and pharmacodynamic study of decitabine in combination with carboplatin in patients with recurrent, platinum-resistant, epithelial ovarian cancer. *Cancer, 116*(17), 4043–4053.

Fang, M. Z., Wang, Y., Ai, N., Hou, Z., Sun, Y., Lu, H., et al. (2003). Tea polyphenol (−)-epigallocatechin-3-gallate inhibits DNA methyltransferase and reactivates methylation-silenced genes in cancer cell lines. *Cancer Research, 63*(22), 7563–7570.

Federico, R., Leone, L., Botta, M., Binda, C., Angelini, R., Venturini, G., et al. (2001). Inhibition of pig liver and *Zea mays* L. polyamine oxidase: A comparative study. *Journal of Enzyme Inhibition, 16*(2), 147–155.

Fitzpatrick, P. F. (2010). Oxidation of amines by flavoproteins. *Archives of Biochemistry and Biophysics, 493*(1), 13–25.

Forneris, F., Binda, C., Adamo, A., Battaglioli, E., & Mattevi, A. (2007). Structural basis of LSD1-CoREST selectivity in histone H3 recognition. *The Journal of Biological Chemistry, 282*(28), 20070–20074.

Forneris, F., Binda, C., Vanoni, M. A., Mattevi, A., & Battaglioli, E. (2005). Histone demethylation catalysed by LSD1 is a flavin-dependent oxidative process. *FEBS Letters, 579*(10), 2203–2207.

Foster, C. T., Dovey, O. M., Lezina, L., Luo, J. L., Gant, T. W., Barlev, N., et al. (2010). Lysine-specific demethylase 1 regulates the embryonic transcriptome and CoREST stability. *Molecular and Cellular Biology, 30*(20), 4851–4863.

Fotheringham, S., Epping, M. T., Stimson, L., Khan, O., Wood, V., Pezzella, F., et al. (2009). Genome-wide loss-of-function screen reveals an important role for the proteasome in HDAC inhibitor-induced apoptosis. *Cancer Cell, 15*(1), 57–66.

Fu, S., Hu, W., Iyer, R., Kavanagh, J. J., Coleman, R. L., Levenback, C. F., et al. (2011). Phase 1b-2a study to reverse platinum resistance through use of a hypomethylating agent, azacitidine, in patients with platinum-resistant or platinum-refractory epithelial ovarian cancer. *Cancer, 117*(8), 1661–1669.

Fujita, N., Watanabe, S., Ichimura, T., Tsuruzoe, S., Shinkai, Y., Tachibana, M., et al. (2003). Methyl-CpG binding domain 1 (MBD1) interacts with the Suv39h1-HP1 heterochromatic complex for DNA methylation-based transcriptional repression. *The Journal of Biological Chemistry, 278*(26), 24132–24138.

Fuks, F., Burgers, W. A., Brehm, A., Hughes-Davies, L., & Kouzarides, T. (2000). DNA methyltransferase Dnmt1 associates with histone deacetylase activity. *Nature Genetics, 24*(1), 88–91.

Fuks, F., Hurd, P. J., Deplus, R., & Kouzarides, T. (2003). The DNA methyltransferases associate with HP1 and the SUV39H1 histone methyltransferase. *Nucleic Acids Research*, *31*(9), 2305–2312.

Ghoshal, K., Datta, J., Majumder, S., Bai, S., Kutay, H., Motiwala, T., et al. (2005). 5-Aza-deoxycytidine induces selective degradation of DNA methyltransferase 1 by a proteasomal pathway that requires the KEN box, bromo-adjacent homology domain, and nuclear localization signal. *Molecular and Cellular Biology*, *25*(11), 4727–4741.

Glozak, M. A., & Seto, E. (2007). Histone deacetylases and cancer. *Oncogene*, *26*(37), 5420–5432.

Goll, M. G., & Bestor, T. H. (2005). Eukaryotic cytosine methyltransferases. *Annual Review of Biochemistry*, *74*, 481–514.

Goll, M. G., Kirpekar, F., Maggert, K. A., Yoder, J. A., Hsieh, C. L., Zhang, X., et al. (2006). Methylation of tRNAAsp by the DNA methyltransferase homolog Dnmt2. *Science*, *311*(5759), 395–398.

Graca, I., Sousa, E. J., Baptista, T., Almeida, M., Ramalho-Carvalho, J., Palmeira, C., et al. (2014). Anti-tumoral effect of the non-nucleoside DNMT inhibitor RG108 in human prostate cancer cells. *Current Pharmaceutical Design*, *20*(11), 1803–1811.

Guenther, M. G., Barak, O., & Lazar, M. A. (2001). The SMRT and N-CoR corepressors are activating cofactors for histone deacetylase 3. *Molecular and Cellular Biology*, *21*(18), 6091–6101.

Gui, C. Y., Ngo, L., Xu, W. S., Richon, V. M., & Marks, P. A. (2004). Histone deacetylase (HDAC) inhibitor activation of p21WAF1 involves changes in promoter-associated proteins, including HDAC1. *Proceedings of the National Academy of Sciences of the United States of America*, *101*(5), 1241–1246.

Guil, S., & Esteller, M. (2009). DNA methylomes, histone codes and miRNAs: Tying it all together. *The International Journal of Biochemistry & Cell Biology*, *41*(1), 87–95.

Hakimi, M. A., Bochar, D. A., Chenoweth, J., Lane, W. S., Mandel, G., & Shiekhattar, R. (2002). A core-BRAF35 complex containing histone deacetylase mediates repression of neuronal-specific genes. *Proceedings of the National Academy of Sciences of the United States of America*, *99*(11), 7420–7425.

Hanka, L. J., Evans, J. S., Mason, D. J., & Dietz, A. (1966). Microbiological production of 5-azacytidine. I. Production and biological activity. *Antimicrobial Agents and Chemotherapy (Bethesda)*, *6*, 619–624.

Hansen, K. D., Timp, W., Bravo, H. C., Sabunciyan, S., Langmead, B., McDonald, O. G., et al. (2011). Increased methylation variation in epigenetic domains across cancer types. *Nature Genetics*, *43*(8), 768–775.

Harris, W. J., Huang, X., Lynch, J. T., Spencer, G. J., Hitchin, J. R., Li, Y., et al. (2012). The histone demethylase KDM1A sustains the oncogenic potential of MLL-AF9 leukemia stem cells. *Cancer Cell*, *21*(4), 473–487.

Hayami, S., Kelly, J. D., Cho, H. S., Yoshimatsu, M., Unoki, M., Tsunoda, T., et al. (2011). Overexpression of LSD1 contributes to human carcinogenesis through chromatin regulation in various cancers. *International Journal of Cancer*, *128*(3), 574–586.

Herman, J. G., & Baylin, S. B. (2003). Gene silencing in cancer in association with promoter hypermethylation. *The New England Journal of Medicine*, *349*(21), 2042–2054.

Hermann, A., Schmitt, S., & Jeltsch, A. (2003). The human Dnmt2 has residual DNA-(cytosine-C5) methyltransferase activity. *The Journal of Biological Chemistry*, *278*(34), 31717–31721.

Hojfeldt, J. W., Agger, K., & Helin, K. (2013). Histone lysine demethylases as targets for anticancer therapy. *Nature Reviews. Drug Discovery*, *12*(12), 917–930.

Hollenbach, P. W., Nguyen, A. N., Brady, H., Williams, M., Ning, Y., Richard, N., et al. (2010). A comparison of azacitidine and decitabine activities in acute myeloid leukemia cell lines. *PLoS One*, *5*(2), e9001.

Huang, Y., Greene, E., Murray Stewart, T., Goodwin, A. C., Baylin, S. B., Woster, P. M., et al. (2007). Inhibition of lysine-specific demethylase 1 by polyamine analogues results in reexpression of aberrantly silenced genes. *Proceedings of the National Academy of Sciences of the United States of America, 104*(19), 8023–8028.

Huang, Y., Marton, L. J., Woster, P. M., & Casero, R. A. (2009). Polyamine analogues targeting epigenetic gene regulation. *Essays in Biochemistry, 46,* 95–110.

Huang, J., Sengupta, R., Espejo, A. B., Lee, M. G., Dorsey, J. A., Richter, M., et al. (2007). p53 is regulated by the lysine demethylase LSD1. *Nature, 449*(7158), 105–108.

Huang, Y., Stewart, T. M., Wu, Y., Baylin, S. B., Marton, L. J., Perkins, B., et al. (2009). Novel oligoamine analogues inhibit lysine-specific demethylase 1 and induce reexpression of epigenetically silenced genes. *Clinical Cancer Research, 15*(23), 7217–7228.

Huang, Y., Vasilatos, S. N., Boric, L., Shaw, P. G., & Davidson, N. E. (2012). Inhibitors of histone demethylation and histone deacetylation cooperate in regulating gene expression and inhibiting growth in human breast cancer cells. *Breast Cancer Research and Treatment, 131*(3), 777–789.

Humphrey, G. W., Wang, Y., Russanova, V. R., Hirai, T., Qin, J., Nakatani, Y., et al. (2001). Stable histone deacetylase complexes distinguished by the presence of SANT domain proteins CoREST/kiaa0071 and Mta-L1. *The Journal of Biological Chemistry, 276*(9), 6817–6824.

Issa, J. P., Baylin, S. B., & Herman, J. G. (1997). DNA methylation changes in hematologic malignancies: Biologic and clinical implications. *Leukemia, 11*(Suppl. 1), S7–S11.

Issa, J. P., Roboz, G., Rizzieri, D., Jabbour, E., Stock, W., O'Connell, C., et al. (2015). Safety and tolerability of guadecitabine (SGI-110) in patients with myelodysplastic syndrome and acute myeloid leukaemia: A multicentre, randomised, dose-escalation phase 1 study. *The Lancet. Oncology, 16*(9), 1099–1110.

Jackson, J. P., Lindroth, A. M., Cao, X., & Jacobsen, S. E. (2002). Control of CpNpG DNA methylation by the KRYPTONITE histone H3 methyltransferase. *Nature, 416*(6880), 556–560.

Jair, K. W., Bachman, K. E., Suzuki, H., Ting, A. H., Rhee, I., Yen, R. W., et al. (2006). De novo CpG island methylation in human cancer cells. *Cancer Research, 66*(2), 682–692.

Jenuwein, T., & Allis, C. D. (2001). Translating the histone code. *Science, 293*(5532), 1074–1080.

Jia, D., Jurkowska, R. Z., Zhang, X., Jeltsch, A., & Cheng, X. (2007). Structure of Dnmt3a bound to Dnmt3L suggests a model for de novo DNA methylation. *Nature, 449*(7159), 248–251.

Jin, L., Hanigan, C. L., Wu, Y., Wang, W., Park, B. H., Woster, P. M., et al. (2013). Loss of LSD1 (lysine-specific demethylase 1) suppresses growth and alters gene expression of human colon cancer cells in a p53- and DNMT1 (DNA methyltransferase 1)-independent manner. *The Biochemical Journal, 449*(2), 459–468.

Jones, P. A., & Baylin, S. B. (2002). The fundamental role of epigenetic events in cancer. *Nature Reviews Genetics, 3*(6), 415–428.

Jones, P. A., & Baylin, S. B. (2007). The epigenomics of cancer. *Cell, 128*(4), 683–692.

Jones, S. F., Infante, J. R., Spigel, D. R., Peacock, N. W., Thompson, D. S., Greco, F. A., et al. (2012). Phase 1 results from a study of romidepsin in combination with gemcitabine in patients with advanced solid tumors. *Cancer Investigation, 30*(6), 481–486.

Jones, P. A., & Taylor, S. M. (1980). Cellular differentiation, cytidine analogs and DNA methylation. *Cell, 20*(1), 85–93.

Juergens, R. A., Wrangle, J., Vendetti, F. P., Murphy, S. C., Zhao, M., Coleman, B., et al. (2011). Combination epigenetic therapy has efficacy in patients with refractory advanced non-small cell lung cancer. *Cancer Discovery, 1*(7), 598–607.

Juo, Y. Y., Gong, X. J., Mishra, A., Cui, X., Baylin, S. B., Azad, N. S., et al. (2015). Epigenetic therapy for solid tumors: From bench science to clinical trials. *Epigenomics*, 7(2), 215–235.

Jurkowska, R. Z., Jurkowski, T. P., & Jeltsch, A. (2011). Structure and function of mammalian DNA methyltransferases. *Chembiochem*, 12(2), 206–222.

Jurkowski, T. P., Meusburger, M., Phalke, S., Helm, M., Nellen, W., Reuter, G., et al. (2008). Human DNMT2 methylates tRNA(Asp) molecules using a DNA methyltransferase-like catalytic mechanism. *RNA*, 14(8), 1663–1670.

Juttermann, R., Li, E., & Jaenisch, R. (1994). Toxicity of 5-aza-2′-deoxycytidine to mammalian cells is mediated primarily by covalent trapping of DNA methyltransferase rather than DNA demethylation. *Proceedings of the National Academy of Sciences of the United States of America*, 91(25), 11797–11801.

Kahl, P., Gullotti, L., Heukamp, L. C., Wolf, S., Friedrichs, N., Vorreuther, R., et al. (2006). Androgen receptor coactivators lysine-specific histone demethylase 1 and four and a half LIM domain protein 2 predict risk of prostate cancer recurrence. *Cancer Research*, 66(23), 11341–11347.

Karytinos, A., Forneris, F., Profumo, A., Ciossani, G., Battaglioli, E., Binda, C., et al. (2009). A novel mammalian flavin-dependent histone demethylase. *The Journal of Biological Chemistry*, 284(26), 17775–17782.

Kauffman, E. C., Robinson, B. D., Downes, M. J., Powell, L. G., Lee, M. M., Scherr, D. S., et al. (2011). Role of androgen receptor and associated lysine-demethylase coregulators, LSD1 and JMJD2A, in localized and advanced human bladder cancer. *Molecular Carcinogenesis*, 50(12), 931–944.

Khan, O., Fotheringham, S., Wood, V., Stimson, L., Zhang, C., Pezzella, F., et al. (2010). HR23B is a biomarker for tumor sensitivity to HDAC inhibitor-based therapy. *Proceedings of the National Academy of Sciences of the United States of America*, 107(14), 6532–6537.

Khoddami, V., & Cairns, B. R. (2013). Identification of direct targets and modified bases of RNA cytosine methyltransferases. *Nature Biotechnology*, 31(5), 458–464.

Kim, K. H., Kim, W., Howard, T. P., Vazquez, F., Tsherniak, A., Wu, J. N., et al. (2015). SWI/SNF-mutant cancers depend on catalytic and non-catalytic activity of EZH2. *Nature Medicine*, 21(12), 1491–1496.

Kim, C. H., Marquez, V. E., Mao, D. T., Haines, D. R., & McCormack, J. J. (1986). Synthesis of pyrimidin-2-one nucleosides as acid-stable inhibitors of cytidine deaminase. *Journal of Medicinal Chemistry*, 29(8), 1374–1380.

Kim, K., Skora, A. D., Li, Z., Liu, Q., Tam, A. J., Blosser, R. L., et al. (2014). Eradication of metastatic mouse cancers resistant to immune checkpoint blockade by suppression of myeloid-derived cells. *Proceedings of the National Academy of Sciences of the United States of America*, 111(32), 11774–11779.

Kim, M., Thompson, L. A., Wenger, S. D., & O'Bryant, C. L. (2012). Romidepsin: A histone deacetylase inhibitor for refractory cutaneous T-cell lymphoma. *The Annals of Pharmacotherapy*, 46(10), 1340–1348.

King, M. Y., & Redman, K. L. (2002). RNA methyltransferases utilize two cysteine residues in the formation of 5-methylcytosine. *Biochemistry*, 41(37), 11218–11225.

Klose, R. J., Kallin, E. M., & Zhang, Y. (2006). JmjC-domain-containing proteins and histone demethylation. *Nature Reviews. Genetics*, 7(9), 715–727.

Kuo, H. K., Griffith, J. D., & Kreuzer, K. N. (2007). 5-Azacytidine induced methyltransferase-DNA adducts block DNA replication in vivo. *Cancer Research*, 67(17), 8248–8254.

Lacoste, N., Utley, R. T., Hunter, J. M., Poirier, G. G., & Cote, J. (2002). Disruptor of telomeric silencing-1 is a chromatin-specific histone H3 methyltransferase. *The Journal of Biological Chemistry*, 277(34), 30421–30424.

Leclercq, S., Gueugnon, F., Boutin, B., Guillot, F., Blanquart, C., Rogel, A., et al. (2011). A 5-aza-2'-deoxycytidine/valproate combination induces cytotoxic T-cell response against mesothelioma. *The European Respiratory Journal, 38*(5), 1105–1116.

Lee, H. Z., Kwitkowski, V. E., Del Valle, P. L., Ricci, M. S., Saber, H., Habtemariam, B. A., et al. (2015). FDA approval: Belinostat for the treatment of patients with relapsed or refractory peripheral T-cell lymphoma. *Clinical Cancer Research, 21*(12), 2666–2670.

Lee, Y. S., Lim, K. H., Guo, X., Kawaguchi, Y., Gao, Y., Barrientos, T., et al. (2008). The cytoplasmic deacetylase HDAC6 is required for efficient oncogenic tumorigenesis. *Cancer Research, 68*(18), 7561–7569.

Lee, M. G., Wynder, C., Cooch, N., & Shiekhattar, R. (2005). An essential role for CoREST in nucleosomal histone 3 lysine 4 demethylation. *Nature, 437*(7057), 432–435.

Lee, M. G., Wynder, C., Schmidt, D. M., McCafferty, D. G., & Shiekhattar, R. (2006). Histone H3 lysine 4 demethylation is a target of nonselective antidepressive medications. *Chemistry & Biology, 13*(6), 563–567.

Li, E., Bestor, T. H., & Jaenisch, R. (1992). Targeted mutation of the DNA methyltransferase gene results in embryonic lethality. *Cell, 69*(6), 915–926.

Li, B., Carey, M., & Workman, J. L. (2007). The role of chromatin during transcription. *Cell, 128*(4), 707–719.

Li, H., Chiappinelli, K. B., Guzzetta, A. A., Easwaran, H., Yen, R. W., Vatapalli, R., et al. (2014). Immune regulation by low doses of the DNA methyltransferase inhibitor 5-azacitidine in common human epithelial cancers. *Oncotarget, 5*(3), 587–598.

Li, L. H., Olin, E. J., Buskirk, H. H., & Reineke, L. M. (1970). Cytotoxicity and mode of action of 5-azacytidine on L1210 leukemia. *Cancer Research, 30*(11), 2760–2769.

Lillico, R., Sobral, M. G., Stesco, N., & Lakowski, T. M. (2016). HDAC inhibitors induce global changes in histone lysine and arginine methylation and alter expression of lysine demethylases. *Journal of Proteomics, 133*, 125–133.

Lim, S., Janzer, A., Becker, A., Zimmer, A., Schule, R., Buettner, R., et al. (2010). Lysine-specific demethylase 1 (LSD1) is highly expressed in ER-negative breast cancers and a biomarker predicting aggressive biology. *Carcinogenesis, 31*(3), 512–520.

Lin, J., Gilbert, J., Rudek, M. A., Zwiebel, J. A., Gore, S., Jiemjit, A., et al. (2009). A phase I dose-finding study of 5-azacytidine in combination with sodium phenylbutyrate in patients with refractory solid tumors. *Clinical Cancer Research, 15*(19), 6241–6249.

Ling, Y., Sankpal, U. T., Robertson, A. K., McNally, J. G., Karpova, T., & Robertson, K. D. (2004). Modification of de novo DNA methyltransferase 3a (Dnmt3a) by SUMO-1 modulates its interaction with histone deacetylases (HDACs) and its capacity to repress transcription. *Nucleic Acids Research, 32*(2), 598–610.

Lombardi, P. M., Cole, K. E., Dowling, D. P., & Christianson, D. W. (2011). Structure, mechanism, and inhibition of histone deacetylases and related metalloenzymes. *Current Opinion in Structural Biology, 21*(6), 735–743.

Lu, L. W., Chiang, G. H., Medina, D., & Randerath, K. (1976). Drug effects on nucleic acid modification. I. A specific effect of 5-azacytidine on mammalian transfer RNA methylation in vivo. *Biochemical and Biophysical Research Communications, 68*(4), 1094–1101.

Lu, L. J., & Randerath, K. (1979). Effects of 5-azacytidine on transfer RNA methyltransferases. *Cancer Research, 39*(3), 940–949.

Lu, Y., Wajapeyee, N., Turker, M. S., & Glazer, P. M. (2014). Silencing of the DNA mismatch repair gene MLH1 induced by hypoxic stress in a pathway dependent on the histone demethylase LSD1. *Cell Reports, 8*(2), 501–513.

Luszczek, W., Cheriyath, V., Mekhail, T. M., & Borden, E. C. (2010). Combinations of DNA methyltransferase and histone deacetylase inhibitors induce DNA damage in small cell lung cancer cells: Correlation of resistance with IFN-stimulated gene expression. *Molecular Cancer Therapeutics, 9*(8), 2309–2321.

Lyko, F., & Brown, R. (2005). DNA methyltransferase inhibitors and the development of epigenetic cancer therapies. *Journal of the National Cancer Institute, 97*(20), 1498–1506.

Maes, T., Mascaro, C., Ortega, A., Lunardi, S., Ciceri, F., Somervaille, T. C., et al. (2015). KDM1 histone lysine demethylases as targets for treatments of oncological and neurodegenerative disease. *Epigenomics, 7*(4), 609–626.

Mann, B. S., Johnson, J. R., Cohen, M. H., Justice, R., & Pazdur, R. (2007). FDA approval summary: Vorinostat for treatment of advanced primary cutaneous T-cell lymphoma. *The Oncologist, 12*(10), 1247–1252.

Mann, B. S., Johnson, J. R., He, K., Sridhara, R., Abraham, S., Booth, B. P., et al. (2007b). Vorinostat for treatment of cutaneous manifestations of advanced primary cutaneous T-cell lymphoma. *Clinical Cancer Research, 13*(8), 2318–2322.

Margueron, R., & Reinberg, D. (2011). The polycomb complex PRC2 and its mark in life. *Nature, 469*(7330), 343–349.

Matei, D., Fang, F., Shen, C., Schilder, J., Arnold, A., Zeng, Y., et al. (2012). Epigenetic resensitization to platinum in ovarian cancer. *Cancer Research, 72*(9), 2197–2205.

McGarvey, K. M., Fahrner, J. A., Greene, E., Martens, J., Jenuwein, T., & Baylin, S. B. (2006). Silenced tumor suppressor genes reactivated by DNA demethylation do not return to a fully euchromatic chromatin state. *Cancer Research, 66*(7), 3541–3549.

McGrath, J., & Trojer, P. (2015). Targeting histone lysine methylation in cancer. *Pharmacology & Therapeutics, 150*, 1–22.

McLean, C. M., Karemaker, I. D., & van Leeuwen, F. (2014). The emerging roles of DOT1L in leukemia and normal development. *Leukemia, 28*(11), 2131–2138.

Metzger, E., Wissmann, M., Yin, N., Muller, J. M., Schneider, R., Peters, A. H., et al. (2005). LSD1 demethylates repressive histone marks to promote androgen-receptor-dependent transcription. *Nature, 437*(7057), 436–439.

Mohammad, H. P., Smitheman, K. N., Kamat, C. D., Soong, D., Federowicz, K. E., Van Aller, G. S., et al. (2015). A DNA hypomethylation signature predicts antitumor activity of LSD1 inhibitors in SCLC. *Cancer Cell, 28*(1), 57–69.

Momparler, R. L., Bouffard, D. Y., Momparler, L. F., Dionne, J., Belanger, K., & Ayoub, J. (1997). Pilot phase I-II study on 5-aza-2'-deoxycytidine (Decitabine) in patients with metastatic lung cancer. *Anticancer Drugs, 8*(4), 358–368.

Morin, R. D., Johnson, N. A., Severson, T. M., Mungall, A. J., An, J., Goya, R., et al. (2010). Somatic mutations altering EZH2 (Tyr641) in follicular and diffuse large B-cell lymphomas of germinal-center origin. *Nature Genetics, 42*(2), 181–185.

Motorin, Y., Lyko, F., & Helm, M. (2010). 5-Methylcytosine in RNA: Detection, enzymatic formation and biological functions. *Nucleic Acids Research, 38*(5), 1415–1430.

Mould, D. P., McGonagle, A. E., Wiseman, D. H., Williams, E. L., & Jordan, A. M. (2015). Reversible inhibitors of LSD1 as therapeutic agents in acute myeloid leukemia: Clinical significance and progress to date. *Medicinal Research Reviews, 35*(3), 586–618.

Murray-Stewart, T., Woster, P. M., & Casero, R. A., Jr. (2014). The re-expression of the epigenetically silenced e-cadherin gene by a polyamine analogue lysine-specific demethylase-1 (LSD1) inhibitor in human acute myeloid leukemia cell lines. *Amino Acids, 46*(3), 585–594.

Nan, X., Ng, H. H., Johnson, C. A., Laherty, C. D., Turner, B. M., Eisenman, R. N., et al. (1998). Transcriptional repression by the methyl-CpG-binding protein MeCP2 involves a histone deacetylase complex. *Nature, 393*(6683), 386–389.

Nervi, C., De Marinis, E., & Codacci-Pisanelli, G. (2015). Epigenetic treatment of solid tumours: A review of clinical trials. *Clinical Epigenetics, 7*, 127.

New, M., Olzscha, H., & La Thangue, N. B. (2012). HDAC inhibitor-based therapies: Can we interpret the code? *Molecular Oncology, 6*(6), 637–656.

Newman, E. M., Morgan, R. J., Kummar, S., Beumer, J. H., Blanchard, M. S., Ruel, C., et al. (2015). A phase I, pharmacokinetic, and pharmacodynamic evaluation of the DNA methyltransferase inhibitor 5-fluoro-2'-deoxycytidine, administered with tetrahydrouridine. *Cancer Chemotherapy and Pharmacology, 75*(3), 537–546.

Nowotarski, S. L., Pachaiyappan, B., Holshouser, S. L., Kutz, C. J., Li, Y., Huang, Y., et al. (2015). Structure-activity study for (bis)ureidopropyl- and (bis)thioureidopropyldiamine LSD1 inhibitors with 3-5-3 and 3-6-3 carbon backbone architectures. *Bioorganic & Medicinal Chemistry, 23*(7), 1601–1612.

O'Hagan, H. M., Mohammad, H. P., & Baylin, S. B. (2008). Double strand breaks can initiate gene silencing and SIRT1-dependent onset of DNA methylation in an exogenous promoter CpG island. *PLoS Genetics, 4*(8), e1000155.

O'Hagan, H. M., Wang, W., Sen, S., Destefano Shields, C., Lee, S. S., Zhang, Y. W., et al. (2011). Oxidative damage targets complexes containing DNA methyltransferases, SIRT1, and polycomb members to promoter CpG Islands. *Cancer Cell, 20*(5), 606–619.

Ohm, J. E., McGarvey, K. M., Yu, X., Cheng, L., Schuebel, K. E., Cope, L., et al. (2007). A stem cell-like chromatin pattern may predispose tumor suppressor genes to DNA hypermethylation and heritable silencing. *Nature Genetics, 39*(2), 237–242.

Ooi, S. K., Qiu, C., Bernstein, E., Li, K., Jia, D., Yang, Z., et al. (2007). DNMT3L connects unmethylated lysine 4 of histone H3 to de novo methylation of DNA. *Nature, 448*(7154), 714–717.

Parry, L., & Clarke, A. R. (2011). The roles of the methyl-CpG binding proteins in cancer. *Genes & Cancer, 2*(6), 618–630.

Pasini, A., Delmonte, A., Tesei, A., Calistri, D., & Giordano, E. (2015). Targeting chromatin-mediated transcriptional control of gene expression in non-small cell lung cancer therapy: Preclinical rationale and clinical results. *Drugs, 75*(15), 1757–1771.

Peng, D., Kryczek, I., Nagarsheth, N., Zhao, L., Wei, S., Wang, W., et al. (2015). Epigenetic silencing of TH1-type chemokines shapes tumour immunity and immunotherapy. *Nature, 527*(7577), 249–253.

Perissi, V., Jepsen, K., Glass, C. K., & Rosenfeld, M. G. (2010). Deconstructing repression: Evolving models of co-repressor action. *Nature Reviews. Genetics, 11*(2), 109–123.

Pohlmann, P., DiLeone, L. P., Cancella, A. I., Caldas, A. P., Dal Lago, L., Campos, O., Jr., et al. (2002). Phase II trial of cisplatin plus decitabine, a new DNA hypomethylating agent, in patients with advanced squamous cell carcinoma of the cervix. *American Journal of Clinical Oncology, 25*(5), 496–501.

Portela, A., & Esteller, M. (2010). Epigenetic modifications and human disease. *Nature Biotechnology, 28*(10), 1057–1068.

Prince, H. M., Bishton, M. J., & Harrison, S. J. (2009). Clinical studies of histone deacetylase inhibitors. *Clinical Cancer Research, 15*(12), 3958–3969.

Prusevich, P., Kalin, J. H., Ming, S. A., Basso, M., Givens, J., Li, X., et al. (2014). A selective phenelzine analogue inhibitor of histone demethylase LSD1. *ACS Chemical Biology, 9*(6), 1284–1293.

Rai, K., Chidester, S., Zavala, C. V., Manos, E. J., James, S. R., Karpf, A. R., et al. (2007). Dnmt2 functions in the cytoplasm to promote liver, brain, and retina development in zebrafish. *Genes & Development, 21*(3), 261–266.

Rao, Z. Y., Cai, M. Y., Yang, G. F., He, L. R., Mai, S. J., Hua, W. F., et al. (2010). EZH2 supports ovarian carcinoma cell invasion and/or metastasis via regulation of TGF-beta1 and is a predictor of outcome in ovarian carcinoma patients. *Carcinogenesis, 31*(9), 1576–1583.

Rao, R., Nalluri, S., Kolhe, R., Yang, Y., Fiskus, W., Chen, J., et al. (2010). Treatment with panobinostat induces glucose-regulated protein 78 acetylation and endoplasmic reticulum stress in breast cancer cells. *Molecular Cancer Therapeutics, 9*(4), 942–952.

Rea, S., Eisenhaber, F., O'Carroll, D., Strahl, B. D., Sun, Z. W., Schmid, M., et al. (2000). Regulation of chromatin structure by site-specific histone H3 methyltransferases. *Nature, 406*(6796), 593–599.

Ren, J., Singh, B. N., Huang, Q., Li, Z., Gao, Y., Mishra, P., et al. (2011). DNA hypermethylation as a chemotherapy target. *Cellular Signalling*, *23*(7), 1082–1093.

Richardson, P. G., Harvey, R. D., Laubach, J. P., Moreau, P., Lonial, S., & San-Miguel, J. F. (2016). Panobinostat for the treatment of relapsed or relapsed/refractory multiple myeloma: Pharmacology and clinical outcomes. *Expert Review of Clinical Pharmacology*, *9*(1), 35–48.

Robertson, K. D., Ait-Si-Ali, S., Yokochi, T., Wade, P. A., Jones, P. L., & Wolffe, A. P. (2000). DNMT1 forms a complex with Rb, E2F1 and HDAC1 and represses transcription from E2F-responsive promoters. *Nature Genetics*, *25*(3), 338–342.

Rodriguez-Paredes, M., & Esteller, M. (2011). Cancer epigenetics reaches mainstream oncology. *Nature Medicine*, *17*(3), 330–339.

Ropero, S., & Esteller, M. (2007). The role of histone deacetylases (HDACs) in human cancer. *Molecular Oncology*, *1*(1), 19–25.

Rose, N. R., & Klose, R. J. (2014). Understanding the relationship between DNA methylation and histone lysine methylation. *Biochimica et Biophysica Acta*, *1839*(12), 1362–1372.

Roulois, D., Loo Yau, H., Singhania, R., Wang, Y., Danesh, A., Shen, S. Y., et al. (2015). DNA-demethylating agents target colorectal cancer cells by inducing viral mimicry by endogenous transcripts. *Cell*, *162*(5), 961–973.

Rountree, M. R., Bachman, K. E., & Baylin, S. B. (2000). DNMT1 binds HDAC2 and a new co-repressor, DMAP1, to form a complex at replication foci. *Nature Genetics*, *25*(3), 269–277.

Sampath, D., Rao, V. A., & Plunkett, W. (2003). Mechanisms of apoptosis induction by nucleoside analogs. *Oncogene*, *22*(56), 9063–9074.

San-Miguel, J. F., Richardson, P. G., Gunther, A., Sezer, O., Siegel, D., Blade, J., et al. (2013). Phase Ib study of panobinostat and bortezomib in relapsed or relapsed and refractory multiple myeloma. *Journal of Clinical Oncology*, *31*(29), 3696–3703.

Santi, D. V., Norment, A., & Garrett, C. E. (1984). Covalent bond formation between a DNA-cytosine methyltransferase and DNA containing 5-azacytosine. *Proceedings of the National Academy of Sciences of the United States of America*, *81*(22), 6993–6997.

Sato, T., Kaneda, A., Tsuji, S., Isagawa, T., Yamamoto, S., Fujita, T., et al. (2013). PRC2 overexpression and PRC2-target gene repression relating to poorer prognosis in small cell lung cancer. *Scientific Reports*, *3*, 1911.

Schaefer, M., Hagemann, S., Hanna, K., & Lyko, F. (2009). Azacytidine inhibits RNA methylation at DNMT2 target sites in human cancer cell lines. *Cancer Research*, *69*(20), 8127–8132.

Schaefer, M., & Lyko, F. (2010). Solving the Dnmt2 enigma. *Chromosoma*, *119*(1), 35–40.

Schenk, T., Chen, W. C., Gollner, S., Howell, L., Jin, L., Hebestreit, K., et al. (2012). Inhibition of the LSD1 (KDM1A) demethylase reactivates the all-trans-retinoic acid differentiation pathway in acute myeloid leukemia. *Nature Medicine*, *18*(4), 605–611.

Schmidt, D. M., & McCafferty, D. G. (2007). trans-2-Phenylcyclopropylamine is a mechanism-based inactivator of the histone demethylase LSD1. *Biochemistry*, *46*(14), 4408–4416.

Schrump, D. S., Fischette, M. R., Nguyen, D. M., Zhao, M., Li, X., Kunst, T. F., et al. (2006). Phase I study of decitabine-mediated gene expression in patients with cancers involving the lungs, esophagus, or pleura. *Clinical Cancer Research*, *12*(19), 5777–5785.

Schulte, J. H., Lim, S., Schramm, A., Friedrichs, N., Koster, J., Versteeg, R., et al. (2009). Lysine-specific demethylase 1 is strongly expressed in poorly differentiated neuroblastoma: Implications for therapy. *Cancer Research*, *69*(5), 2065–2071.

Schwartsmann, G., Schunemann, H., Gorini, C. N., Filho, A. F., Garbino, C., Sabini, G., et al. (2000). A phase I trial of cisplatin plus decitabine, a new DNA-hypomethylating agent, in patients with advanced solid tumors and a follow-up early phase II evaluation in patients with inoperable non-small cell lung cancer. *Investigational New Drugs, 18*(1), 83–91.

Segura-Pacheco, B., Trejo-Becerril, C., Perez-Cardenas, E., Taja-Chayeb, L., Mariscal, I., Chavez, A., et al. (2003). Reactivation of tumor suppressor genes by the cardiovascular drugs hydralazine and procainamide and their potential use in cancer therapy. *Clinical Cancer Research, 9*(5), 1596–1603.

Shao, Y., Gao, Z., Marks, P. A., & Jiang, X. (2004). Apoptotic and autophagic cell death induced by histone deacetylase inhibitors. *Proceedings of the National Academy of Science of the United States of America, 101*(52), 18030–18035.

Sharif, J., Muto, M., Takebayashi, S., Suetake, I., Iwamatsu, A., Endo, T. A., et al. (2007). The SRA protein Np95 mediates epigenetic inheritance by recruiting Dnmt1 to methylated DNA. *Nature, 450*(7171), 908–912.

Sharma, D., Blum, J., Yang, X., Beaulieu, N., Macleod, A. R., & Davidson, N. E. (2005). Release of methyl CpG binding proteins and histone deacetylase 1 from the estrogen receptor alpha (ER) promoter upon reactivation in ER-negative human breast cancer cells. *Molecular Endocrinology, 19*(7), 1740–1751.

Sharma, S. K., Hazeldine, S., Crowley, M. L., Hanson, A., Beattie, R., Varghese, S., et al. (2012). Polyamine-based small molecule epigenetic modulators. *MedChemComm, 3*(1), 14–21.

Sharma, S. K., Wu, Y., Steinbergs, N., Crowley, M. L., Hanson, A. S., Casero, R. A., et al. (2010). (Bis)urea and (bis)thiourea inhibitors of lysine-specific demethylase 1 as epigenetic modulators. *Journal of Medicinal Chemistry, 53*(14), 5197–5212.

Shen, L., & Pili, R. (2012). Class I histone deacetylase inhibition is a novel mechanism to target regulatory T cells in immunotherapy. *Oncoimmunology, 1*(6), 948–950.

Shi, Y. (2007). Histone lysine demethylases: Emerging roles in development, physiology and disease. *Nature Reviews. Genetics, 8*(11), 829–833.

Shi, Y., Lan, F., Matson, C., Mulligan, P., Whetstine, J. R., Cole, P. A., et al. (2004). Histone demethylation mediated by the nuclear amine oxidase homolog LSD1. *Cell, 119*(7), 941–953.

Shi, Y. J., Matson, C., Lan, F., Iwase, S., Baba, T., & Shi, Y. (2005). Regulation of LSD1 histone demethylase activity by its associated factors. *Molecular Cell, 19*(6), 857–864.

Shih, J. C., Chen, K., & Ridd, M. J. (1999). Monoamine oxidase: From genes to behavior. *Annual Review of Neuroscience, 22*, 197–217.

Singal, R., Ramachandran, K., Gordian, E., Quintero, C., Zhao, W., & Reis, I. M. (2015). Phase I/II study of azacitidine, docetaxel, and prednisone in patients with metastatic castration-resistant prostate cancer previously treated with docetaxel-based therapy. *Clinical Genitourinary Cancer, 13*(1), 22–31.

Singh, M. M., Manton, C. A., Bhat, K. P., Tsai, W. W., Aldape, K., Barton, M. C., et al. (2011). Inhibition of LSD1 sensitizes glioblastoma cells to histone deacetylase inhibitors. *Neuro-Oncology, 13*(8), 894–903.

Sorm, F., Piskala, A., Cihak, A., & Vesely, J. (1964). 5-Azacytidine, a new, highly effective cancerostatic. *Experientia, 20*(4), 202–203.

Stathis, A., Hotte, S. J., Chen, E. X., Hirte, H. W., Oza, A. M., Moretto, P., et al. (2011). Phase I study of decitabine in combination with vorinostat in patients with advanced solid tumors and non-Hodgkin's lymphomas. *Clinical Cancer Research, 17*(6), 1582–1590.

Steele, N., Finn, P., Brown, R., & Plumb, J. A. (2009). Combined inhibition of DNA methylation and histone acetylation enhances gene re-expression and drug sensitivity in vivo. *British Journal of Cancer, 100*(5), 758–763.

Stimson, L., & La Thangue, N. B. (2009). Biomarkers for predicting clinical responses to HDAC inhibitors. *Cancer Letters, 280*(2), 177–183.

Stresemann, C., & Lyko, F. (2008). Modes of action of the DNA methyltransferase inhibitors azacytidine and decitabine. *International Journal of Cancer, 123*(1), 8–13.

Tawbi, H. A., Beumer, J. H., Tarhini, A. A., Moschos, S., Buch, S. C., Egorin, M. J., et al. (2013). Safety and efficacy of decitabine in combination with temozolomide in metastatic melanoma: A phase I/II study and pharmacokinetic analysis. *Annals of Oncology*, *24*(4), 1112–1119.

Taylor, S. M., & Jones, P. A. (1982). Mechanism of action of eukaryotic DNA methyltransferase. Use of 5-azacytosine-containing DNA. *Journal of Molecular Biology*, *162*(3), 679–692.

Tellez, C. S., Grimes, M. J., Picchi, M. A., Liu, Y., March, T. H., Reed, M. D., et al. (2014). SGI-110 and entinostat therapy reduces lung tumor burden and reprograms the epigenome. *International Journal of Cancer*, *135*(9), 2223–2231.

Tessarz, P., & Kouzarides, T. (2014). Histone core modifications regulating nucleosome structure and dynamics. *Nature Reviews. Molecular Cell Biology*, *15*(11), 703–708.

Thinnes, C. C., England, K. S., Kawamura, A., Chowdhury, R., Schofield, C. J., & Hopkinson, R. J. (2014). Targeting histone lysine demethylases—Progress, challenges, and the future. *Biochimica et Biophysica Acta*, *1839*(12), 1416–1432.

Van Triest, B., Pinedo, H. M., Giaccone, G., & Peters, G. J. (2000). Downstream molecular determinants of response to 5-fluorouracil and antifolate thymidylate synthase inhibitors. *Annals of Oncology*, *11*(4), 385–391.

Varambally, S., Dhanasekaran, S. M., Zhou, M., Barrette, T. R., Kumar-Sinha, C., Sanda, M. G., et al. (2002). The polycomb group protein EZH2 is involved in progression of prostate cancer. *Nature*, *419*(6907), 624–629.

Vasilatos, S. N., Katz, T. A., Oesterreich, S., Wan, Y., Davidson, N. E., & Huang, Y. (2013). Crosstalk between lysine-specific demethylase 1 (LSD1) and histone deacetylases mediates antineoplastic efficacy of HDAC inhibitors in human breast cancer cells. *Carcinogenesis*, *34*(6), 1196–1207.

Vendetti, F. P., Topper, M., Huang, P., Dobromilskaya, I., Easwaran, H., Wrangle, J., et al. (2015). Evaluation of azacitidine and entinostat as sensitization agents to cytotoxic chemotherapy in preclinical models of non-small cell lung cancer. *Oncotarget*, *6*(1), 56–70.

Venturelli, S., Armeanu, S., Pathil, A., Hsieh, C. J., Weiss, T. S., Vonthein, R., et al. (2007). Epigenetic combination therapy as a tumor-selective treatment approach for hepatocellular carcinoma. *Cancer*, *109*(10), 2132–2141.

Verdin, E., Dequiedt, F., & Kasler, H. G. (2003). Class II histone deacetylases: Versatile regulators. *Trends in Genetics*, *19*(5), 286–293.

Volkel, P., Dupret, B., Le Bourhis, X., & Angrand, P. O. (2015). Diverse involvement of EZH2 in cancer epigenetics. *American Journal of Translational Research*, *7*(2), 175–193.

Vujcic, S., Liang, P., Diegelman, P., Kramer, D. L., & Porter, C. W. (2003). Genomic identification and biochemical characterization of the mammalian polyamine oxidase involved in polyamine back-conversion. *The Biochemical Journal*, *370*(Pt. 1), 19–28.

Walport, L. J., Hopkinson, R. J., & Schofield, C. J. (2012). Mechanisms of human histone and nucleic acid demethylases. *Current Opinion in Chemical Biology*, *16*(5–6), 525–534.

Wang, L., Amoozgar, Z., Huang, J., Saleh, M. H., Xing, D., Orsulic, S., et al. (2015). Decitabine enhances lymphocyte migration and function and synergizes with CTLA-4 blockade in a murine ovarian cancer model. *Cancer Immunology Research*, *3*(9), 1030–1041.

Wang, Y., Devereux, W., Woster, P. M., Stewart, T. M., Hacker, A., & Casero, R. A., Jr. (2001). Cloning and characterization of a human polyamine oxidase that is inducible by polyamine analogue exposure. *Cancer Research*, *61*(14), 5370–5373.

Wang, Y., Hacker, A., Murray-Stewart, T., Frydman, B., Valasinas, A., Fraser, A. V., et al. (2005). Properties of recombinant human N1-acetylpolyamine oxidase (hPAO): Potential role in determining drug sensitivity. *Cancer Chemotherapy and Pharmacology*, *56*(1), 83–90.

Wang, J., Hevi, S., Kurash, J. K., Lei, H., Gay, F., Bajko, J., et al. (2009). The lysine demethylase LSD1 (KDM1) is required for maintenance of global DNA methylation. *Nature Genetics*, *41*(1), 125–129.

Wang, J., Scully, K., Zhu, X., Cai, L., Zhang, J., Prefontaine, G. G., et al. (2007). Opposing LSD1 complexes function in developmental gene activation and repression programmes. *Nature, 446*(7138), 882–887.

Weiss, J. W., & Pitot, H. C. (1975). Effects of 5-azacytidine on nucleolar RNA and the pre-ribosomal particles in Novikoff hepatoma cells. *Biochemistry, 14*(2), 316–326.

Wilson, B. G., Wang, X., Shen, X., McKenna, E. S., Lemieux, M. E., Cho, Y. J., et al. (2010). Epigenetic antagonism between polycomb and SWI/SNF complexes during oncogenic transformation. *Cancer Cell, 18*(4), 316–328.

Witt, O., Deubzer, H. E., Milde, T., & Oehme, I. (2009). HDAC family: What are the cancer relevant targets? *Cancer Letters, 277*(1), 8–21.

Witt, O., & Lindemann, R. (2009). HDAC inhibitors: Magic bullets, dirty drugs or just another targeted therapy. *Cancer Letters, 280*(2), 123–124.

Wong, M. M., Guo, C., & Zhang, J. (2014). Nuclear receptor corepressor complexes in cancer: Mechanism, function and regulation. *American Journal of Clinical and Experimental Urology, 2*(3), 169–187.

Wrangle, J., Wang, W., Koch, A., Easwaran, H., Mohammad, H. P., Vendetti, F., et al. (2013). Alterations of immune response of non-small cell lung cancer with azacytidine. *Oncotarget, 4*(11), 2067–2079.

Xia, C., Leon-Ferre, R., Laux, D., Deutsch, J., Smith, B. J., Frees, M., et al. (2014). Treatment of resistant metastatic melanoma using sequential epigenetic therapy (decitabine and panobinostat) combined with chemotherapy (temozolomide). *Cancer Chemotherapy and Pharmacology, 74*(4), 691–697.

Yang, M., Culhane, J. C., Szewczuk, L. M., Gocke, C. B., Brautigam, C. A., Tomchick, D. R., et al. (2007). Structural basis of histone demethylation by LSD1 revealed by suicide inactivation. *Nature Structural & Molecular Biology, 14*(6), 535–539.

Yang, M., Culhane, J. C., Szewczuk, L. M., Jalili, P., Ball, H. L., Machius, M., et al. (2007). Structural basis for the inhibition of the LSD1 histone demethylase by the antidepressant trans-2-phenylcyclopropylamine. *Biochemistry, 46*(27), 8058–8065.

Yang, M., Gocke, C. B., Luo, X., Borek, D., Tomchick, D. R., Machius, M., et al. (2006). Structural basis for CoREST-dependent demethylation of nucleosomes by the human LSD1 histone demethylase. *Molecular Cell, 23*(3), 377–387.

Yang, D., Torres, C. M., Bardhan, K., Zimmerman, M., McGaha, T. L., & Liu, K. (2012). Decitabine and vorinostat cooperate to sensitize colon carcinoma cells to Fas ligand-induced apoptosis in vitro and tumor suppression in vivo. *Journal of Immunology, 188*(9), 4441–4449.

Yang, W. M., Tsai, S. C., Wen, Y. D., Fejer, G., & Seto, E. (2002). Functional domains of histone deacetylase-3. *The Journal of Biological Chemistry, 277*(11), 9447–9454.

Yao, Y., Chen, P., Diao, J., Cheng, G., Deng, L., Anglin, J. L., et al. (2011). Selective inhibitors of histone methyltransferase DOT1L: Design, synthesis, and crystallographic studies. *Journal of the American Chemical Society, 133*(42), 16746–16749.

Yardley, D. A., Ismail-Khan, R. R., Melichar, B., Lichinitser, M., Munster, P. N., Klein, P. M., et al. (2013). Randomized phase II, double-blind, placebo-controlled study of exemestane with or without entinostat in postmenopausal women with locally recurrent or metastatic estrogen receptor-positive breast cancer progressing on treatment with a nonsteroidal aromatase inhibitor. *Journal of Clinical Oncology, 31*(17), 2128–2135.

Yoo, C. B., Chuang, J. C., Byun, H. M., Egger, G., Yang, A. S., Dubeau, L., et al. (2008). Long-term epigenetic therapy with oral zebularine has minimal side effects and prevents intestinal tumors in mice. *Cancer Prevention Research (Philadelphia), 1*(4), 233–240.

You, A., Tong, J. K., Grozinger, C. M., & Schreiber, S. L. (2001). CoREST is an integral component of the CoREST-human histone deacetylase complex. *Proceedings of the National Academy of Sciences of the United States of America, 98*(4), 1454–1458.

Zhang, J., Kalkum, M., Chait, B. T., & Roeder, R. G. (2002). The N-CoR-HDAC3 nuclear receptor corepressor complex inhibits the JNK pathway through the integral subunit GPS2. *Molecular Cell, 9*(3), 611–623.

Zhang, Y., Ng, H. H., Erdjument-Bromage, H., Tempst, P., Bird, A., & Reinberg, D. (1999). Analysis of the NuRD subunits reveals a histone deacetylase core complex and a connection with DNA methylation. *Genes & Development, 13*(15), 1924–1935.

Zhou, L., Cheng, X., Connolly, B. A., Dickman, M. J., Hurd, P. J., & Hornby, D. P. (2002). Zebularine: A novel DNA methylation inhibitor that forms a covalent complex with DNA methyltransferases. *Journal of Molecular Biology, 321*(4), 591–599.

Zhu, Q., Huang, Y., Marton, L. J., Woster, P. M., Davidson, N. E., & Casero, R. A., Jr. (2012). Polyamine analogs modulate gene expression by inhibiting lysine-specific demethylase 1 (LSD1) and altering chromatin structure in human breast cancer cells. *Amino Acids, 42*(2–3), 887–898.

Zhu, W. G., Lakshmanan, R. R., Beal, M. D., & Otterson, G. A. (2001). DNA methyltransferase inhibition enhances apoptosis induced by histone deacetylase inhibitors. *Cancer Research, 61*(4), 1327–1333.

CHAPTER THREE

Emerging Roles of Epigenetic Regulator Sin3 in Cancer

N. Bansal*, G. David[†], E. Farias*, S. Waxman*[,1]

*The Tisch Cancer Institute, Icahn School of Medicine at Mount Sinai, New York, NY, United States
[†]New York University School of Medicine, New York, NY, United States
[1]Corresponding author: e-mail address: samuel.waxman@mssm.edu

Contents

Abstract

Revolutionizing treatment strategies is an urgent clinical need in the fight against cancer. Recently the scientific community has recognized chromatin-associated proteins as promising therapeutic candidates. However, there is a need to develop more targeted epigenetic inhibitors with less toxicity. Sin3 family is one such target which consists of evolutionary conserved proteins with two paralogues Sin3A and Sin3B. Sin3A/B are global transcription regulators that provide a versatile platform for diverse chromatin-modifying activities. Sin3 proteins regulate key cellular functions that include cell cycle, proliferation, and differentiation, and have recently been implicated in cancer pathogenesis. In this chapter, we summarize the key concepts of Sin3 biology and elaborate the recent advancements in the role of Sin3 proteins in cancer with specific examples in multiple endocrine neoplasia type 2, pancreatic ductal adenocarcinoma, and triple negative breast cancer. Finally, a program to create an integrative approach for screening antitumor agents that target chromatin-associated factors like Sin3 is presented.

Advances in Cancer Research, Volume 130
ISSN 0065-230X
http://dx.doi.org/10.1016/bs.acr.2016.01.006

1. INTRODUCTION

Cancer is second to cardiac diseases as the most common cause of death in the United States and is expected to become the front-runner by 2030 (American Society of Clinical Oncology, 2014). With both genetic and epigenetic origins contributing to its complex and heterogeneous landscape, cancer is a multifaceted disease with numerous yet not absolute treatment options. For this reason there is a constant need to evolve and develop new treatment modalities. Intensive work and advances in cancer research are very promising with the recent report of American Cancer Society showing an increase in the rate of survival and disease prognosis (American Cancer Society, 2015). This is attributed to improved diagnostic measures that enable early detection and introduction of novel drug targets and therapeutic strategies.

Over the last two decades, concept of reprogramming cancer cells by targeting the cancer epigenome and reorganization of chromatin architecture to regulate gene expression has emerged as a promising strategy against cancer (Sharma, Kelly, & Jones, 2010; You & Jones, 2012). Epigenome, in broader terms, refers to reversible and dynamic regulation of gene expression by chromatin-associated factors, independent of primary DNA sequence. These epigenetic factors include proteins that are members of large multiprotein complexes and act as readers or modifiers of numerous epigenetic regulations including DNA methylation, histone modifications, chromatin remodeling, and RNA interference (RNAi) (Ning, Li, Zhao, & Wang, 2015). Recently, intriguing evidence implicate genetic mutations and/or aberrant recruitment of epigenetic regulators in tumorigenesis (reviewed in You & Jones, 2012). More importantly, the reversibility of the chromatin modifications presents targeting the altered epigenetics, an attractive and promising therapeutic strategy in cancer. It is for this reason that intensive research efforts are being made to develop inhibitors that target specific chromatin-associated proteins with several like suberoylanilide hydroxamic acid (SAHA) and azacitidine already in clinical use or undergoing trials (Helin & Dhanak, 2013).

In this chapter, we will focus on a "new kid on the block"—the family of Sin3 proteins. We describe its structure, associated chromatin-remodeling functions, and the advances made in identifying the role of Sin3 in tumorigenesis. Potential of Sin3 as a drug target and development of therapeutic agents is also discussed. Finally, a brief overview on the utility and pitfalls of current methodologies used to study the functions of epigenetic factors and design of effective therapeutics is also presented.

2. STRUCTURE OF SIN3 PROTEIN AND CORE COMPLEX

Sin3 (SWI-independent-3) was identified in 1987 as a large acidic protein (~174.9 kDa), in a genetic screen to study mating-type switching in *Saccharomyces cerevisiae* (Nasmyth, Stillman, & Kipling, 1987; Sternberg, Stern, Clark, & Herskowitz, 1987). Over the next decade Sin3 was recognized as both a negative and positive regulator of gene expression with several aliases (SDI1, UME4, RPD1, CPE1, and SDS16) and homologues conserved from yeast to humans (Silverstein & Ekwall, 2005). Sequence analysis of Sin3 confirmed that it is suited for multiple protein–protein interactions. Sin3 lacks any known DNA-binding motifs or enzymatic activity. Instead it was characterized by the presence of six highly conserved regions (HCRs) (Fig. 1). Four of these include the paired amphipathic α-helices that share structural similarity with helix–loop–helix dimerization domain of Myc family of transcription factors. The other two regions are the histone deacetylase interaction domain and the highly conserved region (HCR). While the basic structure of Sin3 has been conserved in eukaryotes, there

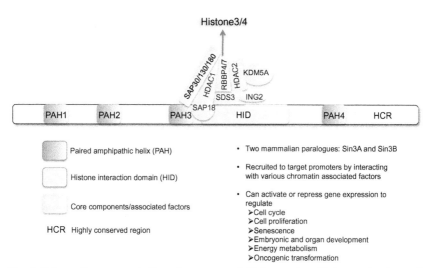

Fig. 1 Schematic representation of structure of Sin3 proteins. Sin3 proteins have six conserved domains from yeast to mammals. These include four PAH domains (1–4), one HID, and one HCR domain. A snapshot of cellular functions of Sin3 proteins is also provided. (See the color plate.)

is evidence of gene duplication giving rise to several homologues in many eukaryotes, an event thought to be essential to achieve functional flexibility (reviewed in detail in Grzenda, Lomberk, Zhang, & Urrutia, 2009; Kadamb, Mittal, Bansal, Batra, & Saluja, 2013). In mammals Sin3 family consists of two members, Sin3A and Sin3B, that have both overlapping and distinct functions (Kadamb et al., 2013). Both Sin3A and Sin3B have all the six conserved domains described earlier and are therefore thought to possess similar scaffolding capabilities. Consistent with this both Sin3A and Sin3B interact with common transcription factors like p53, Mad1, KLF, REST, and ESET (reviewed in Kadamb et al., 2013). In contrast, transcription factor like CIITA has been shown to interact only with Sin3B (Xu, Harton, & Smith, 2008). In another detailed study, investigating functions of Sin3 proteins in muscle development, decreased levels of Sin3A but not Sin3B were associated with defects in the sarcomere structure in the myotubes. In the same study it was also shown that while loss of Sin3B led to compensatory increase in recruitment of Sin3A at target loci, vice versa was not true (van Oevelen et al., 2010). Such studies prompt identification of functionally distinct Sin3A and Sin3B complexes.

The initial genetic screens identified Sin3 in complex with other proteins like Sds3 and Rpd3 (yeast homologue of histone deacetylase) (Silverstein & Ekwall, 2005). Following its structural analysis, it became apparent that the mainstay of Sin3's function as a global transcription regulator was via its multiple protein–protein interactions. Indeed, Sin3 acts as a molecular scaffold for the recruitment of what is called as the Sin3/HDAC (histone deacetylase activity) complex to target loci with or without sequence-specific transcription factors (Grzenda et al., 2009; Kadamb et al., 2013). The Sin3/HDAC complex is a class I HDAC-containing complex consisting of several chromatin-associated factors that include HDAC1/2, RBBP4/7, SDS3, SAP30/130/180, RBP1, BRMS1, FAM60A, ING1/2, PHF12 (Pf1), MRG15, and KDM5A/B (Bansal et al., 2015; Kadamb et al., 2013; Smith et al., 2012). Other than HDAC1/2 activity, the Sin3 complex also interacts with MeCP2 (methylated DNA-binding protein) and HDAC3-associated SMRT and N-CoR corepressor complexes (Silverstein & Ekwall, 2005). Since the aim of this chapter is to illustrate the role of Sin3 in cancer, we direct the readers to other published reviews for a more comprehensive overview of Sin3/HDAC complex (Grzenda et al., 2009; Kadamb et al., 2013; Silverstein & Ekwall, 2005). However, it is important to mention that despite the initial discoveries of Sin3 as positive regulator of transcription in yeast, the mammalian Sin3/HDAC complex is commonly referred to as "corepressor" complex. This is primarily due to recruitment of HDAC activity that is linked to promoter hypoacetylation, chromatin condensation, and gene repression (Baymaz, Karemaker, & Vermeulen, 2015; Laugesen & Helin, 2014). However, in recent times (supporting its initial discovery in yeast), there have been several reports that show recruitment of Sin3/HDAC complex at actively transcribed genes. This in fact is true for several other "corepressor complexes" like N-CoR/SMRT and NuRD complexes (Baymaz et al., 2015).

3. EXPRESSION AND REGULATION

Sin3 proteins are ubiquitously expressed in normal cells. The numbers of studies that investigate per se the regulation of Sin3 proteins are limited; nonetheless they require due attention. At the transcription level, a recent report has shown that Sin3B is repressed by polycomb group protein Bmi-1. In this study the authors show that Bmi-1-driven repression of Sin3B is relieved by oncogenic stress that results in onset of senescence (DiMauro, Cantor, Bainor, & David, 2015). Sin3B also interacts with an E3 ubiquitin ligase, RNF220 that targets Sin3B for ubiquitination and promotes its proteasomal degradation (Kong et al., 2010). Recently microRNA-mediated regulation of Sin3A has also been reported. These include two miRNAs, miR-210 and miR-138 (Ramachandran et al., 2012; Shang, Hong, Guo, Liu, & Xue, 2014). In relation to cancer biology miR-138 is identified as tumor-suppressive microRNA that inhibits cancer stem cell (CSC) phenotype, epithelial-to-mesenchymal transition (EMT), and metastasis in many cancer including lung, colorectal, and pancreas (Cristobal et al., 2015; Gao, Wang, Xie, Zhang, & Dong, 2015; Li et al., 2015; Xu et al., 2015).

4. FUNCTIONS OF SIN3 PROTEIN

In both yeast and mammals, Sin3 proteins have been shown to both activate and repress transcription of target genes to regulate diverse cellular and biological functions in embryonic development, cell cycle, proliferation, senescence, stem cell differentiation, and energy metabolism (Fig. 1; Kadamb et al., 2013). While the mechanism of repression mostly involves deacetylation of histone and nonhistone proteins, the mechanism for gene activation is less clear and may be HDAC independent (Baymaz et al., 2015; Kadamb et al., 2013). The dual regulation of transcription by Sin3 depends on the molecular and cellular conditions. This is best demonstrated by the recruitment of Sin3 at Nanog promoter; wherein recruitment of Sin3A/HDAC complex by p53 in differentiated cells downregulates Nanog, while Sox-2-mediated recruitment in proliferating embryonic stem cells activates Nanog (Baltus, Kowalski, Tutter, & Kadam, 2009; Lin et al., 2005).

The mainstay of Sin3 functions is protein–protein interactions with chromatin-associated factors. These interactions can be direct or indirect mediated by other members of the Sin3 complex. For example, the role of Sin3 in cell cycle progression, differentiation, and senescence is reliant on protein interactions with regulators like E2Fs, retinoblastoma-related proteins (Rb, p107, p130, also known as pocket proteins), ING protein family, MRG15, H3K4 demethylase RBP2 (KDM5A), and deposition of heterochromatin marks like HP1γ and H3K9me3 (David et al., 2008; Grandinetti & David, 2008; Grandinetti et al., 2009; Kadamb et al., 2013; Rayman et al., 2002). Another example of protein interactions as the basis for Sin3 functions is from recent report on the role of Sin3A–Pf1 interaction in EMT and maintenance of CSC-like traits in triple negative breast cancer (TNBC) that has been discussed at length in Section 8 (Bansal et al., 2015).

5. ROLE OF SIN3 IN CANCER-TUMOR SUPPRESSOR OR ONCOGENE

As described, Sin3 is involved in the regulation of critical cellular functions and therefore contribution of aberrant regulation by Sin3 in malignant transformations is obvious. One of the first and pioneering studies by groups of Eisenman (Ayer, Laherty, Lawrence, Armstrong, & Eisenman, 1996; Hurlin, Queva, & Eisenman, 1997; Laherty et al., 1997), DePinho (Rao et al., 1996; Schreiber-Agus et al., 1997), and others (Kasten, Ayer, & Stillman, 1996) found that recruitment of Sin3A/B by the Mad–Max heterodimer was necessary to antagonize the transcriptional activation driven by the proto-oncogene Myc in differentiating cells. Subsequently, further studies established the important role of Sin3A/Sin3B in mediating in gene repression by Myc antagonists (Mad1 and Mnt), inhibition of cell proliferation and transformation (Cultraro, Bino, & Segal, 1997; Hurlin et al., 1997). These studies identified that a specific peptide sequence within the N-terminus of Mad1 (Sin3 interaction domain or SID) interacts with two alpha helices of the PAH2 domain of Sin3 and is sufficient to repress the transcriptional activity of linked VP16 and c-Myc transactivation domains via recruitment of Sin3 complex and associated HDAC1/2

(Ayer et al., 1996; Hurlin et al., 1997; Laherty et al., 1997). Other than Mad–Max-dependent negative regulation of c-Myc, more recently Sin3A/B were also shown to limit c-Myc activity by directly interacting with Myc. Interaction with Sin3/HDAC complex results in deacetylation and degradation of Myc protein (Garcia-Sanz et al., 2014).

Under conditions of cellular stress, an increase in the levels of Sin3 proteins is observed. Overexpression of Ras induces oncogenic stress that leads to an increase in the levels of Sin3B sufficient for onset of oncogene-induced senescence (Grandinetti et al., 2009). The impact of this biological response on tumorigenesis has been studied in detail (Rielland et al., 2014) and elaborated in Section 7. Similarly, levels of both Sin3A and Sin3B increase under conditions of genotoxic stress and have been shown to be important for increasing stability and trans-repressive functions of tumor suppressor TP53 (Bansal et al., 2011; Kadamb, Mittal, Bansal, & Saluja, 2015; Murphy et al., 1999; Zilfou, Hoffman, Sank, George, & Murphy, 2001). Sin3 proteins also interact with retinoblastoma family of tumor suppressors via RBP1 member of the Sin3 complex for repressing transcription of E2F-responsive pro-proliferative genes (Lai et al., 2001). RBP1 directly interacts with another protein called BRMS1 that has been identified in purified Sin3 complexes by several groups and is known to inhibit metastasis in several types of cancer (Hurst, 2012; Meehan et al., 2004; Meehan & Welch, 2003).

Contrary to the apparent tumor suppressor functions of Sin3 described earlier, aberrant regulation of and by Sin3 has also been documented in several types of cancer. For instance in acute promyelocytic leukemia, Sin3A interacts with PLZF–RARα fusion protein that is created by chromosomal translocation (Chen et al., 1993; Lin et al., 1998). In the study by Lin et al. (1998), a complex containing Sin3A, HDAC1, and SMRT was shown to be recruited by PLZF–RARa oncoprotein to repress retinoid-responsive genes, inhibit differentiation, and induce cell transformation. Further, treatment with HDAC inhibitor, trichostatin A, restored sensitivity of leukemic cell lines to all-*trans* retinoic acid (atRA). This study was further substantiated by two independent reports on interaction between Sin3A and a chimeric protein AML–ETO and gene repression in acute myeloid leukemia (Lutterbach et al., 1998; Wang, Hoshino, Redner, Kajigaya, & Liu, 1998). It is of note that although these studies implicated Sin3 as a therapeutic target in leukemia, the use of anticancer agents was limited to the use of HDAC inhibitors and till date Sin3 has not been a direct drug target. Oncogenic role of Sin3 in pancreatic and breast cancer has also been reported and is described in greater details in Sections 7 and 8.

Function of Sin3 as tumor suppressor or oncogene is open for debate. It appears to be context dependent and is subject to the dynamics of its spatio-temporal protein interactome. To this end, studies that specifically focus on Sin3 in development and progression of cancer in specific cancer models will be relevant. To the best of our knowledge, three research groups have addressed this, two in which Sin3 promotes cancer and one that supports tumor suppressor functions of Sin3. These studies are elaborated in Sections 6–9.

6. SIN3 INHIBITS INVASION IN *DROSOPHILA* MEN2 MODEL

Fruitfly or *Drosophila* models have been instrumental in understanding several developmental processes. In recent times, *Drosophila* is recognized as powerful multicellular genetic tool to understand fundamental mechanisms of multiple gene interactions in cancer development and progression. Using one such model system, *Drosophila* homolog of mammalian Sin3A (dSin3) was identified to be an important regulator of EMT in multiple endocrine neoplasia type 2B (MEN2B) (Das, Sangodkar, Negre, Narla, & Cagan, 2013). Gain-of-function, dominant mutations in the receptor tyrosine kinase Ret lead to familial cancer syndromes MEN2A, MEN2B, or familial medullary thyroid carcinoma (MTC). Each of these syndromes is defined by tumors of the endocrine glands arising from neural crest derivatives like MTC, pheochromocytoma, and parathyroid adenomas (Leboulleux, Baudin, Travagli, & Schlumberger, 2004). The authors first established *Drosophila* MEN2 models by introducing mutations analogous to MEN2A or MEN2B in *Drosophila* Ret (dRet) and targeting them to developing eye epithelium in *Drosophila* (Read et al., 2005). The system was validated by measuring multiple signaling pathways like Ras, Src, and JNK that are known to get activated in the presence of mammalian oncogenic Ret isoforms (Read et al., 2005). Next, the authors addressed in detail the role of Sin3A in this model of tumorigenesis by genetically manipulating the *Drosophila* homolog dSin3, in the background of dRet mutations (dRet^{MEN2B}) (Das et al., 2013). Knocking down expression of dSin3 by either deleting single copy of dSin3 (sin3a$^{+/-}$) or RNAi (sin3a^{RNAi}) enhanced the "rough eye phenotype" of targeted dRet^{MEN2B}. In *Drosophila*, "rough eye" is characterized by excess proliferation, cell death, and developmental abnormalities in the eye. Development or enhancement of a "rough eye" is a readout for an oncogenic function, while its suppression is correlated to tumor-suppressive activity. Therefore, enhancement of "rough eye phenotype" in the absence of dSin3 is associated with the role of Sin3 as a tumor suppressor (Das et al., 2013). Further experiments demonstrated that RNAi-mediated depletion of dSin3 led to strong enhancement of cell migration. Interestingly, increased cell migration was observed even by reducing dSin3 alone and was augmented in the presence of caspase inhibitor. EMT and invasive phenotype of these cells were also evaluated in this study (Das et al., 2013). For this, expression of N-cadherin (marker for EMT), cell polarity, and morphology were examined. Increased N-cadherin was observed in dSin3^{RNAi} cells treated with caspase inhibitor p35 in wing pouch region of the fly. dSin3^{RNAi} cells gained more mesenchymal appearance and lost adherens junctions. This was paralleled by an increase in expression of enzymes like MMP1 and MMP2 required by invading cells to degrade the extracellular matrix. At the molecular level, dSin3 was recruited to promoters of genes that counter the "oncogenic module" consisting of multiple signaling pathways (src, jnk, rho, and wnt/B catenin) and cellular functions (cell migration and cytoskeleton remodeling) (Das et al., 2013). Interestingly, at the level of transcription, like the study published by Dynlacht group (van Oevelen et al., 2010), most of these target genes (73%) were activated by dSin3. For example, *Drosophila* C-terminal Scr-kinase (dCsk) inhibits src kinase by phosphorylating it at the C-terminus. In this study (Das et al., 2013), dCsk was among the dSin3-activated loci. The results of this study were validated in patient samples from lung cancer (Das et al., 2013). This also correlated with data extracted from ONCOMINE from specific tumor cohorts (lung, renal, liver, gastric, lymphoma, and breast) (Das et al., 2013). However, it is important to note that there is a great deal of variability in expression of Sin3 proteins in cancer. For instance, extensive data mining in ONCOMINE will reveal that in comparison to normal tissue, expression of Sin3A can be either upregulated or downregulated by severalfolds in different tumor cohorts; this also reflects the open debate of tumor suppressor vs oncogenic role of Sin3A and implicates that complex and often aberrant gene interactions within a heterogeneous landscape of cancer could be important determinants of gene function.

7. Sin3B PROMOTES SENESCENCE-ASSOCIATED INFLAMMATION AND PANCREATIC CANCER PROGRESSION

As mentioned earlier, the contribution of Sin3 proteins in cancer progression has been largely based on correlative studies. The recent development of elegant mouse models that faithfully recapitulate the progression of specific cancers has allowed a direct delineation of the role of specific proteins in these processes (Sharpless & Depinho, 2006). In this regard, the generation of loss-of-function mutations in the mouse for Sin3 proteins has been crucial. Such studies have revealed nonredundant functions for Sin3A and the closely related Sin3B protein (Cowley et al., 2005; Dannenberg et al., 2005; David et al., 2008). Importantly, genetic deletion of either Sin3A or Sin3B is embryonically lethal at different stages of development. Indeed, while Sin3B-null embryos die at late gestation, Sin3A-deleted embryos die as early at 3.5 dpc, at the blastocyst stage (Cowley et al., 2005; Dannenberg et al., 2005; David et al., 2008). This is consistent with the observation that Sin3A inactivation is incompatible with cell survival (Cowley et al., 2005; Dannenberg et al., 2005). The generation of a conditional allele for Sin3B allowed however to test its contribution to cancer progression (David et al., 2008; Grandinetti & David, 2008). Specifically, a previous study has demonstrated that Sin3B levels are upregulated in preneoplastic lesions in both human and mouse pancreata (Grandinetti et al., 2009). When combined with pancreatic-specific expression of oncogenic KRas, genetic inactivation of Sin3B in the pancreas led to a significant decrease of pancreatic cancer progression (Fig. 2) (Rielland et al., 2014). Genetic inactivation of Sin3B did not influence the levels of Sin3A that is expressed at low levels in normal pancreas, Pancreatic intraepithelial neoplasia (PanINs) and pancreatic ductal adenocarcinoma (PDAC) (Rielland et al., 2014, unpublished data). Specifically, Sin3B-deleted pancreata developed KRas-driven early pancreatic lesions with an increased latency compared to their Sin3B-expresing counterparts, and these lesions progressed much more slowly to adenocarcinoma. Importantly, Sin3B inactivation appeared to prevent the occurrence of cellular senescence in early pancreatic preneoplastic lesions, consistent with previous studies demonstrating its central role in oncogene-induced senescence (DiMauro et al., 2015; Grandinetti et al., 2009). Senescent cells are known to secrete a set of inflammatory cytokines collectively referred to as the SASP (or senescence-associated secretory phenotype) (for a review, see Rodier & Campisi, 2011). Consistent with the absence of senescence in Sin3B-deleted pancreas, expression levels of inflammatory cytokines (including IL-1 α and IL-6) were dramatically reduced in Kras-expressing pancreata upon genetic inactivation of Sin3B. Given the well-established contribution of inflammation in pancreatic cancer progression (Ling et al., 2012), it is tempting to speculate that Sin3B promotes PDAC progression by triggering senescence-associated inflammation in KRas-expressing pancreatic lesions. These observations have important implications regarding

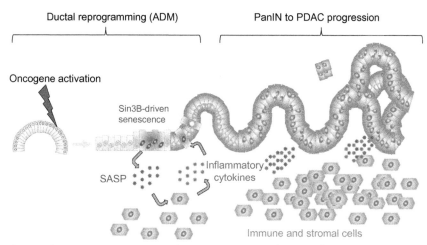

Fig. 2 Schematic representation of the potential contribution of Sin3B in KRas-driven pancreatic cancer progression. Upon oncogene activation, pancreatic acini undergo acinar-to-ductal-metaplasia (ADM) and acquire ductal phenotypes. These cells then enter cellular senescence, in a Sin3B-dependent manner. Senescent preneoplastic lesions, including metaplasia and early Pancreatic intraepithelial neoplasia (PanIN), secrete a set of cytokines collectively referred to as senescence-associated secretory phenotype (SASP), which in turn promotes immune cells' recruitment and activation. These immune cells further promote the generation of a pro-inflammatory environment, which is believed to be detrimental, and favor pancreatic cancer progression. In the absence of Sin3B, no senescence is observed, thus correlating with a reduced inflammation and delayed pancreatic cancer progression. (See the color plate.)

the contribution of Sin3 proteins to cancer progression. First, they establish unequivocally the essential role of Sin3B in oncogene-induced senescence in vivo. Second, they indicate that surprisingly, Sin3B-driven senescence could serve as a tumor-promoting factor in specific contexts, such as inflammation–driven cancers. In this regard, it would be interesting to test whether Sin3B could serve as a therapeutic target to prevent detrimental inflammation in other pathological contexts. Alternatively, it will be important to test whether Sin3B inactivation may promote cancer progression in tumors where senescence is known to serve as a barrier against cancer progression, such as prostate cancer (Perez–Mancera, Young, & Narita, 2014).

8. Sin3A PROMOTES EMT AND CSC-LIKE PHENOTYPE IN TNBC

In recent times, epigenetic deregulation has been associated with aberrant gene expression and tumorigenesis. Fortunately, these changes are reversible that opens a therapeutic window. Exploiting this concept, several drugs called as "epidrugs" are in clinical trials; these include inhibitors of HDACs (HDACi) and DNA methyltransferases (DNMTi). However, such generic inhibitors lack specificity and have several off-target effects. To counter this problem, Farias et al. published the concept of targeting specific protein–protein interactions between the epigenetic regulators (Farias et al., 2010). That this approach can be successful in epigenetic reprogramming of cancer cells was exemplified by disrupting protein interactions mediated by the PAH2 domain of Sin3A in TNBC (Farias et al., 2010). The PAH2 domain of Sin3A is structurally well characterized and known to interact with a small set of transcription and epigenetic factors that contain a conserved sequence called the Sin3 interaction domain or SID (Fig. 3). The prototype SID sequence corresponds to amino acids 5–24 of MAD protein (VRMNIQMLLEAADYLERRER) and was previously used to study

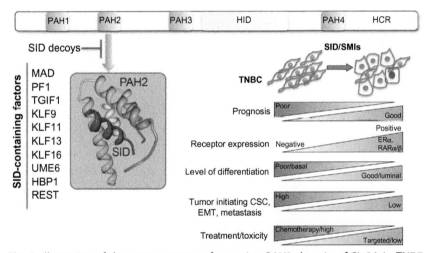

Fig. 3 Illustration of the consequences of targeting PAH2 domain of Sin3A in TNBC. Targeted disruption of protein–protein interactions by using Sin3 interaction domain (SID) decoys that disrupt PAH2 domain-mediated interaction of Sin3A with SID-containing factors leads to epigenetic reprogramming of TNBC cells. The key effects observed include reexpression of clinically relevant genes (ERα and RARα/β), decrease in cancer stem cells (CSCs), reversal of epithelial-to-mesenchymal transition (EMT), and inhibition of metastatic dissemination to distant organ sites. *SMI*, small molecule inhibitor designed to inhibit protein interaction between PAH2 domain of Sin3A and SID-containing factors. *Part of the figure adapted from Kwon, Y. J., Petrie, K., Leibovitch, B. A., Zeng, L., Mezei, M., Howell, L., et al. (2015). Selective inhibition of SIN3 corepressor with avermectins as a novel therapeutic strategy in triple negative breast cancer. Molecular Cancer Therapeutics, 14, 1824–1836.* (See the color plate.)

SID–PAH2 interactions in vitro. In this study (Farias et al., 2010), the authors stably expressed SID as a decoy to interfere with interactions between PAH2 domain of Sin3A and its partner proteins. Their results clearly demonstrated that this strategy was effective in reexpression of several epigenetically silenced genes in TNBC like E-cadherin (CDH1), estrogen receptor alpha (ERα/ESR1), and retinoic acid receptor beta (RARβ). The reexpression was associated with epigenetic marks linked to gene activation like increased promoter H3K4me3 and DNA hypomethylation and decreased H3K27me3 at the *CDH1* and *ESR1* gene promoters. In TNBC cells, introduction of SID decoys induced changes in cells from a basal to a more luminal phenotype. This was associated with expression of markers for cell differentiation and EMT reversal like CDH1, membrane-associated β-catenin, and zona occludens-1. Clinically relevant results of this study included restored sensitivity of TNBC cells to tamoxifen and retinoids. These results were substantiated by a more recent publication from the same group (Bansal et al., 2015), in which instead of using a stably expressing SID decoy, cells were exogenously treated with a competitive SID peptide for 24–72 h periods. In this study the authors also identified that the SID-induced phenotypic changes (Fig. 3) were due to disruption of protein interaction between PAH2 domain of Sin3 and a chromatin-associated factor Pf1 (PHF12). Pf1 is expressed from a locus amplified from breast cancer and links Sin3 PAH2 to a chromatin-modifying protein complex containing MRG15, LID (*Drosophila* homologue of KDM5A and KDM5B), and EMSY (Malovannaya et al., 2011; Moshkin et al., 2009; Yochum & Ayer, 2001, 2002) that has been implicated in breast cancer. In fact, SID treatment not only dissociated Pf1 from Sin3A but also disrupted interactions of Sin3A complex with H3K4 demethylase KDM5B and MRG15 (Bansal et al., 2015). The highlight of this study was the discovery of the role of Sin3A–Pf1 interaction in regulating the EMT and CSC phenotype in TNBC. CSCs or tumor-initiating stem cells constitute a small percentage of the tumor bulk and have been implicated in tumor initiation, metastasis, and resistance to treatment (Pattabiraman & Weinberg, 2014). Identification and evaluation of novel targeted therapies against CSCs are an urgent clinical need. Sin3A–Pf1 complex upregulate activity or expression of several genes associated with EMT and CSC function like ALDH1, CD44, CD24, CD49f, SNAI2, Nanog, Sox2, and Oct4 (Bansal et al., 2015). The predicted decrease in CSC function by SID treatment was corroborated by decrease in tumorsphere formation and more importantly, a dramatic decrease in metastatic dissemination to distant organ sites like lungs and bone marrow

(Bansal et al., 2015). These findings were also in agreement with previous reports on the role of Sin3A complex in positive regulation of pluripotency (Baltus et al., 2009). Together these studies correlate with oncogenic role of Sin3A in epigenetic deregulation that can be corrected by use of SID decoys and provided a rationale for its therapeutic targeting at least in TNBC. Like Sin3, other chromatin repressive complexes like polycomb repressive complexes (PRC1 and PRC2), NuRD, and Co-REST are also known to regulate embryonic and cancer stem cells and their therapeutic targeting in cancer is also an active field of research (reviewed in Helin & Dhanak, 2013; Laugesen & Helin, 2014).

9. TARGETING Sin3A IN BREAST CANCER USING SMALL MOLECULE MIMETICS OF PAH2 DOMAIN-BINDING SID MOTIF

A daunting challenge in breast cancer treatment (and cancer in general) is to overcome dissemination of metastasis and resistance to treatment. Within breast cancer, an estimated 15–20% of total breast cancer cases are diagnosed as triple negative (TNBC), an aggressive poorly differentiated basal subtype of breast cancer for which no targeted therapies are currently available (Abramson & Mayer, 2014; Andre & Zielinski, 2012; Hudis & Gianni, 2011). In TNBC, the estrogen (ERα) and progesterone receptors are not expressed, making hormonal therapy ineffective. In these cancers, the HER2 oncogene is not overexpressed, making HER2-targeted therapies irrelevant, hence the term "triple negative" (Hudis & Gianni, 2011) The current standard of care in TNBC is limited to cytotoxic chemotherapeutic regimens and development of neoadjuvant/adjuvant targeted therapies is an urgent clinical need (Abramson & Mayer, 2014; Hudis & Gianni, 2011).

To address this, one of the most recent advancements is the prospect of targeting metastatic progression of TNBC in adjuvant settings by using small molecule inhibitors that block PAH2 domain-mediated protein interactions of Sin3A (Kwon et al., 2015). As discussed in Section 8, SID decoys were shown to be very effective in reprogramming TNBC cells toward a more differentiated phenotype with significantly decreased metastatic potential (Fig. 3) (Bansal et al., 2015; Farias et al., 2010). To evaluate the relevance of translating this strategy from bench to bedside, an in silico screen for PAH2 domain-binding compounds led to identification several candidate compounds, one of them being avermectin macrocyclic lactone derivatives selamectin and ivermectin (Mectizan, an FDA approved drug for the treatment of River Night Blindness) (Kwon et al., 2015). Both selamectin and ivermectin phenocopied SID decoys and modulated the expression of therapeutically targetable genes. Selamectin also inhibited invasion and downregulated expression of genes like *MMP9* and *MT1-MMP/MMP14* that are associated with invasion and metastasis. Although avermectins had a very modest effect on primary tumor growth, in postsurgical adjuvant settings severalfold decrease in metastatic dissemination to the lungs was reported (Kwon et al., 2015). These are clinically significant results since 90% of morbidity and mortality in cancer patients is due to metastasis of the primary tumor cells (Mehlen & Puisieux, 2006; Nguyen, Bos, & Massague, 2009). Therefore, strategies to counteract metastatic spread of breast cancer are absolutely required to make significant progress in the strategy to cure breast cancer. The translational relevance of SID small molecule mimetics is further underlined by the results of a drug screen in which selamectin sensitized TNBC cells to a number of drugs that are clinically being used to treat metastatic breast cancer (Kwon et al., 2015). These results strongly encourage repurposing avermectins as anticancer drugs and also evaluate additional small molecule mimetics of SID for improved efficacy and specificity.

10. CONCLUDING REMARKS: CHALLENGES AND ROADBLOCKS IN DEVELOPING CHROMATIN MODIFIERS AS DRUG TARGETS

With plethora of groundbreaking studies to back them up, epigenetic regulators have emerged as front-runners in cancer therapeutic discovery and development. DNMTi like azacitidine and decitabine are already used in clinic as first-line treatment for myelodysplastic syndrome. Similarly, HDACi like SAHA is an approved treatment for cutaneous T-cell lymphoma. However, despite their promise of a targeted, minimally toxic therapy, the field of epigenetic drug development faces numerous scientific challenges.

Central to the concept of targeting epigenetic regulators in cancer is that a given drug target (for instance Sin3A) is a subunit of one or more multiprotein transcription complexes that exert differential regulation in multiple molecularly and phenotypically heterogeneous populations within a given tumor. This combined with inherent differences between each cancer type and subtype makes data interpretation complex and requires implementation of innovative and integrative approaches to identify candidate drug targets, precise mechanisms of action, and reliable biomarkers.

The classical way of identifying a gene function in tumorigenesis is by genetic manipulations. While the use of robust techniques of gene deletion, overexpression, or RNAi has led to groundbreaking discoveries in the past, these may not be applicable to every gene. This is especially true for proteins like Sin3 that engage in multiple protein–protein interactions and have multiple paralogs with overlapping functions. Deleting Sin3 (or reducing its level by RNAi) can have a fundamentally different effect on the function of the residual complex in comparison to interfering with only specific protein interactions of Sin3 proteins. Currently, studies directly addressing this issue in the same model system are lacking but can be valuable in addressing the contrasting results and questionable status of Sin3A as tumor suppressor (in *Drosophila* MEN2 model; Das et al., 2013) or as oncogene (in human TNBC cell models; Bansal et al., 2015).

Another challenging aspect in cancer treatment is tumor heterogeneity (Marusyk & Polyak, 2010); this is especially relevant in studies investigating the mechanism of drug action, identifying the target cells and response to therapy. Within a given tumor there can be distinct populations of cells that are unique in their morphology, gene expression, and metabolome. Current methodologies and techniques that are being widely used, including genome-wide profiling like Chip-seq and RNA-seq, measure parameters of the bulk population in which signals from minority population (for example, the CSCs discussed earlier) may be obscured by stronger signals from the bulk population. The net result can compromise data interpretation and conclusions. Cancer treatment is not a number's game; the key is to hit the right cell not the maximum number of cells. Understanding the tumor heterogeneity, therefore, is the next big question in cancer and technologies to measure cellular variations at the single cell level (instead of mixed cell population) are gaining momentum (Bendall & Nolan, 2012; Saadatpour, Lai, Guo, & Yuan, 2015).

An additional point that needs to be emphasized is that tumor microenvironment and molecular changes within the cancer cells are important determinants of the overall outcome of a therapeutic agent (Stadler et al., 2015; Sun, 2015), and in contrast to cytotoxic agents, 2D cultures may not be the ideal yardsticks for evaluation of agents that target chromatin modifiers whose antitumor activity is based on gene reprogramming and phenotypic changes; instead studies on 3D Matrigel or in vivo may be better suited. In addition to classical MTT assay, screening for anticancer agents in

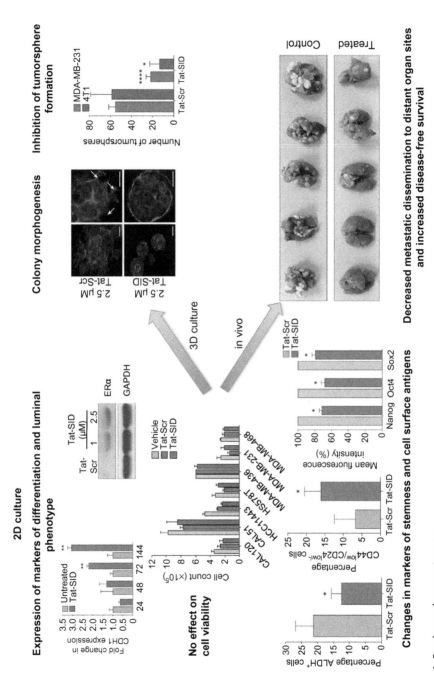

2D culture

Expression of markers of differentiation and luminal phenotype

No effect on cell viability

Colony morphogenesis

3D culture

in vivo

Inhibition of tumorsphere formation

Changes in markers of stemness and cell surface antigens

Decreased metastatic dissemination to distant organ sites and increased disease-free survival

Fig. 4 See legend on next page.

2D cultures should include additional profiling like markers for differentiation and stemness. This is best demonstrated in studies describing the use of SID decoys as potential therapy in TNBC (Bansal et al., 2015; Kwon et al., 2015). As illustrated in Fig. 4, SID decoys produce significant anticancer effects but without any evident cytotoxicity in 2D cultures. Instead in 2D cultures, changes in expression of several CSC and differentiation markers are observed. Importantly in 3D cultures dramatic effects on cell differentiation and morphogenesis are observed. Correlating with the effect of SID decoys on cell viability in 2D cultures, SID decoys are modest agents to treat the primary tumors. In contrast, treatments with SID decoys in postsurgical adjuvant settings show a remarkable decrease in lung metastasis and disseminated tumor cells in bone marrow (Bansal et al., 2015; Kwon et al., 2015); a clinical scenario related with cancer-associated morbidity and mortality (Gupta & Massague, 2006; Mehlen & Puisieux, 2006; Nguyen et al., 2009). Thus for screening antitumor agents there is an urgent need to employ techniques that measure cell status beyond cell viability either in vitro or in primary tumors in vivo.

ACKNOWLEDGMENTS

This study was supported by grants from the National Institute of Health-National Cancer Institute (R01CA158121), Samuel Waxman Cancer Research Foundation, Triple Negative Breast Cancer Foundation, and the Chemotherapy Foundation.

Conflict of Interest: None declared.

Fig. 4 Techniques to evaluate antitumor agents. Techniques to screen antitumor agents, especially drugs whose expected mode of action is cellular reprogramming, should include an integrative approach that combines 2D cultures with 3D cultures and in vivo evaluation. As an example, the scheme illustrates effects of SID decoys (Tat-SID in comparison to the scrambled control, Tat-Scr or untreated) in 2D and 3D cultures as well as in vivo experiments. In 2D cultures, SID decoys have no effect on cell viability (as assessed by MTT assays) in a range of TNBC lines tested; however, these cells show reexpression of markers of differentiation and luminal phenotype (CDH1 and ERα). Changes in expression of cell surface antigen and other cancer stem cell markers are also observed. In 3D Matrigel cultures, SID decoy treatment induces differentiation and colony morphogenesis. In suspension cultures antitumor potential of SID decoys is reflected by decrease in the formation of tumorspheres. The most promising and impressive results are obtained in in vivo models where significant decrease is observed in metastatic dissemination to distant organ sites like the lungs and bone marrow. $*p < 0.05$; $**p < 0.01$; $****p < 0.0001$. *Adapted from data published in Bansal, N., Petrie, K., Christova, R., Chung, C. Y., Leibovitch, B. A., Howell, L., et al. (2015). Targeting the SIN3A-PF1 interaction inhibits epithelial to mesenchymal transition and maintenance of a stem cell phenotype in triple negative breast cancer. Oncotarget, 6, 34087–34105. (See the color plate.)*

REFERENCES

Abramson, V. G., & Mayer, I. A. (2014). Molecular heterogeneity of triple negative breast cancer. *Current Breast Cancer Reports*, *6*, 154–158.

American Cancer Society. (2015). *Cancer facts & figures 2015*. Atlanta: American Cancer Society.

American Society of Clinical Oncology. (2014). The state of cancer care in America, 2014: A report by the American Society of Clinical Oncology. *Journal of Oncology Practice*, *10*, 119–142.

Andre, F., & Zielinski, C. C. (2012). Optimal strategies for the treatment of metastatic triple-negative breast cancer with currently approved agents. *Annals of Oncology*, *23*(Suppl. 6). vi46–51.

Ayer, D. E., Laherty, C. D., Lawrence, Q. A., Armstrong, A. P., & Eisenman, R. N. (1996). Mad proteins contain a dominant transcription repression domain. *Molecular and Cellular Biology*, *16*, 5772–5781.

Baltus, G. A., Kowalski, M. P., Tutter, A. V., & Kadam, S. (2009). A positive regulatory role for the mSin3A-HDAC complex in pluripotency through Nanog and Sox2. *Journal of Biological Chemistry*, *284*, 6998–7006.

Bansal, N., Kadamb, R., Mittal, S., Vig, L., Sharma, R., Dwarakanath, B. S., et al. (2011). Tumor suppressor protein p53 recruits human Sin3B/HDAC1 complex for down-regulation of its target promoters in response to genotoxic stress. *PLoS One*, *6*, e26156.

Bansal, N., Petrie, K., Christova, R., Chung, C. Y., Leibovitch, B. A., Howell, L., et al. (2015). Targeting the SIN3A-PF1 interaction inhibits epithelial to mesenchymal transition and maintenance of a stem cell phenotype in triple negative breast cancer. *Oncotarget*, *6*, 34087–34105.

Baymaz, H. I., Karemaker, I. D., & Vermeulen, M. (2015). Perspective on unraveling the versatility of 'co-repressor' complexes. *Biochimica et Biophysica Acta*, *1849*, 1051–1056.

Bendall, S. C., & Nolan, G. P. (2012). From single cells to deep phenotypes in cancer. *Nature Biotechnology*, *30*, 639–647.

Chen, S. J., Zelent, A., Tong, J. H., Yu, H. Q., Wang, Z. Y., Derre, J., et al. (1993). Rearrangements of the retinoic acid receptor alpha and promyelocytic leukemia zinc finger genes resulting from t(11;17)(q23;q21) in a patient with acute promyelocytic leukemia. *Journal of Clinical Investigation*, *91*, 2260–2267.

Cowley, S. M., Iritani, B. M., Mendrysa, S. M., Xu, T., Cheng, P. F., Yada, J., et al. (2005). The mSin3A chromatin-modifying complex is essential for embryogenesis and T-cell development. *Molecular and Cellular Biology*, *25*, 6990–7004.

Cristobal, I., Torrejon, B., Gonzalez-Alonso, P., Manso, R., Rojo, F., & Garcia-Foncillas, J. (2015). Downregulation of miR-138 as a contributing mechanism to Lcn-2 over-expression in colorectal cancer with liver metastasis. *World Journal of Surgery*. http://dx.doi.org/10.1007/s00268-015-3241-z. Epub ahead of print.

Cultraro, C. M., Bino, T., & Segal, S. (1997). Function of the c-Myc antagonist Mad1 during a molecular switch from proliferation to differentiation. *Molecular and Cellular Biology*, *17*, 2353–2359.

Dannenberg, J. H., David, G., Zhong, S., van der Torre, J., Wong, W. H., & Depinho, R. A. (2005). mSin3A corepressor regulates diverse transcriptional networks governing normal and neoplastic growth and survival. *Genes & Development*, *19*, 1581–1595.

Das, T. K., Sangodkar, J., Negre, N., Narla, G., & Cagan, R. L. (2013). Sin3a acts through a multi-gene module to regulate invasion in Drosophila and human tumors. *Oncogene*, *32*, 3184–3197.

David, G., Grandinetti, K. B., Finnerty, P. M., Simpson, N., Chu, G. C., & Depinho, R. A. (2008). Specific requirement of the chromatin modifier mSin3B in cell cycle exit and cellular differentiation. *Proceedings of the National Academy of Sciences of the United States of America*, *105*, 4168–4172.

DiMauro, T., Cantor, D. J., Bainor, A. J., & David, G. (2015). Transcriptional repression of Sin3B by Bmi-1 prevents cellular senescence and is relieved by oncogene activation. *Oncogene, 34*, 4011–4017.

Farias, E. F., Petrie, K., Leibovitch, B., Murtagh, J., Chornet, M. B., Schenk, T., et al. (2010). Interference with Sin3 function induces epigenetic reprogramming and differentiation in breast cancer cells. *Proceedings of the National Academy of Sciences of the United States of America, 107*, 11811–11816.

Gao, S., Wang, J., Xie, J., Zhang, T., & Dong, P. (2015). Role of miR-138 in the regulation of larynx carcinoma cell metastases. *Tumour Biology.* http://dx.doi.org/10.1007/s13277-015-4244-y. Epub ahead of print.

Garcia-Sanz, P., Quintanilla, A., Lafita, M. C., Moreno-Bueno, G., Garcia-Gutierrez, L., Tabor, V., et al. (2014). Sin3b interacts with Myc and decreases Myc levels. *Journal of Biological Chemistry, 289*, 22221–22236.

Grandinetti, K. B., & David, G. (2008). Sin3B: An essential regulator of chromatin modifications at E2F target promoters during cell cycle withdrawal. *Cell Cycle, 7*, 1550–1554.

Grandinetti, K. B., Jelinic, P., DiMauro, T., Pellegrino, J., Fernandez Rodriguez, R., Finnerty, P. M., et al. (2009). Sin3B expression is required for cellular senescence and is up-regulated upon oncogenic stress. *Cancer Research, 69*, 6430–6437.

Grzenda, A., Lomberk, G., Zhang, J. S., & Urrutia, R. (2009). Sin3: Master scaffold and transcriptional corepressor. *Biochimica et Biophysica Acta, 1789*, 443–450.

Gupta, G. P., & Massague, J. (2006). Cancer metastasis: Building a framework. *Cell, 127*, 679–695.

Helin, K., & Dhanak, D. (2013). Chromatin proteins and modifications as drug targets. *Nature, 502*, 480–488.

Hudis, C. A., & Gianni, L. (2011). Triple-negative breast cancer: An unmet medical need. *The Oncologist, 16*(Suppl. 1), 1–11.

Hurlin, P. J., Queva, C., & Eisenman, R. N. (1997). Mnt, a novel Max-interacting protein is coexpressed with Myc in proliferating cells and mediates repression at Myc binding sites. *Genes & Development, 11*, 44–58.

Hurst, D. R. (2012). Metastasis suppression by BRMS1 associated with SIN3 chromatin remodeling complexes. *Cancer Metastasis Reviews, 31*, 641–651.

Kadamb, R., Mittal, S., Bansal, N., Batra, H., & Saluja, D. (2013). Sin3: Insight into its transcription regulatory functions. *European Journal of Cell Biology, 92*, 237–246.

Kadamb, R., Mittal, S., Bansal, N., & Saluja, D. (2015). Stress-mediated Sin3B activation leads to negative regulation of subset of p53 target genes. *Bioscience Reports, 35*, e00234.

Kasten, M. M., Ayer, D. E., & Stillman, D. J. (1996). SIN3-dependent transcriptional repression by interaction with the Mad1 DNA-binding protein. *Molecular and Cellular Biology, 16*, 4215–4221.

Kong, Q., Zeng, W., Wu, J., Hu, W., Li, C., & Mao, B. (2010). RNF220, an E3 ubiquitin ligase that targets Sin3B for ubiquitination. *Biochemical and Biophysical Research Communications, 393*, 708–713.

Kwon, Y. J., Petrie, K., Leibovitch, B. A., Zeng, L., Mezei, M., Howell, L., et al. (2015). Selective inhibition of SIN3 corepressor with avermectins as a novel therapeutic strategy in triple negative breast cancer. *Molecular Cancer Therapeutics, 14*, 1824–1836.

Laherty, C. D., Yang, W. M., Sun, J. M., Davie, J. R., Seto, E., & Eisenman, R. N. (1997). Histone deacetylases associated with the mSin3 corepressor mediate mad transcriptional repression. *Cell, 89*, 349–356.

Lai, A., Kennedy, B. K., Barbie, D. A., Bertos, N. R., Yang, X. J., Theberge, M. C., et al. (2001). RBP1 recruits the mSIN3-histone deacetylase complex to the pocket of retinoblastoma tumor suppressor family proteins found in limited discrete regions of the nucleus at growth arrest. *Molecular and Cellular Biology, 21*, 2918–2932.

Laugesen, A., & Helin, K. (2014). Chromatin repressive complexes in stem cells, development, and cancer. *Cell Stem Cell*, *14*, 735–751.

Leboulleux, S., Baudin, E., Travagli, J. P., & Schlumberger, M. (2004). Medullary thyroid carcinoma. *Clinical Endocrinology*, *61*, 299–310.

Li, J., Wang, Q., Wen, R., Liang, J., Zhong, X., Yang, W., et al. (2015). MiR-138 inhibits cell proliferation and reverses epithelial-mesenchymal transition in non-small cell lung cancer cells by targeting GIT1 and SEMA4C. *Journal of Cellular and Molecular Medicine*, *19*(12), 2793–2805.

Lin, T., Chao, C., Saito, S., Mazur, S. J., Murphy, M. E., Appella, E., et al. (2005). p53 induces differentiation of mouse embryonic stem cells by suppressing Nanog expression. *Nature Cell Biology*, *7*, 165–171.

Lin, R. J., Nagy, L., Inoue, S., Shao, W., Miller, W. H., Jr., & Evans, R. M. (1998). Role of the histone deacetylase complex in acute promyelocytic leukaemia. *Nature*, *391*, 811–814.

Ling, J., Kang, Y., Zhao, R., Xia, Q., Lee, D. F., Chang, Z., et al. (2012). KrasG12D-induced IKK2/beta/NF-kappaB activation by IL-1alpha and p62 feedforward loops is required for development of pancreatic ductal adenocarcinoma. *Cancer Cell*, *21*, 105–120.

Lutterbach, B., Westendorf, J. J., Linggi, B., Patten, A., Moniwa, M., Davie, J. R., et al. (1998). ETO, a target of t(8;21) in acute leukemia, interacts with the N-CoR and mSin3 corepressors. *Molecular and Cellular Biology*, *18*, 7176–7184.

Malovannaya, A., Lanz, R. B., Jung, S. Y., Bulynko, Y., Le, N. T., Chan, D. W., et al. (2011). Analysis of the human endogenous coregulator complexome. *Cell*, *145*, 787–799.

Marusyk, A., & Polyak, K. (2010). Tumor heterogeneity: Causes and consequences. *Biochimica et Biophysica Acta*, *1805*, 105–117.

Meehan, W. J., Samant, R. S., Hopper, J. E., Carrozza, M. J., Shevde, L. A., Workman, J. L., et al. (2004). Breast cancer metastasis suppressor 1 (BRMS1) forms complexes with retinoblastoma-binding protein 1 (RBP1) and the mSin3 histone deacetylase complex and represses transcription. *Journal of Biological Chemistry*, *279*, 1562–1569.

Meehan, W. J., & Welch, D. R. (2003). Breast cancer metastasis suppressor 1: Update. *Clinical & Experimental Metastasis*, *20*, 45–50.

Mehlen, P., & Puisieux, A. (2006). Metastasis: A question of life or death. *Nature Reviews. Cancer*, *6*, 449–458.

Moshkin, Y. M., Kan, T. W., Goodfellow, H., Bezstarosti, K., Maeda, R. K., Pilyugin, M., et al. (2009). Histone chaperones ASF1 and NAP1 differentially modulate removal of active histone marks by LID-RPD3 complexes during NOTCH silencing. *Molecular Cell*, *35*, 782–793.

Murphy, M., Ahn, J., Walker, K. K., Hoffman, W. H., Evans, R. M., Levine, A. J., et al. (1999). Transcriptional repression by wild-type p53 utilizes histone deacetylases, mediated by interaction with mSin3a. *Genes & Development*, *13*, 2490–2501.

Nasmyth, K., Stillman, D., & Kipling, D. (1987). Both positive and negative regulators of HO transcription are required for mother-cell-specific mating-type switching in yeast. *Cell*, *48*, 579–587.

Nguyen, D. X., Bos, P. D., & Massague, J. (2009). Metastasis: From dissemination to organ-specific colonization. *Nature Reviews. Cancer*, *9*, 274–284.

Ning, B., Li, W., Zhao, W., & Wang, R. (2015). Targeting epigenetic regulations in cancer. *Acta Biochimica et Biophysica Sinica (Shanghai)*, *48*, 97–109.

Pattabiraman, D. R., & Weinberg, R. A. (2014). Tackling the cancer stem cells—What challenges do they pose? *Nature Reviews. Drug Discovery*, *13*, 497–512.

Perez-Mancera, P. A., Young, A. R., & Narita, M. (2014). Inside and out: The activities of senescence in cancer. *Nature Reviews. Cancer*, *14*, 547–558.

Ramachandran, S., Karp, P. H., Jiang, P., Ostedgaard, L. S., Walz, A. E., Fisher, J. T., et al. (2012). A microRNA network regulates expression and biosynthesis of wild-type and DeltaF508 mutant cystic fibrosis transmembrane conductance regulator. *Proceedings of the National Academy of Sciences of the United States of America, 109*, 13362–13367.

Rao, G., Alland, L., Guida, P., Schreiber-Agus, N., Chen, K., Chin, L., et al. (1996). Mouse Sin3A interacts with and can functionally substitute for the amino-terminal repression of the Myc antagonist Mxi1. *Oncogene, 12*, 1165–1172.

Rayman, J. B., Takahashi, Y., Indjeian, V. B., Dannenberg, J. H., Catchpole, S., Watson, R. J., et al. (2002). E2F mediates cell cycle-dependent transcriptional repression in vivo by recruitment of an HDAC1/mSin3B corepressor complex. *Genes & Development, 16*, 933–947.

Read, R. D., Goodfellow, P. J., Mardis, E. R., Novak, N., Armstrong, J. R., & Cagan, R. L. (2005). A Drosophila model of multiple endocrine neoplasia type 2. *Genetics, 171*, 1057–1081.

Rielland, M., Cantor, D. J., Graveline, R., Hajdu, C., Mara, L., Diaz Bde, D., et al. (2014). Senescence-associated SIN3B promotes inflammation and pancreatic cancer progression. *Journal of Clinical Investigation, 124*, 2125–2135.

Rodier, F., & Campisi, J. (2011). Four faces of cellular senescence. *Journal of Cell Biology, 192*, 547–556.

Saadatpour, A., Lai, S., Guo, G., & Yuan, G. C. (2015). Single-cell analysis in cancer genomics. *Trends in Genetics, 31*, 576–586.

Schreiber-Agus, N., Alland, L., Muhle, R., Goltz, J., Chen, K., Stevens, L., et al. (1997). A biochemical and biological analysis of Myc superfamily interactions. *Current Topics in Microbiology and Immunology, 224*, 159–168.

Shang, C., Hong, Y., Guo, Y., Liu, Y. H., & Xue, Y. X. (2014). MiR-210 up-regulation inhibits proliferation and induces apoptosis in glioma cells by targeting SIN3A. *Medical Science Monitor, 20*, 2571–2577.

Sharma, S., Kelly, T. K., & Jones, P. A. (2010). Epigenetics in cancer. *Carcinogenesis, 31*, 27–36.

Sharpless, N. E., & Depinho, R. A. (2006). The mighty mouse: Genetically engineered mouse models in cancer drug development. *Nature Reviews. Drug Discovery, 5*, 741–754.

Silverstein, R. A., & Ekwall, K. (2005). Sin3: A flexible regulator of global gene expression and genome stability. *Current Genetics, 47*, 1–17.

Smith, K. T., Sardiu, M. E., Martin-Brown, S. A., Seidel, C., Mushegian, A., Egidy, R., et al. (2012). Human family with sequence similarity 60 member A (FAM60A) protein: A new subunit of the Sin3 deacetylase complex. *Molecular & Cellular Proteomics, 11*, 1815–1828.

Stadler, M., Walter, S., Walzl, A., Kramer, N., Unger, C., Scherzer, M., et al. (2015). Increased complexity in carcinomas: Analyzing and modeling the interaction of human cancer cells with their microenvironment. *Seminars in Cancer Biology, 35*, 107–124.

Sternberg, P. W., Stern, M. J., Clark, I., & Herskowitz, I. (1987). Activation of the yeast HO gene by release from multiple negative controls. *Cell, 48*, 567–577.

Sun, Y. (2015). Tumor microenvironment and cancer therapy resistance. *Cancer Letters.* http://dx.doi.org/10.1016/j.canlet.2015.07.044. Epub ahead of print.

van Oevelen, C., Bowman, C., Pellegrino, J., Asp, P., Cheng, J., Parisi, F., et al. (2010). The mammalian Sin3 proteins are required for muscle development and sarcomere specification. *Molecular and Cellular Biology, 30*, 5686–5697.

Wang, J., Hoshino, T., Redner, R. L., Kajigaya, S., & Liu, J. M. (1998). ETO, fusion partner in t(8;21) acute myeloid leukemia, represses transcription by interaction with the human N-CoR/mSin3/HDAC1 complex. *Proceedings of the National Academy of Sciences of the United States of America, 95*, 10860–10865.

Xu, Y., Harton, J. A., & Smith, B. D. (2008). CIITA mediates interferon-gamma repression of collagen transcription through phosphorylation-dependent interactions with co-repressor molecules. *Journal of Biological Chemistry, 283*, 1243–1256.

Xu, R., Zeng, G., Gao, J., Ren, Y., Zhang, Z., Zhang, Q., et al. (2015). miR-138 suppresses the proliferation of oral squamous cell carcinoma cells by targeting Yes-associated protein 1. *Oncology Reports, 34*, 2171–2178.

Yochum, G. S., & Ayer, D. E. (2001). Pf1, a novel PHD zinc finger protein that links the TLE corepressor to the mSin3A-histone deacetylase complex. *Molecular and Cellular Biology, 21*, 4110–4118.

Yochum, G. S., & Ayer, D. E. (2002). Role for the mortality factors MORF4, MRGX, and MRG15 in transcriptional repression via associations with Pf1, mSin3A, and Transducin-Like Enhancer of Split. *Molecular and Cellular Biology, 22*, 7868–7876.

You, J. S., & Jones, P. A. (2012). Cancer genetics and epigenetics: Two sides of the same coin? *Cancer Cell, 22*, 9–20.

Zilfou, J. T., Hoffman, W. H., Sank, M., George, D. L., & Murphy, M. (2001). The corepressor mSin3a interacts with the proline-rich domain of p53 and protects p53 from proteasome-mediated degradation. *Molecular and Cellular Biology, 21*, 3974–3985.

CHAPTER FOUR

PAKs in Human Cancer Progression: From Inception to Cancer Therapeutic to Future Oncobiology

R. Kumar[*,†,1], D.-Q. Li[‡,§,¶,1]

*School of Medicine and Health Sciences, George Washington University, Washington, DC, United States
†Rajiv Gandhi Center of Biotechnology, Thiruvananthapuram, India
‡Fudan University Shanghai Cancer Center and Institutes of Biomedical Sciences, Shanghai Medical College, Fudan University, Shanghai, China
§Key Laboratory of Breast Cancer in Shanghai, Shanghai Medical College, Fudan University, Shanghai, China
¶Key Laboratory of Epigenetics in Shanghai, Shanghai Medical College, Fudan University, Shanghai, China
1Corresponding authors: e-mail address: bcmrxk@gwu.edu; daqiangli1974@fudan.edu.cn

Contents

Advances in Cancer Research, Volume 130
ISSN 0065-230X
http://dx.doi.org/10.1016/bs.acr.2016.01.002

Abstract

Since the initial recognition of a mechanistic role of p21-activated kinase 1 (PAK1) in breast cancer invasion, PAK1 has emerged as one of the widely overexpressed or hyper-activated kinases in human cancer at-large, allowing the PAK family to make in-roads in cancer biology, tumorigenesis, and cancer therapeutics. Much of our current under-standing of the PAK family in cancer progression relates to a central role of the PAK family in the integration of cancer-promoting signals from cell membrane receptors as well as function as a key nexus-modifier of complex, cytoplasmic signaling network. Another core aspect of PAK signaling that highlights its importance in cancer progres-sion is through PAK's central role in the cross talk with signaling and interacting proteins, as well as PAK's position as a key player in the phosphorylation of effector substrates to engage downstream components that ultimately leads to the develop-ment cancerous phenotypes. Here we provide a comprehensive review of the recent advances in PAK cancer research and its downstream substrates in the context of invasion, nuclear signaling and localization, gene expression, and DNA damage response. We discuss how a deeper understanding of PAK1's pathobiology over the years has widened research interest to the PAK family and human cancer, and position-ing the PAK family as a promising cancer therapeutic target either alone or in combi-nation with other therapies. With many landmark findings and leaps in the progress of PAK cancer research since the infancy of this field nearly 20 years ago, we also discuss postulated advances in the coming decade as the PAK family continues to shape the future of oncobiology.

1. INTRODUCTION

One of the earliest phenotypic responses of living cells to extracellular signals is remodeling of the actin cytoskeleton system and formation of dynamic motile structures by engaging the Rho GTPases and its effector proteins (Nobes & Hall, 1995). In addition, cytoskeleton remodeling and signaling are also fundamental for conferring an invasive behavior to cancer cells (Kumar & Hall, 2009; Vadlamudi & Kumar, 2003), an essential com-ponent for a productive cancer progression. The p21-activated kinases (PAKs) were first discovered by Manser and colleagues in 1994 as down-stream effectors of the Rho GTPases in rat brain (Manser, Leung, Salihuddin, Zhao, & Lim, 1994). This was followed by the characterization of PAK1–3 as effectors of Cdc42/Rac GTPases (Bagrodia, Taylor, Creasy, Chernoff, & Cerione, 1995; Knaus, Morris, Dong, Chernoff, & Bokoch, 1995; Martin, Bollag, McCormick, & Abo, 1995). The core structure and functions of PAKs are evolutionary conserved from protozoa to mammals (Kumar et al., 2009). The PAK family of serine/threonine protein

Group I

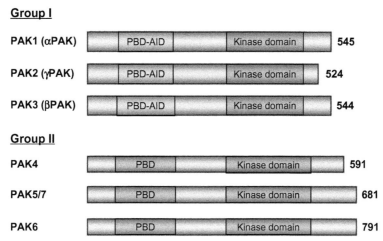

Fig. 1 Schematic representation of the PAK family members. *PBD*, p21-binding domain; *AID*, autoinhibitor domain. (See the color plate.)

kinases consists of group I PAKs (PAK1–3) and group II PAKs (PAK4–6) (Fig. 1). The functions of PAKs are germane to its kinase activity and/or scaffolding activity. A large body of growing literature has established that PAKs are widely overexpressed in human cancer (Table 1) and serve as integrators of cell surface signaling to a variety of hallmarks of cancer progression and metastasis (Tables 2–4).

Historically, PAKs are known as effectors of the Rho GTPases with a role in cell motility and cytoskeleton remodeling. However, since the first demonstration of a mechanistic role of PAK1 in human cancer cell invasion as a component of ErbB2 growth factor receptor signaling (Adam et al., 1998), PAK1 upregulation in breast tumors (Vadlamudi et al., 2000), and PAK1 overexpression in human cancer at-large (Kumar, Gururaj, & Barnes, 2006; Radu, Semenova, Kosoff, & Chernoff, 2014) (Table 1), the focus of PAK research has changed to connect the PAK family—as a converging nexus for a variety of extracellular and intracellular cancer promoting signals—to cancer phenotypes. This is achieved through PAK interacting proteins and downstream substrates which provide necessary signals to phenotypic responses, including proliferation, invasion, metastasis, cell survival, epithelial-to-mesenchymal transition (EMT), therapeutic resistance, angiogenesis, cell-cycle progression, mitosis, DNA repair, and gene expression (Fig. 2). Many of these functions are mediated by PAK's substrates and/or genomic targets (Tables 3 and 4).

Table 1 PAKs Expression and Correlation with Clinicopathological Features of Human Cancer

Categories	PAKs	Cancer Types	Expression Status	Clinicopathological Features	References
Group I	PAK1	Ovarian cancer	Amplification	High tumor grade and poor prognosis	Brown et al. (2008), Schraml et al. (2003), and Siu, Wong, et al. (2010)
		Breast caner	Upregulation	Tamoxifen resistance and poor outcome	Balasenthil, Sahin, et al. (2004), Bostner, Skoog, Fornander, Nordenskjold, and Stal (2010), Kok et al. (2011), and Ong et al. (2015)
			Amplification	Tamoxifen resistance, disease progression, and poor outcome	Bostner et al. (2007), Ong et al. (2011, 2015), and Shrestha et al. (2012)
		Colorectal cancer	Upregulation	Malignant progression and poor prognosis	Carter et al. (2004), Qing et al. (2012), Song, Wang, Zheng, Yang, and Xu (2015), and Zhu et al. (2012)
		Hepatocellular carcinoma	Upregulation	Metastasis, poor prognosis, and HBV infection	Ching et al. (2007) and Xu et al. (2012)
		Renal cancer	Upregulation	Tumor growth and resistance to 5-fluorouracil	O'Sullivan et al. (2007)
		Bladder cancer	Upregulation	Tumor development and progression	Huang, Chen, Luo, Zhang, and Xu (2015) and Ito et al. (2007)
		Glioblastoma	Upregulation	Shorter survival	Aoki et al. (2007)

Gestational trophoblastic disease	Upregulation	Aggressive phenotype, proliferation, and invasion	Siu, Yeung, et al. (2010)
Upper urinary tract cancer	Upregulation	Invasion and metastasis	Kamai et al. (2010)
Thyroid cancer	Upregulation	Migration and invasion	McCarty et al. (2010)
Oral carcinoma	Amplification	Tumor progression	Tu et al. (2011)
Non-small cell lung cancer	Upregulation	Cell survival and proliferation	Ong et al. (2011)
Gastric cancer	Upregulation	Metastasis and poor prognosis	Li, Luo, et al. (2012) and Wang et al. (2015)
	Amplification	Tumor growth	Qian et al. (2014)
Skin cancer	Upregulation	Advanced grade	Chow et al. (2012)
Prostate cancer	Upregulation	Tumor growth and microinvasion	Goc et al. (2013)
Endometrial cancer	Upregulation	Progression and metastasis	Lu, Qu, et al. (2013)
Melanoma	Upregulation	Tumor growth	Ong et al. (2013)
Gastroesophageal junction adenocarcinoma	Upregulation	Invasion and metastasis	Li, Zou, et al. (2013, 2015)

Continued

Table 1 PAKs Expression and Correlation with Clinicopathological Features of Human Cancer—cont'd

Categories	PAKs	Cancer Types	Expression Status	Clinicopathological Features	References
		Pancreatic cancer	Upregulation	Tumorigenesis and invasion	Jagadeeshan et al. (2015) and Zhou et al. (2014)
		Head and neck cancer	Upregulation	Tumor aggressiveness and poor prognosis	Park et al. (2015)
		Esophageal small cell carcinoma	Upregulation	Metastasis and poor prognosis	Gan et al. (2015)
	PAK2	Breast cancer	Upregulation	Chemotherapeutic resistance	Li, Wen, et al. (2011)
		Hepatocellular carcinoma	Upregulation	Cell migration	Sato et al. (2013)
		Gastric cancer	Upregulation	Tumor progression and poor prognosis	Gao, Ma, Pang, and Xie (2014)
	PAK3	Thymic neuroendocrine tumor	Upregulation	Migration and invasion	Liu et al. (2010)
Group II	PAK4	Pancreatic cancer	Amplification	Tumorigenesis and progression	Chen et al. (2008), Kimmelman et al. (2008), and Mahlamaki et al. (2004)
		Oral cancer	Overexpression	Poor prognosis	Begum et al. (2009)
		Ovarian cancer	Upregulation	Cancer progression and poor prognosis	Siu, Chan, et al. (2010)
			Amplification	Poor prognosis	Davis et al. (2013)
		Choriocarcinoma	Upregulation	Proliferation, migration, and invasion	Zhang et al. (2011)

	Cancer type	Regulation	Effect	Reference
	Hepatocellular carcinoma	Upregulation	Cancer metastasis	Mak et al. (2011)
	Gastric cancer	Upregulation	Tumorigenesis and metastasis	Ahn et al. (2011) and Guo et al. (2014)
	Glioma	Upregulation	Anoikis resistance and metastases	Kesanakurti, Chetty, Rajasekhar Maddirela, Gujrati, and Rao (2012)
	Endometrial cancer	Upregulation	Migration and invasion	Lu, Xia, et al. (2013)
	Breast cancer	Upregulation	Disease progression	Li, Wang, et al. (2013)
	Colorectal cancer	Upregulation	Metastasis and infiltration	Song, Wang, et al. (2015)
	Non-small cell lung cancer	Upregulation	Invasion, metastasis, and poor prognosis	Cai, Ye, et al. (2015)
	Cervical cancer	Upregulation	Cisplatin resistance	Shu, Wu, Sun, Chi, and Wang (2015)
PAK5	Gastric cancer	Upregulation	Disease progression	Gu et al. (2013)
	Hepatocellular carcinoma	Upregulation	Disease initiation and progression	Fang et al. (2014)
	Non-small cell lung cancer present	Gain-of-function mutations	Cell viability	Fawdar et al. (2013)
	Ovarian cancer	Upregulation	Paclitaxel chemoresistance	Li, Yao, et al. (2013)
	Osteosarcoma	Upregulation	Tumorigenesis	Han et al. (2014)
	Esophageal cancer	Upregulation	Chemoresistance to cisplatin	He et al. (2014)
	Glioma	Upregulation	Tumor growth	Gu et al. (2015)

Continued

Table 1 PAKs Expression and Correlation with Clinicopathological Features of Human Cancer—cont'd

Categories	PAKs	Cancer Types	Expression Status	Clinicopathological Features	References
	PAK6	Prostate cancer	Upregulation	Tumorigenesis, progression, and chemoresistance	Kaur, Yuan, Lu, and Balk (2008) and Wen et al. (2009)
		Hepatocellular carcinoma	Upregulation	Poor prognosis	Chen et al. (2014)
			Downregulation	Tumor suppressive function	Liu, Liu, et al. (2015)
		Clear cell renal cell cancer	Downregulation	Poor prognosis	Liu et al. (2014)
		Colon cancer	Upregulation	Chemoresistance to 5-fluorouracil	Chen et al. (2015)

Table 2 Upstream Activators and Signals of PAKs in Human Cancer Cells

Categories	PAKs	Activators	Functions	References
Group I	PAK1	Heregulin	Migration and invasion	Adam et al. (1998) and Bagheri-Yarmand, Vadlamudi, Wang, Mendelsohn, and Kumar (2000)
		Rac3	Proliferation	Mira, Benard, Groffen, Sanders, and Knaus (2000)
		PDGF	–	He et al. (2001)
		Etk/Bmx	Mammary tumorigenesis	Bagheri-Yarmand et al. (2001)
		Cdc2	Cell division	Thiel et al. (2002)
		CXCL1	Chemotaxis	Wang, Sai, and Richmond (2003)
		Estrogen	Cell survival	Mazumdar and Kumar (2003)
		VEGF	Neovasculature	Wary (2003)
		bFGF	Neovasculature	Wary (2003)
		BCAR3	Antiestrogen resistance	Cai et al. (2003)
		KSHV-GPCR	Cell transformation	Dadke, Fryer, Golemis, and Field (2003)
		LPA	Cell motility	Jung et al. (2004)
		Akt	Cell survival	Yuan et al. (2005)
		ArgBP2γ	Cell survival	Yuan et al. (2005)
		JAK2	Cell survival and motility	Hammer et al. (2013) and Rider, Shatrova, Feener, Webb, and Diakonova (2007)
		ERK	Cell migration	Yuan, Santi, Rushing, Cornelison, and MacDonald (2010)
		Phosphoinositides	Upregulating Pak1 activity in cancer cells	Strochlic, Viaud, Rennefahrt, Anastassiadis, and Peterson (2010)

Continued

Table 2 Upstream Activators and Signals of PAKs in Human Cancer Cells—cont'd

Categories	PAKs	Activators	Functions	References
		HBx	Resistance to anoikis	Xu et al. (2012)
		STRADα	Cell polarity and invasion	Eggers, Kline, Zhong, Zhou, and Marcus (2012)
		RhoJ	Melanoma chemoresistance	Ho et al. (2012)
		Klotho	Resistance to anoikis	Chen et al. (2013)
		MGAT5	Anoikis resistance	Liu, Liu, et al. (2013)
		CK2	Malignant transformation of prostate epithelial cells	Shin, Kim, and Kim (2013)
		BRAF	Thyroid cancer cell motility	McCarty et al. (2014)
		CKIP1	Migration and invasion	Kim, Shin, Roy, and Kim (2015)
	PAK2	TGF-β	Morphological alteration	Wilkes, Murphy, Garamszegi, and Leof (2003)
		A2M	Cancer metastatic potential	Misra, Deedwania, and Pizzo (2005)
		AMPK	Mitotic progression	Banko et al. (2011)
		miR-23b	Cytoskeletal remodeling, motility, and metastasis	Pellegrino et al. (2013)
	PAK3	AP1	Actin organization and migration	Holderness Parker, Donninger, Birrer, and Leaner (2013)

Table 2 Upstream Activators and Signals of PAKs in Human Cancer Cells—cont'd

Categories	PAKs	Activators	Functions	References
Group II	PAK4	HGF	Actin organization and cell adhesion	Wells, Abo, and Ridley (2002)
		CDK5RAP3	Hepatocellular carcinoma metastasis	Mak et al. (2011)
		PKD	Cell migration	Bastea et al. (2013) and Spratley, Bastea, Doppler, Mizuno, and Storz (2011)
		PKA	Prostate cancer progression	Park et al. (2013)
		SH3RF2	Stabilization of PAK4 protein	Kim, Kang, et al. (2014)
	PAK5	Aurora-A	Cisplatin resistance of esophageal cancer	He et al. (2014)
	PAK6	MAPK6	Stress-related signals	Kaur et al. (2005)
		MAPK14	Stress-related signals	Kaur et al. (2005)
		Androgen	Prostate cancer cells motility and invasion	Liu, Busby, et al. (2013)

Abbreviations: *A2M*, α2-macroglobulin; *AMPK*, 5-AMP-activated protein kinase; *ArgBP2γ*, ARG-binding protein 2γ; *AP1*, activating protein 1; *bFGF*, basic fibroblast growth factor; *BCAR3*, breast cancer antiestrogen resistance 3; *BRAF*, B-Raf proto-oncogene; *CDK5RAP3*, CDK5 regulatory subunit associated protein 3; *CK2*, casein kinase II; *CKIP1*, casein kinase 2-interacting protein 1; *CXCL1*, chemokine (C–X–C motif) ligand 1; *Hbx*, hepatitis B virus X protein; *KSHV-GPCR*, Kaposi's sarcoma-associated herpesvirus-G protein-coupled receptor; *HGF*, hepatocyte growth factor; *LPA*, lysophosphatidic acid; *MAPK6*, mitogen-activated protein kinase 6; *MAPK14*, mitogen-activated protein kinase 14; *MGAT5*, N-acetylglucosaminyl transferase V; *miR*, microRNA; *PDGF*, platelet-derived growth factor; *PKA*, protein kinase A; *PKD*, protein kinase D; *STRADα*, STE20-related kinase adaptor protein α; *TGF-β*, transforming growth factor β; *SH3RF2*, SH3 domain containing ring finger 2.

Table 3 PAK Effector Substrates in Human Cancer Cells

Categories	PAKs	Substrates	Phosphorylation Sites	Functions	References
Group I	PAK1	Stathmin	S16	Microtubule dynamics	Daub, Gevaert, Vandekerckhove, Sobel, and Hall (2001)
		Merlin	S518	Inhibition of Merlin	Shrestha et al. (2012) and Xiao, Beeser, Chernoff, and Testa (2002)
		Vimentin	S25, S38, S50, S65, and S72	Reorganization of vimentin filaments	Goto et al. (2002)
		Histone H3	S10	Mitotic events	Li et al. (2002)
		FLNA	S2152	Cytoskeletal reorganization	Hammer et al. (2013) and Vadlamudi et al. (2002)
		ERα	S305	Breast cancer development and tamoxifen resistance	Bostner et al. (2010), Kok et al. (2011), Rayala, Talukder, et al. (2006), and Wang, Mazumdar, Vadlamudi, and Kumar (2002)
		Stat5a	S779	Stimulating β-casein promoter activity	Wang, Vadlamudi, et al. (2003)
		CtBP	S158	Functional inactivation of CtBP	Barnes et al. (2003)
		Raf-1	S338 and 339	Tumor vasculature	Wary (2003)
		p41-Arc	T21	Cell motility	Vadlamudi, Li, Barnes, Bagheri-Yarmand, and Kumar (2004)

DLC1	S88	Cancerous phenotypes and macropinocytosis	Vadlamudi, Bagheri-Yarmand, et al. (2004) and Yang, Vadlamudi, and Kumar (2005)
PGM1	T466	Glucose metabolism	Gururaj, Barnes, Vadlamudi, and Kumar (2004)
SHARP	S3486 and T3568	Modulating Notch signaling	Vadlamudi, Manavathi, et al. (2005)
TBCB	S65 and S128	Microtubule dynamics	Vadlamudi, Barnes, et al. (2005)
Snail	S246	Epithelial–mesenchymal transition	Yang, Rayala, et al. (2005)
VE-cadherin	S665	VEGF-dependent endocytosis	Gavard and Gutkind (2006)
PCBP1	T60 and T127	Transcription, splicing, and translation	Meng et al. (2007)
ILK	T173 and S246	Nuclear localization and functions of ILK	Acconcia, Barnes, Singh, Talukder, and Kumar (2007)
ESE-1	S207	Transformation potential	Manavathi, Rayala, and Kumar (2007)
EBP1	T261	Tumor growth and tamoxifen resistance	Akinmade et al. (2008)
NRIF3	S28	Enhancing NRIF3 coactivator activity	Talukder, Li, Manavathi, and Kumar (2008)

Continued

Table 3 PAK Effector Substrates in Human Cancer Cells—cont'd

Categories	PAKs	Substrates	Phosphorylation Sites	Functions	References
		SRC-3 Delta4	T56A, S659A, and S676A	Cell migration	Long et al. (2010)
		β-catenin	S675	Proliferation	Zhu et al. (2012)
		BAD	S111	Cell survival	Ye, Jin, Zhuo, and Field (2011)
		RAF1	S338	Anchorage-independent growth	Shrestha et al. (2012)
		MEK1	S298	Anchorage-independent growth	Shrestha et al. (2012)
		CRK-II	S41	Migration and invasion	Rettig et al. (2012)
		MORC2	S739	Genomic stability and gastric tumorigenesis	Li, Nair, et al. (2012) and Wang et al. (2015)
		Paxillin	S258	Activation and secretion of TACE/ADAM10 proteases	Lee et al. (2013)
		STAT5	S779	Leukemogenesis	Berger et al. (2014)
	PAK2	Merlin	S518	Protein relocalization and intramolecular association	Kissil, Johnson, Eckman, and Jacks (2002) and Rong, Surace, Haipek, Gutmann, and Ye (2004)
		Myc	T358, S373, and T400	Negative regulation of Myc	Huang, Traugh, and Bishop (2004)
		LIMK1	—	Metastatic potential	Misra et al. (2005)

	c-Jun	T2, T8, T89, T93, and T286	Proliferation and transformation	Li, Zhang, et al. (2011)
	Caspase-7	S30, T173, and S239	Chemotherapeutic resistance	Li, Wen, et al. (2011)
	Paxillin	S272/274	Activation and secretion of TACE/ADAM10 proteases	Lee et al. (2013)
	STAT5	S779	Leukemogenesis	Berger et al. (2014)
Group II PAK4	LIMK1	T508	Cell migration	Ahmed, Shea, Masters, Jones, and Wells (2008)
	Integrin β5	S759 and S762	Cell migration	Li, Zhang, et al. (2010)
	p120-catenin	S288	Cytoskeletal reorganization	Wong, Reynolds, Dissanayaka, and Minden (2010)
	β-catenin	S675	Modulating intracellular translocation and signaling of β-catenin	Li, Shao, et al. (2012)
	SCG10	S50	Gastric cancer metastasis	Guo et al. (2014)
	Smad2	S465	Gastric tumorigenesis	Wang et al. (2014)

Continued

Table 3 PAK Effector Substrates in Human Cancer Cells—cont'd

Categories	PAKs	Substrates	Phosphorylation Sites	Functions	References
	PAK5	BAD	S112	Inhibiting apoptosis	Cotteret, Jaffer, Beeser, & Chernoff, 2003 and Wang, Gong, et al. (2010)
		p120-catenin	S288	Cytoskeletal reorganization	Wong et al. (2010)
		GATA1	S161 and S187	Epithelial–mesenchymal transition in breast cancer	Li, Ke, et al. (2015)
		E47	S39	Colon cancer metastasis	Zhu et al. (2015)
	PAK6	AR	S578	Tumor growth	Liu, Li, et al. (2013)
			S308, 346, 360 and T326, 354	Prostate cancer cell migration and invasion	Liu, Busby, et al. (2013)
		MDM2	T158, S186	Tumor growth	Liu, Li, et al. (2013)
		LIMK1	T508	Prostate cancer metastasis	Cai, Chen, et al. (2015)

Abbreviations: *AR*, androgen receptor; *CtBP*, C-terminal binding protein; *DLC1*, deleted in liver cancer 1; *ERα*, estrogen receptor α; *EBP1*, ErbB3 binding protein 1; *ESE-1*, epithelium-specific Ets transcription factor 1; *FLNA*, Filamin A; *GATA1*, GATA binding protein 1; *PCBP1*, poly(RC) binding protein 1; *ILK*, integrin-linked kinase; *LIMK1*, LIM domain kinase 1; *MDM2*, mouse double minute 2; *MORC2*, MORC family CW-type zinc finger 2; *NRIF3*, nuclear receptor-interacting factor 3; *PGM1*, phosphoglucomutase 1; *SHARP*, SMART/HDAC1-associated repressor protein; *SRC-3Delta4*, SRC-3Delta4, a splicing isoform of the SRC-3 oncogene; *STAT5A*, signal transducer and activator of transcription 5A; *TBCB*, tubulin cofactor B; *VE-cadherin*, vascular endothelial-cadherin.

Table 4 Genomic Targets of PAKs in Human Cancer Cells

Categories	PAKs	Substrates	Functions	References
Group I	PAK1	VEGF	Angiogenesis	Bagheri-Yarmand et al. (2000)
		Cyclin D1	Mammary tumorigenesis	Balasenthil, Sahin, et al. (2004) and Tao, Oladimeji, Rider, and Diakonova (2011)
		PFKM	–	Singh, Song, Yang, and Kumar (2005)
		NFAT1	–	Singh et al. (2005)
		Cyclin B1	Proliferation and tumor growth	Liu et al. (2009)
		Tissue factor	Procoagulant activity	Sanchez-Solana, Motwani, Li, Eswaran, and Kumar (2012)
		TFPI	Procoagulant activity	Sanchez-Solana et al. (2012)
		MMP9	Motility and invasion	Goc et al. (2013)
		TGF-β	Motility and invasion	Goc et al. (2013)
		Fibronectin	Pancreatic tumorigenesis	Jagadeeshan et al. (2015)
	PAK2	LIMK1	Cancer metastasis	Misra et al. (2005)
Group II	PAK4	MT1-MMP	Migration and invasion	Zhang et al. (2011)
		p57^{kip2}	Breast cancer progression	Li, Wang, et al. (2013)
	PAK6	MMP9	Motility and invasion	Goc et al. (2013)

Abbreviations: *MMP9*, Metalloproteinase 9; *MT1-MMP*, membrane-type 1 matrix metalloproteinase; *NFAT1*; nuclear factor of activated T-cell; *PFKM*, phosphofructokinase-muscle isoform; *TFPI*, tissue factor pathway inhibitor; *TGF-β*, transforming growth factor β; *VEGF*, vascular endothelial growth factor.

.The high mortality of cancer patients is largely attributed to the ability of primary tumor cells to metastasize to distant organs while the primary tumors could be effectively managed by surgery or tumor-directed treatment modalities. At the cellular level, for a productive invasion and

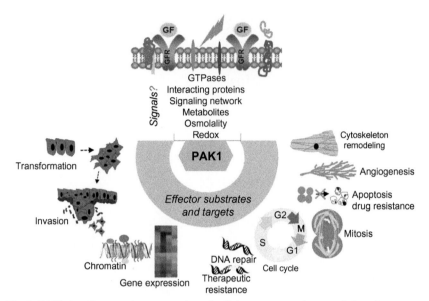

Fig. 2 PAK1 signaling regulates a number of cellular processes characteristics of oncogenesis and cancer progression. ?, potential upstream PAK1 activators. (See the color plate.)

metastasis, cancer cells must undergo an extensive cytoskeleton remodeling (ie, polymerization and depolymerization of microtubules and actin filaments, disruption of focal adhesions, cell spreading, etc.), ensure expression of appropriate genes in response to dynamic extracellular milieu and upstream signals, engage growth and cell-cycle machineries, and acquire a better survival skill to resist apoptotic signals in the primary tumors and on their way to metastatic locations. In addition, cancer cells travel to distant metastatic sites by degrading the extracellular matrix (ECM) by proteases such as urokinase-type plasminogen activator (uPA) and matrix metalloproteases (MMPs). Interestingly, PAK1 signaling and its downstream targets contribute to all of these cellular processes and hence, explain the excitement and hope for PAKs in cancer biology and therapeutics (Table 5).

Most of our current understanding of PAKs in cancer has been shaped by the lessons learned with PAK1, the founding member of the family. As PAKs continue to make in-roads and recognition of prominence in the field of cancer biology, here we will bring out the major advances in the area of PAK1 and its target substrates—the focus of the authors' laboratories, in the context of invasion, nuclear signaling and localization, gene expression, and DNA damage response (DDR). We will also discuss how our enhanced

Table 5 Inhibitors of PAK Activation in Human Cancer Cells

Categories	PAKs	Inhibitors	Functions	References
Group I	PAK1	PP1	Inhibition of malignant transformation	He, Hirokawa, Levitzki, and Maruta (2000)
		hPIP1	A negative regulator of PAK	Xia et al. (2001)
		NESH	Cell motility	Ichigotani, Yokozaki, Fukuda, Hamaguchi, and Matsuda (2002)
		Merlin	Tumorigenesis	Hirokawa et al. (2004) and Kissil et al. (2003)
		CRIPak	Modulation of Pak1-mediated ERα transactivation	Talukder, Meng, and Kumar (2006)
		OSU-03012	Inhibiting migration	Porchia et al. (2007)
		IPA-3	Inhibiting PAK1-mediated signaling	Deacon et al. (2008) and Viaud and Peterson (2009)
		MicroRNA-7	Tumorigenesis and progression	Reddy, Ohshiro, Rayala, and Kumar (2008)
		Curcumin	Proliferation and invasion	Cai et al. (2009)
		LKB1	Cell migration	Deguchi et al. (2010)
		Mesalamine	Intracellular adhesion	Khare et al. (2013)
		miR-let-7	Cell motility	Hu et al. (2013)

Continued

Table 5 Inhibitors of PAK Activation in Human Cancer Cells—cont'd

Categories	PAKs	Inhibitors	Functions	References
		FRAX597	Tumorigenesis	Licciulli et al. (2013)
		Glaucarubinone	Pancreatic cancer growth	Yeo et al. (2014)
		miR–145	Bladder cancer invasion	Kou et al. (2014)
		Derivatives of hispidin and mimosine	Inhibition of PAK1 activity	Nguyen, Taira, and Tawata (2014)
		FRAX1036	Breast cancer apoptosis	Ong et al. (2015)
		Myricetin	Hepatocellular carcinoma apoptosis	Iyer, Gopal, and Halagowder (2015)
		β-elemene	Radiosensitivity of gastric cancer	Liu, Che, et al. (2015)
	PAK2	FRAX597	Tumorigenesis	Licciulli et al. (2013)
		FRAX1036	Breast cancer apoptosis	Ong et al. (2015)
		miR–137	Melanoma proliferation	Hao et al. (2015)
	PAK3	FRAX597	Tumorigenesis	Licciulli et al. (2013)
Group II	PAK4	PF-3758309	Tumor growth	Murray et al. (2010)
		LCH-7749944	Proliferation and invasion	
		miR–145	Tumor growth	Wang et al. (2012)
		Glaucarubinone	Pancreatic cancer growth	Yeo et al. (2014)

KY-04031	Tumor growth and invasion	Ryu et al. (2014)
miR-433	Proliferation of hepatocellular carcinoma	Xue et al. (2015)
1-Phenanthryl-tetrahydroisoquinoline derivatives	Cell proliferation	Song, Li, et al. (2015)
miR-126	Downregulation of PAK4 in ovarian cancer	Luo, Fei, Zhou, and Zhang (2015)
PAK5 miR-129	Hepatocellular carcinoma growth and invasion	Zhai et al. (2015)
PAK6 miR-23a	Prostate cancer metastasis	Cai, Chen, et al. (2015)

Abbreviation: *CRIPak*, cysteine-rich inhibitor of Pak1.

understanding of PAK1 biology in cancer cells has broaden the research interest to other PAK family members, and positioned the PAKs as potential drug targets in cancer therapeutics.

2. MECHANISM OF ACTION

Although groups I and II PAKs share structural features, the two groups have overlapping and nonoverlapping functions and are activated by distinct mechanisms. As opposed to group I PAKs, group II PAKs lack an autoinhibitory domain and PXXP motifs and are constitutively activated. Here we limit our discussion to group I PAKs with a particular emphasis on PAK1. As there are many excellent, recent reviews about the mechanism of PAK activation (Jha & Strauss, 2012; Rane & Minden, 2014), our discussion of this aspect of the PAK story will be brief. The PAK proteins contain a C-terminal catalytic kinase domain and N-terminal regulatory p21-binding domain (PBD) which interacts with the Rho GTPases and/or guanine exchange nucleotide factors. PAK1 exists in a closed, inactive conformation as homodimer wherein the kinase domain of one molecule binds to an autoinhibitory domain (AID) of another molecule. PAK1 activates by the interaction of the p21-GTPase binding domain with GTP-loaded Rho GTPases and phosphoinositide binding to neighboring basic amino acids, triggering a conformational change and autophosphorylation of two PAK1 molecules due to the inactivation of an autoinhibitory switch. In general, group I PAKs are activated by the inactivation of their autoinhibitory activity through multiple mechanisms.

PAK1 is activated by both GTPase-dependent and -independent manner through the integration of multiple signals from cell membrane receptors with proximal cytoplasmic signaling components. The GTPase-independent mechanisms of PAK activation include SH3-adaptor proteins which bind to PXXP motifs in PAKs (Galisteo, Chernoff, Su, Skolnik, & Schlessinger, 1996; Puto, Pestonjamasp, King, & Bokoch, 2003), and cross-phosphorylation of PAKs by kinases such as AKT (Zhou et al., 2003), ETK/BMX (Bagheri-Yarmand et al., 2001), JAK2 (Tao et al., 2011), or 3-phosphoinositide-dependent kinase-1 (Bokoch, 2003) (Table 2). Once activated, the PAK kinases mediate their cellular functions by phosphorylating downstream effector proteins and/or by exercising its scaffolding activity (Table 3). The broad significance of PAK1 activation in cancer cells is a reflection of its ability to funnel a whole range of upstream signals, not necessarily dependent of the Rho GTPases. Thus, the ability PAK1 to impact regulatory processes in cancer cells may be attributed to largely non-GTPase-dependent activation of its kinase activity, in addition to GTPase-dependent mechanisms. Further an optimal stimulation of PAK1 kinase activity is likely to be the result of a combination of more than one mode of PAK activation and its cross talk with signaling cascades in cancer cells.

3. EARLY STUDIES CONNECTING THE PAK FAMILY TO HUMAN CANCER

The process of tumor progression requires among other steps, increased invasion and an appropriate modulation for the expression of genes with roles in oncogenesis. Our interest in the cytoskeleton remodeling in cancer research began with PAK1 in late 1996, when for the first time, Rakesh Kumar and colleagues postulated that PAK1 signaling may control the invasiveness of human tumor cells. Since then, the laboratory has vigorously pursued this hypothesis and discovered new downstream targets and facets of PAK1 biology and functions in human cancer cells and human tumors (Table 3).

Because PAK1 is a downstream effector of a variety of upstream signals triggered by cell membrane receptors, initial laboratory studies in cancer cells in this new frontier during the period of 1996–1998 were focused on PAK1 activation by ErbB2 signaling by heregulin-β1, a ligand for ErbB3 and ErbB that stimulates ErbB2 phosphorylation via heterodimerization with ErbB3 or ErbB4. The laboratory was the first to recognize a mechanistic role of PAK1 signaling in transducing ErbB2-triggered signals in the formation of motile structures and conferring an invasive behavior to cancer cells using breast cancer as a model (Adam et al., 1998). Using the loss- or gain-of-functional studies, the team established that PAK1 inactivation in highly invasive breast cancer cells blunts their invasiveness due to increased cell attachment through the formation of stable focal adhesion points and long less-dynamic stress fibers (Adam, Vadlamudi, Mandal, Chernoff, & Kumar, 2000). In contrast, expression of a hyperactive PAK1 in noninvasive breast cancer cells promotes anchorage-independent growth and invasiveness and as a correlate, PAK1 is also overexpressed in human breast tumors (Vadlamudi et al., 2000). The team also demonstrated for the first time that hyperactivated PAK1 leads to a defective mitosis as well as the landmark finding of PAK1's localization in the nucleus and interaction with chromatin, providing clues about yet-to-be, recognized nuclear functions of PAK1 in human cancer cells (see following sections). This was followed by the creation of the first set of PAK murine models, showing that conditional inactivation or hyperactivation of PAK1 in mammary glands leads to a defective lobular development or epithelium hyperplasia, respectively; thus, revealed the impact of PAK1 signaling on the development of the mammary gland as well as tumorigenesis using whole animal models (see following sections).

In the next phase, the team identified several downstream interacting substrates as mediators of PAK1's action and connected these newly discovered PAK1 effectors beyond cytoskeleton remodeling to invasion, tumorigenesis, nuclear signaling, mitotic progression, DNA damage, and chromatin remodeling (see following sections)—all relevant for the development and maintenance of cancerous phenotypes. These early discoveries spurred a great interest in other laboratories around the globe and led to widespread cumulative documentation of PAK1 overexpression and hyperactivation in human cancer at-large, as well as revealing new aspects of PAKs pathobiology using human cancer cell lines, xenografts, animal models, and tumor specimens as model systems, cumulating to a growing list of a few hundreds of publications in the area of PAKs in cancer. For example, PAK4 overexpression stimulated an anchorage-independent growth of fibroblasts, suggesting a role in transformation (Callow et al., 2002; Qu et al., 2001). Over the years, the status of PAK4 has been found to be closely associated with cancer progression by multiple laboratories (see later). PAK5 levels gradually increase during colon cancer progression from adenoma to invasive to metastatic stages, as well as from well-differentiated to a poorly differentiated phenotypes (Gong et al., 2009). Interesting, PAK5 is also involved in supporting cell survival, possibly associated with its ability to localize in mitochondria (Cotteret & Chernoff, 2006). The PAK6 is an androgen receptor (AR) interacting protein and inhibits AR's transactivation activity in reporter-based assays (Lee et al., 2002). In brief, the lessons from PAK1 cancer research spurred the expansion of related research to other family members, bringing prominence to the PAK family in the scientific map of cancer biology.

4. SUBSTRATES PROMOTING CYTOSKELETON DYNAMIC INVASION AND TUMORIGENESIS

The ability of cancer cells to invade ECM and metastasize is partly controlled by motile structures resulting from signal-dependent cytoskeleton remodeling and by pathways contributing to the degradation of ECM. Here we will discuss a few representative PAK1 substrates with roles

not only in cytoskeleton dynamics but also in invasion and conferring oncogenic phenotypes during cancer progression (Table 3). For example, PAK1
phosphorylation of LIM-kinase (LIMK) on T508 activates LIMK's activity,
resulting in Cofilin-S3 phosphorylation and in-turn, interfering with the
ability of Cofilin to depolymerize F-actin (Edwards, Sanders, Bokoch, &
Gill, 1999). Relevant to the process of cancer progression, LIMK1
upregulates the expression and secretion of uPA and invasion of breast cancer cells, and promotes the ability of LIMK1-overexpressing cells to form
tumor xenografts and metastasize to other organs (Bagheri-Yarmand,
Mazumdar, Sahin, & Kumar, 2006). Interestingly, LIMK also participates
in the degradation of ECM and formation of invadopodia in invading breast
cancer cells (Scott et al., 2010). In addition, the levels of MMP proteases are
regulated by PAK1 signaling in breast and ovarian cancer cells (Gonzalez-
Villasana et al., 2015; Hammer & Diakonova, 2015) as well as potentiated
by PAK5 signaling in breast cancer cells (Wang et al., 2013), and by
PAK4 signaling in glioma cells (Kesanakurti et al., 2012). Although
co-overexpression of LIMK1 and uPA receptor (uPAR) have been noticed
in a small number of human breast tumors (Bagheri-Yarmand et al., 2006),
it will be important to re-evaluate the status of LIMK1, uPAR, MMPs in
the context of PAKs overexpression in human cancer.

　　PAK1 signaling also stimulates cytoskeleton dynamics by supporting
actin nucleation as PAK1 phosphorylation of p41-Arc (also known as
Arpc1b)-T21 is an essential step for its interaction with, and stability of,
the Arp2/2 complex for its actin nucleation activity (Vadlamudi, Li,
et al., 2004). The PAK1 regulation of Arpc1b-T21 phosphorylation also
supports cancer cell invasion through the expression of p41-Arc/Arpc1b
or its phosphorylation mimicking T21E mutant but not phosphorylation-
defective T21A mutants (Vadlamudi, Li, et al., 2004). Further Arpc1b overexpression in breast cancer cells stimulates anchorage-independent growth
and the ability of cells to form tumor xenografts (Molli et al., 2010). Since
Arpc1b may be upregulated in pancreatic cancer cells (Mahlamaki et al.,
2004) and breast tumors (Molli et al., 2010), and because Arpc1b status
may have a predictive value for radiosensitivity of malignant melanomas
(Kumagai et al., 2006), it is possible that the PAK1-Arpc1b pathway may
have cancer-promoting functions that are independent of its role in actin
nucleation.

　　Filamin A (FLAa) binds to actin to orchestrate the branching pattern
of FLNa which acts as a support structure for the cytoskeleton network.
The PAK1 kinase phosphorylates FLAa-S2152 and regulates PAK1-induced

ruffle-forming and cytoskeletal reorganization in growth factor stimulated cells (Vadlamudi et al., 2002). Over the years, FLAa has made several connections with cancer: interaction with CDK4 regulates breast cancer invasion (Zhong et al., 2010); interaction with MMP9 regulates invasion of renal cell carcinoma (Sun, Wei, Jing, & Hu, 2014); its status correlates well with the invasive phenotype of metastatic melanoma (Zhang et al., 2014); and acts as an effector of mTORC2 signaling in invasiveness of glioblastoma cells (Chantaravisoot, Wongkongkathep, Loo, Mischel, & Tamanoi, 2015).

PAK1 signaling is an important modifier of dynein light chain 1 (DLC1), a shared component of the dynein and myosin motor complexes, functions in cancer cells (Vadlamudi, Bagheri-Yarmand, et al., 2004). PAK1 phosphorylation of DLC1-S88 contributes to an enhanced cell survival through interacting and modifying the function of proapoptotic BimL. In addition to DLC1, PAK1 also phosphorylates BimL which antagonizes PAK1 interaction with Bcl2, leading to a better cell survival. Surprisingly, DLC1 was found to be overexpressed in breast tumors and overexpression of DLC1, but not DLC1-S88A mutant, in breast cancer cells promotes cancerous phenotypes in cell- and mice-based models (Vadlamudi, Bagheri-Yarmand, et al., 2004; Vadlamudi, Li, et al., 2004). DLC1-mediated cancer phenotypes may also be affected by its interaction with Cdk2 and Ciz1 to support the cell-cycle progression (den Hollander & Kumar, 2006) and by the ability of DLC1 to stimulate microtubule (MT) stability and assembly of bipolar spindles in cancer cells (Asthana, Kuchibhatla, Jana, Ray, & Panda, 2012).

PAK1 phosphorylation of integrin-linked kinase (ILK) on T173 and S246 regulates its subcellular localization and its interaction with target gene chromatin (Acconcia et al., 2007). Overexpression of activated ILK in experimental systems leads to transformation and confers invasive characteristics (McDonald, Fielding, & Dedhar, 2008). ILK upregulation in breast cancer correlates well the tumor aggression and poor prognosis (Yang et al., 2013). ILK is overexpressed in several human cancer types and inhibits the activity of Hippo tumor suppressor (Serrano, McDonald, Lock, Muller, & Dedhar, 2013) and stimulates IL-6 regulation of Notch1 pathway in breast cancer (Hsu et al., 2015). Interestingly, NOTCH signaling may also exert an inhibitory feedback control on PAK1 signaling as NOTCH1 intracellular domain has been shown to interact with PAK1 and influence its distribution in the nucleus and cytoplasmic compartments (Yoon et al., 2015).

In addition to actin remodeling, cancer cell invasion is equally regulated by the status of MT dynamics. PAK1 signaling may influence MT biogenesis via tubulin cofactor B (TCoB) or MT-destabilizing protein Stathmin. PAK1 phosphorylation of TCoB-S65 and S128 is required for

MT regrowth as overexpression of TCoB but not PAK1 phosphorylation-inactive mutant supports the biogenesis of new MT (Vadlamudi, Barnes, et al., 2005). Interestingly, TCoB overexpression in experimental breast cancer models lead to the appearance of multiple microtubule-organizing center (MTOCs) (Vadlamudi, Barnes, et al., 2005). In contrast, PAK1 phosphorylation of Stathmin abolishes its function to inhibit MT and stimulates MT stabilization at the leading edge (Wittmann, Bokoch, & Waterman-Storer, 2004). Stathmin may be also overexpressed in certain cancers and stimulate tumor invasion (Belletti et al., 2008). Cortactin is another actin binding PAK1 substrate with a role in membrane ruffling and amplified in breast, as well as head and neck cancers (Buday & Downward, 2007; Moshfegh, Bravo-Cordero, Miskolci, Condeelis, & Hodgson, 2014).

5. NUCLEAR SIGNALING, LOCALIZATION, AND FUNCTIONS

To develop and sustain oncogenic phenotypes, cancer cells respond to the dynamic extracellular milieu by modifying the expression of relevant target genes. In general, signaling-dependent gene expression could be influenced by kinases, its substrates and effectors, and through the physical translocation of activated kinases and substrates to the nucleus leading to interaction with the regulatory elements of target genes. In this context, genetic depletion of PAK1 in murine embryonic fibroblasts is accompanied by a substantial differential upregulation or downregulation of genes as compared to their levels in fibroblasts with PAK1, revealing a broader role of PAK1 signaling in gene expression and not just gene stimulation (Motwani, Li, Horvath, & Kumar, 2013). Although PAK1 was originally thought to be a cytoplasmic kinase with a role in cytoskeleton remodeling, the PAK family also possesses distinct nuclear functions.

One of the most exciting phases in the area of PAKs in cancer was the discovery of the nuclear functions and localization of PAK1 in human cancer cells as PAK1 was previously thought to be a cytoplasmic kinase—"It has been known for some time that activated PAK affects centrosome number. In 2000, Rakesh Kumar's group showed that overexpression of activated PAK1 in MCF7 cells led to the accumulation of centrosomes and aberrant mitoses" (Cotteret & Chernoff, 2005; Vadlamudi et al., 2000). Additionally, PAK1 was also found in the nucleus of interphase cells (Li et al., 2002), thus providing an important early clue to the yet to be discovered nuclear functions of PAK1 in human cancer cells. Consistent with this concept, growth factor signaling promotes the nuclear translocation of activated PAK1 in cancer cells (Singh et al., 2005). Interestingly, these studies discovered that activated PAK1 also interacts with the DNase insensitive chromatin, nuclear matrix and chromatin, presumably through DNA-interacting factors (Fig. 3A), and revealed a potential role of PAK1 in the modulation of target

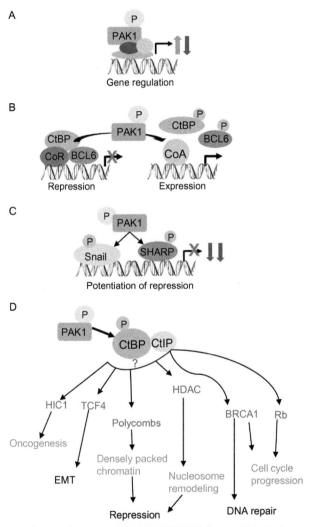

Fig. 3 PAK1 regulation of gene expression. (A) Modulation of target gene expression by activated PAK1 through phosphorylating and/or interacting with DNA-binding factors. (B) Gene expression via PAK1-signaling-dependent derepression of target genes due to decruitment of corepressors such as CtBP and BCL6. (C) Potentiation of target gene repression by PAK1 phosphorylation of Snail or SHARP. (D) PAK1 phosphorylation of CtBP1 is being hypothesized to potentially modulate the functions of downstream targets. (See the color plate.)

gene transcription and expression (Table 4). PAK1 interacts with the chromatin of *PFKM* (muscle-type phosphofructokinase) or *NFAT1* (nuclear factor of activated T-cell 1) and stimulates or represses gene transcription, respectively. In addition, PAK1-Gal4 DNA-binding domain fusion also stimulates the transcription from the Gal4-luciferase reporter (Singh et al., 2005). Nuclear PAK1 also participates in the coagulation cascade wherein the PAK1/c-Jun complex promotes the transcription of tissue factor (*TF*) while repressing the expression of tissue factor pathway inhibitor (*TFPI*), leading to a net stimulation of TF's coagulant activity (Sanchez-Solana et al., 2012). The PAK1/NF-κB complex stimulates the expression of fibronectin in pancreatic cancer cells (Jagadeeshan et al., 2015). More recently, the authors recognized a role of PAK1 signaling in the regulatory interplay between PAK1-phosphorylation-dependent MORC2's ATPase activity and its significance in chromatin dynamics and maintenance of genomic integrity in response to DNA damage and cell membrane generated responses (Li, Nair, et al., 2012, see later).

In addition to PAK1, other members of the PAK family also translocate to the nucleus upon stimulation with appropriate signals. For example, PAK4 shuttles between the cytoplasm and nucleus through nuclear export and localization signals (Li, Shao, et al., 2012), and therefore, may potentially regulate gene expression (Table 4). While examining the significance of PAKs in endometrial cancer, Siu et al. found that PAK4 localizes in both cytoplasm and nucleus. The levels of PAK1 and PAK4 negatively associate with endometrial cancer histological grade, and PAK4 cytoplasmic status inversely associates with invasiveness of myometrium while a reduced PAK4 cytoplasmic level may correlate well with a poor survival of endometrial cancer patients (Siu et al., 2015).

6. SIGNALING REGULATION OF GENE EXPRESSION

In addition to the nuclear translocation, activated PAK1 also participates in gene expression by regulating the phosphorylation-dependent nuclear translocation and/or retention of its direct substrates. PAK1 signaling also regulates gene expression by modifying the function of corepressors on its targets, thereby stimulating the expression of target genes by derepression. One of the first examples of such a mechanism includes PAK1 phosphorylation of a master corepressor C-terminal binding protein 1 (CtBP1) on S158 within its regulatory loop. PAK1 phosphorylation of CtBP1 inhibits its dehydrogenase function, accumulates CtBP1 in the cytoplasm, leading to the loss of CtBP1 corepressor function in the nucleus and consequently, stimulation of target genes (Fig. 3B) (Barnes et al., 2003). The significance of PAK1 regulation of CtBP1 is not limited to cancer biology as the PAK1–CtBP1 pathway also participates in the regulation of presynaptic neuronal control of muscle genes as PAK1 phosphorylation of CtBP1-S158 leads to its decruitment and loss of CtBP1-corepressive complex from its target genes such as myogenin and acetylcholine (Thomas et al., 2015) (Fig. 3B). The principle of PAK1-mediated derepression of target genes is presumed to have a wider implication in cancer biology because activated nuclear PAK1 interacts and phosphorylates chromatin-bound B-cell lymphoma-6 (BCL6), leading to the decruitment of the BCL6 repressor from target promoters and modulation of gene expression in colon cancer cells (Fig. 2B) (Barros, Lam, Jordan, & Matos, 2012). Because CtBP regulates a variety of cancerous phenotypes through specific molecular pathways (Chinnadurai, 2009), the PAK1-dependent phosphorylation of CtBP1 is being hypothesized to be an important upstream modifier of CtBP functions, at-large, in addition to gene expression (Fig. 3D).

In contrast to derepression of target genes, there are also examples of enhanced repression of target gene expression by PAK1 phosphorylation of corepressors (Fig. 3C). For example, PAK1 phosphorylation of EMT regulator Snail-S246 promotes its nuclear translocation and transcription repression of its target genes such as E-cadherin and aromatase (Yang, Rayala, et al., 2005). Another example of PAK1 participation in gene repression includes PAK1 phosphorylation of SHARP—a component of the NOTCH signaling, on S3486 and T3468, leading to further repression of NOTCH target genes in a PAK1-dependent manner (Vadlamudi, Manavathi, et al., 2005).

7. COORDINATED REGULATION OF TRANSLATION, TRANSCRIPTION, AND SPLICING

One of the most exciting frontiers in current science research is unlocking the nature of coordinated pathways that cumulatively regulate signal- and temporospatial-dependent homoeostasis in efficient and highly functional manners. Essential to cellular homeostasis is the efficient control of the gene expression machinery, which consists of three principal components each with its own control mechanism: nuclear transcription; precursor mRNA processing in the nucleus; and mRNA translation in the cytoplasm. Because signaling regulated cascades are primarily modulated by phosphorylation of target substrates, the notion of signaling-dependent coordinated regulation of cytoplasmic and nuclear components of gene expression were thought to be an important question for investigation. In this context, PAK1 signaling could regulate translation, transcription and splicing by phosphorylating a single novel coregulatory polyC-RNA binding protein 1 (PCBP1) on T60 and T127 in growth factor-stimulated eukaryotic cells (Meng et al., 2007). PAK1 activation leads to an increased accumulation of PCBP1 is the nucleus and its recruitment onto the promoter of eukaryotic translation initiation factor 4E (*eIF4E*), and an increased eIF4E expression in PAK1–PCBP1 dependent manner. Interestingly, this process is coordinately accomplished by derepression of translation inhibition due to release of unphosphorylated PCBP1 from the 3′-untranslated mRNA templates containing the DICE sequence. Because PAK1 interacts with several splicing proteins in a yeast two-hybrid screening (Meng et al., 2007), activated PAK1 was also found to promote pre-mRNA splicing from a CD44 splicing-minigene system in a PCBP1-dependent manner, and thus, revealing a role of PAK1 phosphorylation of PCBP1 in mRNA splicing. Since activated PAK1 exists in both cytoplasmic and nuclear compartments, PCBP1 could be phosphorylated PAK1 in both compartments. Therefore we suggest that PAK1 signaling could phosphorylate different pools of PCBP1 as well as promote the nuclear translocation of activated PCBP1 in a coordinated manner in growth factor stimulated cancer cells. The significance of these findings is that coordinated regulation of distinct components of gene expression machinery may ensure an economic biologic system while maintaining the reversibility of the phosphorylation cascade for controlling translation, transcription, and alternative splicing through a shared coregulator.

8. MODIFIER OF ErbB2- AND WNT-SIGNALING

The activation of Wnt-β-catenin signaling represents one of the most deregulated pathways in human cancer with components of the Wnt signaling—Wnt ligands, coreceptors and downstream targets being widely overexpressed or mutated in human cancer. The Wnt signaling targets downstream components through modifying the binding of β-catenin to lymphoid enhancing factor (LEF)/T-cell factor (TCF) transcriptional complex and resulting target gene expression. PAK1 phosphorylates β-catenin on S675 which promotes its stability, nuclear accumulation, transcription activity through the TCF/LEF complex (Zhu et al., 2012). As PAK1 activation leads to hyperactivated β-catenin and PAK1 overexpression correlates well with the levels of β-catenin in cancer cells, PAK1-β-catenin-S675 pathway may be required for a full Wnt signaling (Zhu et al., 2012). In addition to S675, PAK1 signaling also contributes to the transcription activity of β-catenin by phosphorylating S663 residue (Park et al., 2012). PAK1-mediated TCF/LEF transactivation could be effectively blocked by using phosphorylation-inactive mutants of β-catenin-S663A or –S675A or –S663A/S675A mutants; while phosphorylation mimicking mutants β-catenin-S675D or –S663D or –S663D/S675D stimulate TCF/LEF transactivation functions (Park et al., 2012). Because PAK1 is an important mediator of ErbB2 signaling in breast cancer cells stimulated by polypeptide growth factors (Adam et al., 1998; Wang, Shin, Wu, Friedman, & Arteaga, 2006) and given the fact that PAK1 phosphorylates β-catenin-S675 and S663 along with our understanding that ErbB2 signaling also targets and stabilizes β-catenin in human cancer (Ding et al., 2005), PAK1 was thought to be a potential mediatory component to connect ErbB2 signaling with β-catenin-S675. In this context, using MMTV-ErbB2-transgenic/PAK-knockout murine models, Arias-Romero et al. provided elegant evidence to support a role of PAK1 signaling in ErbB2-PAK1-β-catenin axis and its role in mammary gland tumorigenesis (Arias-Romero, Villamar-Cruz, Huang, Hoeflich, & Chernoff, 2013).

Similar to the PAK1 cancer biology, upon activation and nuclear translocation PAK4 phosphorylates β-catenin-S675 and promotes the transcriptional activity of the TCF/LEF complex in cancer cells (Li, Shao, et al., 2012). However, the function of PAK4 in cancer cells may be further modulated in a context-dependent manner as metastasis suppressor NDRG1 antagonizes transforming growth factor β-induced EMT by suppressing the nuclear localization of PAK4 as well as β-catenin-S33/S37 phosphorylation, implying a potential role of PAK4 in modulating β-catenin functions in prostate and colon cancer cells (Jin et al., 2014).

9. MODULATION OF ANGIOGENESIS SIGNALING

The process of angiogenesis is regulated by the combined action of tumor-derived secreted factors such as vascular endothelial growth factor (VEGF) acting on the endothelial cells as well as by endothelial-specific molecules or pathways. Growth factor stimulation of breast cancer cells leads to activation of ErbB2-PAK1 signaling which in-turn, upregulates the transcription, expression, and secretion of VEGF from epithelial cells and promotes angiogenesis in endothelial cells. Interestingly, ErbB2-mediated stimulation of VEGF expression as well as angiogenesis in endothelial cells could be effectively blocked by Herceptin, which targets ErbB2, as well as by dominant-negative PAK1 (Bagheri-Yarmand et al., 2000). Additional evidence of a possible role for PAK1 signaling in angiogenesis are derived from a peptide mimicking the proline-rich region of PAK1, showing that the PAK-peptide interacts with NCK and inhibits the migration of endothelial cells, tube-formation and angiogenesis in in vivo assays (Kiosses et al., 2002). Similarly, a 16-kDa prolactin fragment, which inhibits angiogenesis by blocking the migration of endothelial cells, also inhibits PAK1 activation and its accumulation at the leading edge in endothelial cells (Lee, Kunz, Lin, & Yu-Lee, 2007). Angiopoietin-1, a ligand for Dok receptors in endothelial cells, also stimulates PAK1 activity and promotes the recruitment of the Dok-R-Nck-Pak complex to the activated Tek receptor in endothelial cells (Master et al., 2001). Interestingly, endothelial-specific depletion of PAK2 suggests that PAK2 may be an important mediator of endothelial cell function more so than Pak1, as the loss of PAK2 in endothelial cells was associated with an embryonic lethality associated with defective formation of blood vessels. Further, PAK2 appears to be the major Pak isoforms in endothelial cells (Radu et al., 2015). PAK1 also phosphorylates Tie1 endothelial receptor tyrosine kinase on T794 and regulates vascular development in a zebrafish model (Reinardy et al., 2015). More recently, Zoledronic acid, an antitumor drug, has been shown to inhibit the expression of proangiogenic cytokines in ovarian cancer cells and angiogenesis in vivo murine models, through a mechanism involving PAK1/p38/MMP2 (Gonzalez-Villasana et al., 2015). In brief, PAK1 signaling may regulate angiogenesis at multiple levels involving cooperative interactions of pathways operating in both tumor and endothelial cells.

10. MODIFIER OF DNA DAMAGE RESPONSE AND RADIOSENSITIVITY

The sensitivity of cancer cells to the most widely used form of radiotherapy and other forms of chemotherapy that act by promoting DNA damage or preventing DNA repair, are influenced by the status of cell cycle, apoptotic vs cell survival signaling, growth factors, oncogenes and tumor suppressors, and signaling-dependent phosphorylation of molecules with roles in DDR. A previous study has shown PAK2 activation by ionizing radiation (IR) in leukemia cells (Roig & Traugh, 1999). In an effort to search for a broader impact of PAK1 signaling in DDR, the authors provided the first clue about the nature of genome-wide PAK1 targets that were also responsive to IR using the wild-type and PAK1-null fibroblasts as a model system (Motwani et al., 2013). This study identified about 199 genes that were differentially regulated by PAK1 as well as by IR. Interestingly, many such IR responsive, PAK1-dependent genes belong to the cell-cycle arrest, DNA repair, DNA replication, and cell death pathways; thus, opening up an exciting research avenue to explore the role of PAK1 signaling in DDR.

Because PAK1 signaling plays an important role in the survival of cancer cells, PAK1 signaling or its direct substrate(s) may counteract DNA damage-linked cell death and thus, postulated to contribute to DDR (Fig. 4A). Consistent with this hypothesis, Kumar and colleagues discovered that

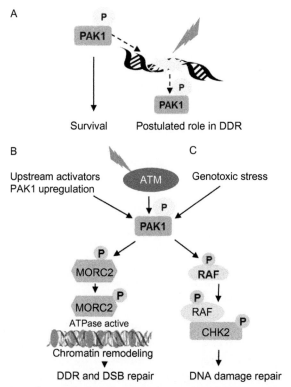

Fig. 4 PAK1 in DNA damage response. (A) PAK1 activation was postulated to be a component of DNA damage response. (B) PAK1 activation by IR or other pathways contributes to DDR and DNA repair through PAK1 phosphorylation-dependent ATPase activity feeding into chromatin remodeling. (C) Genotoxic stress-mediated PAK1 activation stimulates CRAF phosphorylation, leading to CHK2 activation and engagement, and DNA damage response as suggested by Advani et al. (2015). (See the color plate.)

the PAK1 signaling utilizes a novel substrate microrchidia CW-type zinc finger 2 (MORC2) to modulate the process of DNA repair following double-stranded DNA damage (Li, Nair, et al., 2012). It was found that IR stimulates PAK1 kinase activity in an ATM-dependent manner and promotes the accumulation of activated PAK1 in the nucleus and colocalization with MORC2, and thus, revealing a mechanistic role of PAK1 signaling in early DDR. At the molecular level, PAK1 phosphorylates MORC2-S739 and sequentially regulates phosphorylation-dependent MORC2's ATPase activity as well as downstream chromatin remodeling (Fig. 4B). Upon PAK1 signaling, MORC2-S739 contributes to the stimulation of γH2AX phosphorylation and DNA double-strand break (DSB) repair. The significance of PAK1-MORC2 signaling in DSB repair was further revealed with the observation that cells expressing phosphorylation inactive mutant MORC2-S739A exhibit an enhanced DNA damage and reduced clonogenic survival as compared to cells with the wild-type MORC2.

As the levels of PAK1 are upregulated in human cancer due to its widespread overexpression or amplification and the because PAK1 is a signaling nexus, Li et al. provided evidence to implicate a role of PAK1 activation, independent of IR/ATM pathway, in promoting the engagement of the PAK1–MORC2 axis during growth factor stimulation of γH2AX activation and DSB repair. These findings imply an interesting possibility that PAK1 activation may have an inherent role in protecting the genome against spontaneous DNA damage. We hypothesized that targeting the PAK1 phosphorylation site in MORC2 may turn-out to be a superior approach than targeting the PAK1 itself to enhance the sensitivity of cancer cells to DSB-inducing therapies.

The RAS family of GTPases represents one of most commonly overexpressed oncogenes in human cancer and confers cell survival and therapeutic resistance to tumor cells (Li, Luo, et al., 2012; Li, Nair, et al., 2012; Li, Shao, et al., 2012; Nazarian et al., 2010; Seguin et al., 2014; Wilson et al., 2012). In this context, Advani et al. discovered that CARF phosphorylation on Ser338 plays an essential role in protecting cancer cells from DNA damaging agents (Advani et al., 2015). The authors found that DNA damaging agents or genotoxic drug etoposide stimulates PAK1 activity as well as PAK1-mediated phosphorylation of CRAF-S338, resulting in the activation of and interaction with checkpoint kinase 2 and an enhanced DNA repair, conferring radio-resistance to DNA damaging agents (Advani et al., 2015). Consistent with a role of CRAF S338 phosphorylation in the noted modulation of radiosensitivity, targeting CRAF-S338 promoted IR-induced DNA damage (Fig. 4B). This offers another targeted opportunity to sensitize cancer cells to the DNA damaging therapeutics by targeting a specific PAK1 substrate.

In addition to exterior signals, mammalian cells experience spontaneous double-strand breaks which overtime could promote genomic instability—an important component of cancer development. Recent studies suggest that patient tumor cells show evidence of γH2AX phosphorylation, an indicator of DDR, suggesting the involvement of DNA repair pathways in the tumor pathobiology (Brustmann, Hinterholzer, & Brunner, 2011; Sedelnikova & Bonner, 2006; Warters, Adamson, Pond, & Leachman, 2005; Yu, MacPhail, Banath, Klokov, & Olive, 2006). Further, elevated levels of γH2AX are also proposed to be an indicator of poor prognosis in certain cancer subtypes (Brunner et al., 2011; Matthaios et al., 2012; Nagelkerke et al., 2011; Wasco & Pu, 2008). PAK1 overexpression in the primary esophageal small cell carcinomas correlates well with metastasis and reduced overall patient survival. The noted increased levels of γH2AX may offer circumstantial evidence to support a potential connection between the status and/or activation of PAK1 and DDR in human cancer (Gan et al., 2015). These findings suggest that PAK1 upregulation in human cancer may either protect the genome or promote genomic instability or paradoxically, participate in both processes in a context-dependent manner. These hypotheses are likely to be investigated in future mechanistic studies in cancer cell lines and further validate the resulting conclusions in human tumor specimens.

11. SIGNALING DEREGULATION, DEFECTIVE MITOTIC AND HUMAN CANCER

The process of tumor development is profoundly affected by the status of aberrant mitosis, centrosome amplification, DNA ploidy, and genomic instability. Aberrant mitosis may result, in–part, from deregulated segregation of chromosomes and encoded genomic information and abnormal MT dynamics. As mitosis involves signaling-dependent phosphorylation of regulatory proteins/complexes and because PAK1 overexpression in human cancer was just beginning to emerge in the late 1990s, the authors explored the impact of PAK1 overexpression upon mitotic events in human cancer cells. The rationale of these studies was also supported from studies in *Saccharomyces cerevisiae* and *Xenopus* showing the role of PAK homologs Ste20p and Cla4p in the cell-cycle progression and G2/M transition, respectively (Benton, Tinkelenberg, Gonzalez, & Cross, 1997; Cau et al., 2000;

Faure, Vigneron, Doree, & Morin, 1997; Faure et al., 1999; Verde, Wiley, & Nurse, 1998). For the first time, Kumar and colleagues demonstrated that inducible expression of hyperactivated PAK1 in human cancer cells leads to multipolar spindle orientations and centrosomes, revealing unfaithful segregation of mitotic spindles and chromosomes (Li et al., 2002)—all indicators of aberrant mitosis and aneuploidy. To this end, activated PAK1 accumulates in the nucleus before cells enter mitosis, PAK1 localizes on the chromosome during prophase, on centrosome in metaphase/anaphase cells, and on the mid-body in telophase cells in fibroblasts and human breast cancer cells. Further localization studies suggested that activated PAK1 transiently associates with kinetochores in an MT-dependent manner (Li et al., 2002). These early findings opened up a new research avenue to explore the significance of PAK1 activation in mitosis in mammalian and cancer cells.

The noted PAK1 phenotypes during mitosis were thought to be mediated by PAK1 putative substrates with a role in MT dynamics (Fig. 5). Accordingly, Li et al. used a cDNA expression library from G2/M synchronized HeLa cells to search for novel PAK1 substrates with roles in mitosis, and identified histone H3.3A as a novel PAK1 substrate (Li et al., 2002). Because histone 3.3A contains an additional first initiation codon for methionine and may or may not retain the first methionine, the

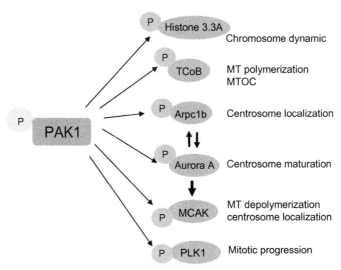

Fig. 5 PAK1 signaling regulates the process of mitosis at multiple levels by phosphorylating its downstream effectors and their cross-regulation. (See the color plate.)

study chose to refer the histone H3.3A as histone H3. As histone H3 phosphorylation is essential for chromosome condensation and cell cycle (Cheung, Allis, & Sassone-Corsi, 2000), PAK1 signaling or more specifically its mitotic substrates such as H3.3A/H3 may be involved in the condensation or other aspects of chromosomes during mitosis (Fig. 5). Interestingly, another family member PAK2 also phosphorylates histone H4-Ser47 to facilitate the formation of H3.3–H4 nucleosome by during DNA replication (Kang et al., 2011). PAK1 signaling also regulates the spindle assembly during mouse oocyte meiotic maturation (Lin et al., 2010). Similar to PAK1, another family member, PAK2, is also recruited to G2 centrosomes and participates in mitotic spindle orientation (Bompard et al., 2013; Nekrasova & Minden, 2011).

Mitotic Cdk2 kinase phosphorylates PAK1 on T212 in fibroblasts and affects postmitotic cell spreading (Thiel et al., 2002). Because cell spreading is regulated by MT dynamics, PAK1 modulates the formation of astral microtubules during metaphase (Banerjee, Worth, Prowse, & Nikolic, 2002). As mitosis is affected by the MT dynamics and stabilizing/ destabilizing proteins, PAK1 signaling may also regulate mitotic MT dynamics. For example, PAK1 phosphorylation of TCoB-S65 and S128 supports the polymerization of newly synthesized MT (Fig. 4). Interestingly, experimental depletion of PAK1 or TCoB could impair MT polymerization while TCoB overexpression leads to multiple MTOCs phenotypes (Vadlamudi, Barnes, et al., 2005)—a phenotype earlier noticed in breast cancer cells with catalytically active PAK1 (Vadlamudi et al., 2000). As PAK1 colocalizes with TCoB on MTs and centrosomes, hyperactive PAK1 signaling may also utilize TCoB to confer multipolar gamma-tubulin containing MTOC phenotypes in human cancer cells (Vadlamudi, Barnes, et al., 2005). More recently, PAK1 phosphorylation of MT-destabilizing protein, the mitotic centromere-associated kinesin (MCAK), on S192 and S111 regulates MCAK's depolymerization activity on MT and centrosome localization (Pakala, Nair, Reddy, & Kumar, 2012).

Although PAK1 resides on centrosomes (Li et al., 2002), the mechanism of PAK1 activation at the centrosome remains unclear until Zhao et al. found that PAK1 became activated in fibroblasts by binding to GIT1/PIX in a GTPase-independent manner. Once activated, PAK1 interacts with and phosphorylates Aurora-A on T288 and S342, playing a role in centrosome maturation (Zhao, Lim, Ng, Lim, & Manser, 2005). Molecular insights of PAK1 activation during mitosis suggest that PAK1 activation in prophase in MDCK II cells depends on Cdk1 phosphorylation of Tiam1-S1466, that in-turn, activates the Rac pathway (Whalley et al., 2015). However, the observed Tiam1-Rac-PAK signaling during mitosis was independent of Aurora-A in MDCK II cells. It is possible that the noted differences in the dependency of PAK1 activation on GTPases in these two studies may be due to the use of distinct model systems and experimental conditions.

In addition to the above molecules, PAK1 signaling in mitotic cells also utilizes Arpc1b, a novel PAK1 substrate identified from the cDNA library prepared from mitotic HeLa cells. Overexpression of Arpc1b, but not its PAK1 phosphorylation-defective Arpc1b-T21A, leads to abnormal centrosome amplification in cancer cells—mimicking the phenotypes previously observed with PAK1 hyperactivation (Vadlamudi et al., 2000). Surprisingly, overexpression of Arpc1b but not Arpc1b-T21A in both PAK1 and PAK1-null cells leads to centrosome amplification and multipolar spindles, suggesting that Arpc1b-T21 may be phosphorylated in PAK1-null cells by a mitotic kinase other than PAK1. To this context, Arpc1b localizes onto centrosomes with Aurora-A, stimulates Aurora-A kinase activity, and successively, Aurora-A phosphorylates Arpc1b on T21 and regulates the cell-cycle progression through mitosis (Molli et al., 2010). These findings revealed a new mitotic function of Arpc1b, independent of its role in the Arp2/3 complex. In addition to PAK1, Arpc1b can be also phosphorylated by Aurora-A and may participate in the mitotic functions of Aurora-A in mammalian cells (Fig. 5). The role of PAK1 signaling in spindle polarity may be further underlined by its ability to phosphorylate both MCAK and Aurora-A (Fig. 5) (Pakala et al., 2012; Zhao et al., 2005). It is interesting to note that Aurora-A can also phosphorylate MCAK, a complex dynamic that ultimately leads to successful spindle bipolarity (Braun et al., 2014; Zhang, Ems-McClung, & Walczak, 2008). In addition, PAK1 signaling may also modulate mitotic progression by modulating the activity of polo-like kinase 1 during mitosis (Maroto, Ye, von Lohneysen, Schnelzer, & Knaus, 2008). Although we have learned a great deal of new knowledge about the significance of PAK1 signaling in orchestrating multiple processes during mitosis in mammalian cells since the original demonstration of a defective mitosis by activated PAK1, one of the continuing gaps in this area is the lack of an integrated model inclusive of PAK1's upstream activators and known effectors in the context of MT dynamics during mitosis in human cancer cells.

12. REGULATION OF NUCLEAR RECEPTOR SIGNALING AND HORMONAL RESPONSE

As PAK1 is amplified and overexpressed in breast cancer (Kumar et al., 2006), PAK1 hyperactivation by upstream signals in estrogen receptor-α (ERα)-positive breast cancer cells is accompanied by PAK1 stimulation of ERα-S305 phosphorylation. PAK1 regulation of ERα phosphorylation enhances ER's transactivation activity on its target genes (ie, cyclin D1) in the absence of a ligand for ER (Rayala, Molli, & Kumar, 2006; Tharakan, Lepont, Singleton, Kumar, & Khan, 2008; Wang et al., 2002). PAK1 stimulation of cyclin D1 expression in cultured cells also requires NF-κB pathway (Balasenthil, Barnes, Rayala, & Kumar, 2004) and could be experimentally achieved by the expression of phosphorylation mimicking ERα-S305E mutant (Balasenthil, Sahin, et al., 2004). Interestingly, PAK1 and cyclin D1 are located on the 11q13–q14 region that is frequently amplified in breast tumors (Bekri et al., 1997). The levels of PAK1 and cyclin D1 are co-upregulated in human breast tumors (Balasenthil, Barnes, et al., 2004; Bostner et al., 2007).

In addition to serine and threonine phosphorylation, PAK1 phosphorylation on Y153, T201, and T285 by JAK2 kinase also regulates PAK1's nuclear translocation and stimulation of *cyclin D1* promoter activity in prolactin-stimulated cells (Tao et al., 2011). Because PAK1 regulation of ER's transactivation is achieved in the absence of estrogen stimulation of ERα, PAK1 overexpression or hyperactivation in ERα-positive breast cancer cells or breast tumors is accomplished by the development of ERα-independent phenotypes (Fig. 6A). Consistent with this finding, patients with ERα-positive breast tumors with the nuclear PAK1 tend to be insensitive to tamoxifen treatment as compared to breast tumors without nuclear PAK1 (Holm et al., 2006).

Interestingly, the level of nuclear PAK1 increases progressively from hyperplasia to carcinoma to adenocarcinoma in a murine model of spontaneous breast tumors driven by the polyoma-middle T-antigen (Wang, Zhang, Balasenthil, Medina, & Kumar, 2006). Therefore, both PAK1 overexpression and its nuclear localization may be associated with a reduced response to tamoxifen and the development of hormone-independence phenotype (Bostner et al., 2007; Rayala, Talukder, et al., 2006). Consistent with a role of nuclear PAK1 in the development of hormone-independent phenotypes, an analysis of 912 tumors from node-negative breast cancer

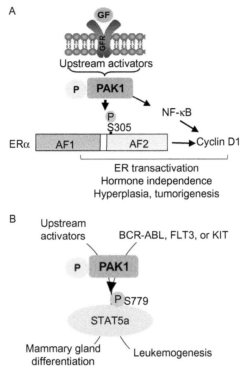

Fig. 6 PAK1 phosphorylation of ER and STAT5a. (A) PAK1 phosphorylation of ER-S305 stimulates its transactivation activity, target gene expression, and resulting associated functions. (B) PAK1 phosphorylation of STAT5a-S779 modulates its transcription activity and differentiation in mammary epithelial cells. In addition, stimulation of PAK1>STAT5-Ser779 regulates leukemogenesis by BCR-ABL, FLT3, or KIT oncogenes. (See the color plate.)

patients treated with or without tamoxifen demonstrated that tamoxifen therapy may not be sufficient for patients with breast tumors with PAK1 and phosphorylated ERα-S305 and further suggests that PAK1 localization may also have some prognostic value in breast cancer (Bostner et al., 2010). However, in contrast to breast tumors, there is no relationship between the levels of activated nuclear PAK1 and survival of glioblastoma patients while the levels of activated PAK1 in the cytoplasm correlated well with a shorter survival of patients (Aoki et al., 2007).

Hormone response of breast cancer cells is also modulated by PAK1 phosphorylation of ERα coactivators which help in the recruitment of ER-coactivator complexes to the target chromatin. PAK1 phosphorylation of coactivator NRIF3-S28 stimulates its coactivator activity for ERα transactivation activity, presumably due to cooperative interaction between

NRIF3-S28 and ERα-S305 (Talukder et al., 2008); estrogen induces the expression of DLC1 which interacts with ERα to stimulate its transactivation activity in ligand-stimulated breast cancer cells (Rayala et al., 2005). Interestingly, a DLC1 interacting protein Cip-interacting zinc finger protein 1 (Ciz1) is also an estrogen inducible gene and stimulates ERα transactivation activity (den Hollander & Kumar, 2006; den Hollander, Rayala, Coverley, & Kumar, 2006), suggesting that DLC1–Ciz1 may be involved in amplifying ERα transaction functions in ERα positive breast cancer cells with PAK1 overexpression.

Another PAK family member, the PAK6, regulates the function of the androgen receptor (AR), a molecule important in the development of prostate cancer. Specifically, PAK6 interacts with AR and translocate PAK6 to the nucleus along with AR upon androgen stimulation of prostate cancer cells. However, as opposed to PAK1 stimulation of ERα transactivation, PAK6 inhibits AR's transactivation activity (Yang et al., 2001). PAK6 phosphorylation of AR-S578 enhances its degradation by E3-ligase Mdm2 in ligand-stimulated cells, implying an inhibitory role of PAK6 in the biology of prostate cancer. In addition, experimental downregulation of PAK6 enhances the growth of prostate tumor xenografts and cytoplasmic PAK6 status may be inversely related with the level of AR in prostate cancer cells (Liu, Busby, et al., 2013; Liu, Li, et al., 2013; Liu, Liu, et al., 2013).

13. SIGNALING, MAMMARY GLAND DEVELOPMENT, AND BREAST CANCER

The first conclusive evidence of a suggestive role of PAK1 hyperactivation in breast cancer biology came from physiologically relevant whole animal systems. Expression of catalytically active PAK1 under the control of a developmentally regulated beta-lactoglobulin promoter in mammary glands leads to apocrine metaplasia and hyperplasia (Wang et al., 2002) as well as intra-ductal tumors, adenoma, and malignant breast tumors in older animals (Wang, Zhang, et al., 2006). Consistent with a role of PAK1 signaling in breast cancer progression, the levels of PAK1 gradually increases as a function of tumor grades in breast cancer patients (Holm et al., 2006; Van Tine and Ellis, 2011). In contrast to studies with catalytically active PAK1, expression of a dominant-negative PAK1-mutant transgene in mammary glands leads to a defective lobuloalveolar morphogenesis and differentiation. Mechanistically, these phenotypic effects of PAK1 were at least in–part, due to the loss of STAT5-S779 phosphorylation by PAK1 (Wang, Vadlamudi, et al., 2003). Thus PAK1 phosphorylation of Stat5a-S779 regulates its transcription activity in mammary epithelial cells. These studies suggest a role of PAK1 signaling in the normal alveolar morphogenesis and lactation during mammary gland development (Fig. 6B). Interestingly, the PAK1-STAT5a axis also plays an important role in leukemogenesis (Fig. 6B) as PAK1 controls the nuclear accumulation of STAT5 in response to oncogenic BCR-ABL (Berger et al., 2014) or FLT3- and KIT pathways (Chatterjee et al., 2014).

14. CLINICOPATHOLOGICAL FEATURES IN HUMAN CANCER

As emphasized throughout our review, PAK family members have been found to be overexpressed and/or hyperactivated in human cancers (Table 1). In general, increased PAK1 activity promotes a number of cancer hallmarks including cancer initiation, growth and spread, and ultimately progression to more aggressive phenotypes. Among the group I and group II PAKs, PAK1 and PAK4 have emerged as highly studied family members in cancer (Table 1). For example, PAK1 gene amplification and/or transcription, but not exclusively other group elements, are upregulated in breast cancer (Wang, Zhang, et al., 2006), ovarian carcinoma (Schraml et al., 2003), colorectal carcinoma (Li, Zheng, et al., 2010), uveal melanoma (Pavey et al., 2006), hepatocellular carcinoma (Ching et al., 2007), renal cell carcinoma (O'Sullivan et al., 2007), bladder cancer (Huang et al., 2015), upper urinary tract cancer (Kamai et al., 2010), gastric carcinoma (Wang, Zhou, Zou, Ren, & Zhang, 2010), prostate cancer (Al-Azayzih, Gao, & Somanath, 2015), oral carcinomas (Tu et al., 2011), non-small cell lung cancer (Ong et al., 2011), skin cancer (Chow et al., 2012), and endometrial cancer (Lu, Qu, et al., 2013). More recently, polymorphism in *PAK1* gene has been also documented in certain ethnic population that might be susceptible to lung cancer (Zheng et al., 2015). In general, PAK1 expression closely correlates with the clinicopathologic features of human cancer such as enhanced tumorigenicity, invasion, metastasis, decreased therapeutic response and poor prognosis (Table 1). In addition to PAK1, other members of the PAK family, including PAK2-6, are now understood to be upregulated or amplified in human cancer and are positively associated with the development and progression of cancer, as well as with poor clinical outcomes (Table 1). However, it is noteworthy to mention that as opposed to the general expression of PAKs, PAK6 is downregulated in hepatocellular carcinoma (Liu, Liu, et al., 2015) and clear cell renal cell cancer (Liu et al., 2014), exerting a tumor suppressor function; thus, reflects the complexity of cancer biology in a context-dependent manner.

14.1 Inflammation-Driven Cancers

In recent years, it is increasingly accepted that persistent stress or inflammation may be an important modifier of early stages of cancer development in some if not all organ systems (Coussens, Zitvogel, & Palucka, 2013; Marx, 2004). Because of the central role of PAK1 signaling in modulating cell survival including the NF-κB pathway, a target and component of proinflammatory cytokines, PAK1 signaling is just beginning to find a place in inflammation-driven cancer. Interestingly, PAK1 activation has been well documented in inflammatory pathologic conditions such as rheumatoid arthritis and asthma (McFawn et al., 2003; Neumann, Foryst-Ludwig, Klar, Schweitzer, & Naumann, 2006). The case of PAK1 signaling and inflammation-driven cancer is best exemplified by inflammatory bowel diseases (IBD) and colitis-associated cancer (CAC) which are largely driven by NF-κB target genes and cytokines which in-turn amplify PAK1 activation and the resulting signals (reviewed by Dammann, Khare, & Gasche, 2014). For example, in addition to activating the NF-κB pathway, *Helicobacter pylori* infection also leads to the stimulation of PAK1 activity and resulting responses. Interestingly, *H. pylori* infection stimulates a direct interaction between the PAK1 and NF-κB-inducing kinase (NIK) (Neumann et al., 2006).

More recently, Khare et al. revealed a role of PAK1 signaling in the action of mesalamine (5-aminosalicylic acid, 5-ASA), a drug used in the treatment of ulcerative colitis. The authors found that the levels of PAK1 expression and activation increases from IBD and CAC as well as stimulation of the survival signaling cascades as compared to the respective levels of these endpoints in normal mucosa (Khare et al., 2015). Treatment with 5-ASA interferes with the level of PAK1 activation and its ability to interact with β-catenin. A number of NF-κB target cytokines, including TNFα, stimulate PAK1 activation as well as NF-κB activation in intestinal organoids derived from the wild-type mice but not from *Pak1*-null mice, with these events effectively blocked by kinase-dead PAK1 in model systems. TNFα also increases PAK1 activation in intestinal organoids from the wild-type but not PAK1-null mice; PAK1 upregulation promotes an enhanced PAK1-p65/c-Rel interaction associated with NF-κB transactivation activity in a kinase-dependent manner. The significance of PAK1 in IBD and CAC is also supported by the finding that PAK1-mediated inhibition of PPARγ in these models could be effectively rescued by 5-ASA treatment while keeping PAK1 activation inhibited (Dammann et al., 2015). These studies suggest a role of PAK1 or its effector components in inflammatory cascades relevant to the development of IBD and CAC.

14.2 Amplification

PAK1 resides at the 11q13–q14 amplicon in the company of other onco-genes such as CCND1, EMSY, FGF4, GARP, FGF3, FGF19, RSF1, GAB2, RAD9A, RPS6KB2 (Wilkerson & Reis-Filho, 2013). Interestingly, many of the genes are co-overexpressed with PAK1, in addition to cyclin D1 in human cancer. While characterizing the details of the 11q13–11q14 region which is commonly amplified in ERα-positive meta-static breast cancer, Bekri et al. identified a core 350-kb interest region within the 11q13–q14 amplicon and placed the *Pak1, Cbp2, Uvrag,* and *Clns1a* genes within this region (Bekri et al., 1997). Breast tumors with an amplified 11q13–q14 amplicon have a tendency to metastasize and are resistant to tamoxifen antihormone therapy (Bostner et al., 2007). In addition to breast cancer, the 11q13–q14 amplicon was found to be frequently amplified in human cancer including ovarian, liver, oral squamous cell carcinoma, and esophageal cancer (Brown et al., 2006; Chattopadhyay et al., 2010; Huang, Gollin, Raja, & Godfrey, 2002; Schraml et al., 2003; Zucman-Rossi, Villanueva, Nault, & Llovet, 2015). Because tumorigenesis is a mutagenic process involving coamplification and mutations of multiple genes or amplicons, one must not exclude the possibility of functional interactions between PAK1 amplification with other coamplified genes or amplicons. For example, the 11q13 region in certain breast cancers is coamplified with the 8p12 amplicon which contains 4EBP1 oncogene (Karlsson et al., 2011). In this context, it is worthwhile to note that PAK1 signaling regulates the transcription of 4EBP1 through phosphorylation of PCBP1 coregulator (Meng et al., 2007).

A recent proteomic analysis suggests that breast as well as head and neck cancer cells with an amplified 11q13 amplicon also exhibit differential expression of three cancer-relevant membrane proteins (Hoover et al., 2015). These proteins include myoepithelial-associated desmosomal cadherin DSG3 associated with myoepithelial cells; TGF-β coreceptor CD109, which is differentially expressed during early stages of tumori-genesis, and also upregulated in triple-negative breast cancer (TNBC)

(Tao, Li, Li, & Yang, 2014) and pancreatic cancer (Haun, Fan, Mackintosh, Zhao, & Tackett, 2014); and CD14 differentiation marker, which was previously thought be expressed in monocytes and tumor-associated macrophages (Ziegler-Heitbrock & Ulevitch, 1993). These findings raise the exciting possibility that PAK1 signaling may be preferentially coregulated by signals initiated through these newly identified membrane proteins. Based on these observations and yet-to-be discovered additional cell membranous proteins, we suggest that PAK1-dependent cancer progression is likely to be dependent on coregulated genes localized on the q11.13–q14 and coamplified amplicons.

14.3 Co-overexpression

Although PAK1 was the first family member found to be frequently upregulated in human cancer, PAK2 and PAK4 are also widely overexpressed in human cancer as per the analysis carried out using the cBioPortal database (Cerami et al., 2012; Gao et al., 2013). However the extent of PAK's overexpression varies widely across cancer types and depends on the nature of the dataset and the specific study used in a given analysis. In the cBioPortal database, PAK1 is the most upregulated family member in ovarian and breast cancer, PAK2 is the most upregulated family member in esophageal and lung cancer, and PAK4 is the most upregulated family member in uterine and ovarian cancer (Fig. 7). Furthermore, PAKs are frequently mutated in human cancer (Fig. 8), though the functional significance of naturally occurring mutations in PAK family remains poorly understood unclear at this time. As of November 8, 2015, no mutations have been found in PAK1's seven autophosporylation sites (Ser21, Ser57, Ser144, Ser149, Ser198, Ser203, and Thr423) in human cancer with the exception of a rare amino acid change in Ser203 (AA Change: R203W) in colon cancer as per the cBioPortal database.

In general, PAK overexpression in human cancer appears to be due to gene amplification or mRNA upregulation, or both. In this context, the availability of mRNA, copy number variations and sequencing data from the same tumor has allowed us to tentatively conclude that PAKs are upregulated in human cancer with or without gene amplification and more than one PAK family member(s) may be co-upregulated in the same tumor (Fig. 9, representative examples). The authors believe that this is a highly relevant point for the clinical development of PAK-inhibitors as the issue of co-overexpression of PAKs opens up a debate about the therapeutic

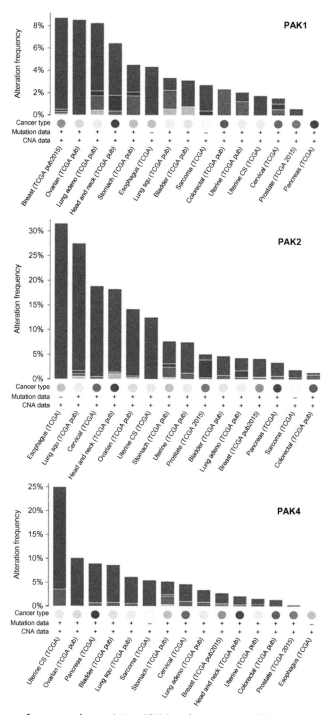

Fig. 7 Status of copy number variation (CNV) and mutations in PAK1, PAK2, and PAK4 in 15 human cancers as analyzed using the cBioPortal database. (See the color plate.)

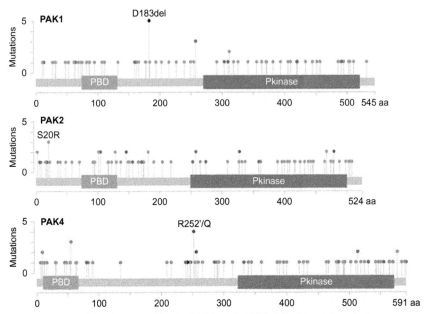

Fig. 8 Mutational landscape of PAK1, PAK2, and PAK4. Point mutations in human cancer as reported in cBioPortal database. Missense mutations are in green, truncating mutations are shown in red, and different mutations at the same ratio are in purple. (See the color plate.)

efficacy of targeting a selective PAK family member vs cotargeting PAKs, and thus, likely to influence the development of a selective vs a dual or Pan PAK-inhibitor for cancer.

15. CANCER THERAPEUTICS ADVANCES

Positioned at the intersection of multiple signal transduction pathways, the PAK family members play an essential role in many human disorders including cancer, mental retardation and allergy, suggesting a role for PAKs as potentially drug targets for various illnesses (Table 5). Yi et al. discerned the development of therapeutic targets of PAK1 by dividing them into two generations (Yi, Maksimoska, Marmorstein, & Kissil, 2010). Early attempts to explore PAK inhibitors were based on the similarities among ATP-bind kinase domains and led to the development of competitive ATP inhibitors such as staurosporine and its derivatives, K252a and CEP-1347 (Kaneko et al., 1997; Nheu et al., 2002; Yi et al., 2010). Following these earlier efforts, in the next phase, instead of focusing on developing

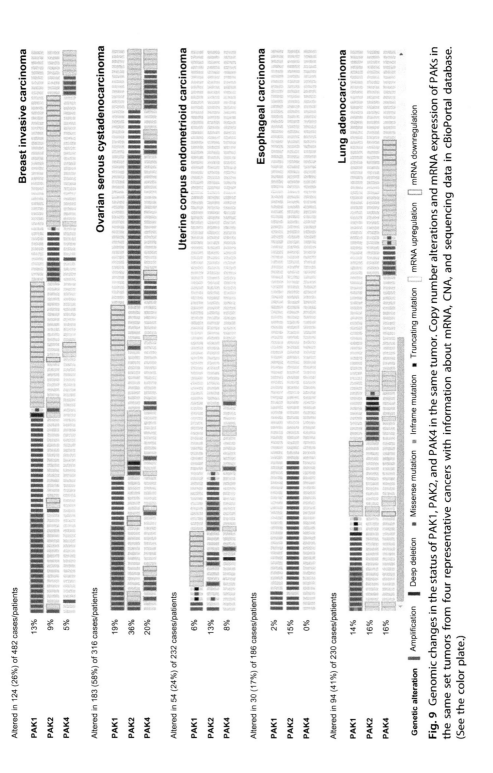

Fig. 9 Genomic changes in the status of PAK1, PAK2, and PAK4 in the same tumor. Copy number alterations and mRNA expression of PAKs in the same set tumors from four representative cancers with information about mRNA, CNA, and sequencing data in cBioPortal database. (See the color plate.)

broad range kinase inhibitors, more attention was paid to search for PAK-specific inhibitors, such as OSU-03012 (Zhu et al., 2004). More recently, attempts were also made to develop selective PAK1 inhibitors by applying the knowledge of structure–functional relationships and small-molecule screenings (Yi et al., 2010).

As oncogenic RAS mutations are detected in about 30% of all human cancers and more than 90% in human pancreatic cancers, it is highly desirable to develop "signal therapeutics" to selectively inhibit or reverse aberrantly activated RAS signaling pathways. As an essential effector for RAS-mediated signaling pathway, PAK1 is often chosen as a therapeutic target for RAS-driven tumors. For example, FK228 or combined tyrosine kinase inhibitors have been shown to inhibit RAS-induced PAK1 activation and rescue Capan-1 human pancreatic cancer xenograft, as well as hormone-independent proliferation of MDA-MB-231 cells resistant to FK228 (Hirokawa et al., 2007). Three additional direct or indirect PAK1 inhibitors, FK228, a CAPE (caffeic acid phenethyl ester)-based propolis extract called "Bio 30" and an ARC (artepillin C)-based green propolis extract (GPE), have been used to treat neurofibromatosis (NF), tuberous sclerosis (TSC), breast and pancreatic cancers (Maruta, 2011). In addition, a list of herbal derived inhibitors of PAK1 are summarized by Hiroshi Maruta in 2014 (Maruta, 2014). More recently, Nguyen et al. has explored the effectiveness of a simple methodology to quickly identify and assess the potency of PAK1 inhibitors by using a combination of immunoprecipitation and a kinase assay (Nguyen, Be Tu, Tawata, & Maruta, 2015).

In addition to radioresistance, upregulation or hyperactivation of PAKs has been implicated to enhanced resistance to chemotherapy and molecular targeting therapy. For instance, elevated PAK1 expression in colorectal cancer cells associates with chemosensitivity to 5-fluorouracil (5-FU) (Qing et al., 2012) and resistance to PI3K inhibitors. Similarly, PAK1 upregulation in B-cell lymphomas and pancreatic cancer cells also contributes to the development of resistance to PI3K inhibitors (Walsh et al., 2013) and MET inhibitors (Zhou et al., 2014), respectively. Likewise, an aberrant expression or activation of PAK4 results in resistance to docetaxel, paclitaxel, and doxorubicin in prostate cancer (Park et al., 2013), cisplatin (CDDP) in gastric cancer (Fu et al., 2014) and cervical cancer (Shu et al., 2015), as well as gemcitabine in pancreatic cancer (Moon et al., 2015). Consistently, PAK4 harboring a somatic mutation, E329K, exhibits increased kinase activity and confers resistance to competitive ATP inhibitors (Whale, Dart, Holt, Jones, & Wells, 2013). In addition, PAK5 upregulation leads to resistance to paclitaxel in epithelial ovarian cancer (Li, Yao, & Zhang, 2013) and mediates cisplatin resistance in esophageal squamous carcinoma cells (He et al., 2014) and hepatocellular carcinoma cells (Zhang et al., 2015). However, gain-of-function mutations in PAK5 enhance activation of the ERK pathway in non-small cell lung cancer and thus, lung cancer cells with PAK5 mutation are sensitive to MEK inhibition (Fawdar et al., 2013). In the same vein, PAK6 inhibits chemosensitivity of prostate cancer cells to docetaxel (Wen et al., 2009) and increases chemoresistance of patients with colon cancer to 5-FU based chemotherapy (Chen et al., 2015).

With PAK1 correlating well with cell survival and therapeutic resistance, targeting PAK1 (and perhaps other family members), as well as PAK1 substrates, represents an obvious next generation of approaches to sensitive cancer cells to IR and genotoxic agents. In addition to serine and threonine phosphorylation, IR also increases PAK1 activity via JAK2-dependent tyrosine phosphorylation of PAK1 (Kim, Youn, et al., 2014). From the therapeutic point of view, IR-induced PAK1 tyrosine phosphorylation could be blocked by pharmacological inhibition of JAK2 by TG101209, which also enhances radiosensitivity of lung cells to IR (Kim, Youn, et al., 2014). It remains unclear whether JAK2 targeting by TG101209 in IR-exposed tumors utilizes IR-regulated pathways other than PAK1. Similarly, PAK1 targeting by β-elemene or the PAK1 inhibitor IPA-3 enhances radiosensitivity of gastric cancer cells to IR-induced apoptosis (Liu, Che, et al., 2015). Similar to PAK1, experimental inhibition of PAK6 also sensitizes prostate cancer cells to IR-induced cell death (Zhang et al., 2010).

Positioned at the intersection of multiple signal transduction pathways, the PAK family members are essentially involved in several human disorders including, cancer, mental retardation, and allergy, and this make the PAKs as potentially drug targets for these illnesses (Table 5). Yi et al. discerned the development of therapeutic targets of PAK1 by dividing them into two generations (Yi et al., 2010). Early attempts to explore PAKs inhibitors were based on the similarities among ATP-bind kinase domains and led to the development of competitive ATP inhibitors such as staurosporine and its derivative K252a and CEP-1347 (Kaneko et al., 1997; Nheu et al., 2002; Yi et al., 2010). In the next phase, instead of focusing on developing a broad range kinase inhibitors, more attention was paid to search for PAK-specific inhibitors, such as OSU-03012 (Zhu et al., 2004). Recently, attempts were also made to develop selective PAK1 inhibitors by applying the knowledge of structure–functional relationship and small-molecule screening (Yi et al., 2010).

Taken together, dysregulation of PAK signaling in human cancer is closely linked with cellular resistance to radiotherapy, chemotherapy, and molecular target therapy. Therefore, targeting PAKs is likely to sensitize cancer cells to radiotherapy or chemotherapy and PAK-directed therapies are promising candidates for combinational target therapeutics.

16. CONCLUSIONS AND PROSPECTIVE

Since the initial placement of PAK1 on the amplified q11.13–q14 amplicon in conjunction with the recognition of a mechanistic role of PAK1 signaling in controlling the invasiveness on cancer cells upon ErbB2 stimulation and PAK1 upregulation in breast cancer, we have gained substantial insight into the nature of effector substrates and downstream cascades that are responsible for executing tumorigenic properties of PAK1 pathway. These advancements have allowed PAK1 to emerge as one of most frequently upregulated pathways in human cancer, bring interest in the role of other PAK family members in cancer biology, and evolve the PAK family as cancer therapeutic targets.

The PAK1 pathway promotes the process of cancer progression by using a variety of cellular strategies including cytoskeleton remodeling to generate motile structures, degrading extracellular matrix via proteases, promoting cell survival while antagonizing apoptotic pathways, promoting angiogenesis, phosphorylating effector substrates, and modulating the expression of gene products with regulatory roles in cancer progression, and metastasis. Below, the authors have put together a partial list of the major advances in the area of PAKs in human cancer:

- Upregulation of the PAK1 pathway in human cancer could be with or without amplification of the 11q.13-11.4 amplicon; PAK1 hyperactivation by upstream activators or yet-to-be functionally characterized mutations.
- Among PAK family, PAK1, PAK2, and PAK5 are overexpressed in human cancer; human cancer may have co-overexpression of more than one family member in the same tumors.
- PAK1 integrates a variety of cancer-relevant signals triggered by cell membrane receptors and molecules proximal to the cell membrane.
- PAK1 is at the nexus of phenotypic signaling and feed into cellular processes leading to several hallmarks of cancer progression and metastasis.

- PAK1 signaling promotes tumorigenesis by phosphorylating its down-stream substrates which were previously thought to be involved in actin- or MT-based cytoskeleton remodeling.
- PAK1 signaling plays an inherent role the development of the mammary gland and confers a hormone-independent phenotype to ERα-positive breast cancer cells and breast tumors.
- Upon stimulation with appropriate signals, activated PAK translocates to the nucleus, interacts with the chromatin—often as a complex with a DNA-binding protein, and modulates the expression of target genes.
- Activated PAK1 regulates gene expression as a result of cross talks with other signaling pathways, phosphorylating DNA-binding factors, or regulating the nuclear translocation of its substrates.
- The hyperactivated PAK1 pathway in cancer cells leads to a defective mitosis and multipolar spindle orientations; PAK localizes on the centro-some; PAK's mitotic functions might be also affected by PAK-phosphorylation of mitotic proteins.
- PAK1 signaling participates in the DDR and targeting PAK may enhance the sensitivity of cancer cells to IR or other chemotherapy.
- Targeting PAK may be particularly beneficial in cells with certain activated pathways, especially in-combination of other targeted therapeutics.

Looking at the progress made since its cloning and connection with human cancer, the nature of tools available, and the knowledge acquired during the last two decades, the authors anticipate that the PAK family will continue to influence cancer biology and therapeutics and shape the future oncobiology in a significant manner. The following is a partial list of postulated advances in PAK-centered cancer research in the coming decade.

- Further advancement of the concept of codependent and/or coordi-nated regulation of different arms of PAK action to gain insights in PAK-regulated cancer phenotypes.
- New facets of PAKs nuclear signaling and functions in cancer and normal cells.
- Identification and characterization of cancer relevant, class-specific substrates of groups I and II PAKs.
- Insights into the off-mechanisms of group II PAKs and how exactly these PAKs respond to extra- and intracellular signals.
- As the scientific community continues to develop PAK-isoform specific inhibitors, we may start witnessing the clinical development of PAN

and/or multifunctional PAK-inhibitors because most of human tumors co-overexpress more than one PAKs.

- Because the PAK1 phosphorylation site in several substrates with roles in tumorigenesis could be also phosphorylated by kinases other than PAK1, we anticipate an enhanced focus for targeting PAK-phosphorylation site(s) of effector substrates rather than PAKs per se. For example, ERα-S305 and β-catenin-S675 are activated by PAK1 and PKA, and Arpc1b-T21 phosphorylated by PAK1 and Aurora-A.
- Status of nuclear PAK1 activation and its specific substrates as potential determinants of radio- or chemosensitivity in cancer therapy; targeting PAK1 or its selective substrates to overcome resistance to DNA damaging agents.
- Since NF-κB is at the center of innate immunity and given the fact that NF-κB signaling and functions are comodulated by PAK1, PAK1 or its targets may have a role in immune surveillance and the tumor escape mechanism.
- Inflammation-driven cancer may soon join the rapidly growing list of candidate human cancers with PAK's overexpression for PAK-directed therapies.
- Potential influence of PAK-signaling nodule on gut microbiome in appropriate models to better appreciate the role of PAK signaling into inflammation-driven cancer.
- More integration of spontaneous animal tumor models to evaluate the efficacy of PAK-directed therapies and less reliance on the cell culture-based preclinical development.
- As certain plants or plant-derived materials inhibit the PAK activity and exhibit antitumor properties, we might see substantial progress in the development of phyto-derived anticancer agents for PAK-overexpressed tumors.
- The PAK-directed therapies may advance into the clinical setting, perhaps in combination with other pathway-directed therapies or radiation. And components of PAK-pathways may emerge as bystander endpoints of other targeted therapies.

ACKNOWLEDGMENTS

We are indebted to several of our colleagues in the field whose deserving work could not be discussed here due to space limitations. The authors thank the previous and current lab members of Prof. Kumar and Prof. Li's Laboratories for their contributions to the PAK field and for assisting in the preparation of this chapter. We gratefully appreciate the

support by the National Institutes of Health grants CA090970 (to R.K.), and the National Natural Science Foundation of China (Nos. 81372847 and 81572584), the Program for Professor of Special Appointment (Eastern Scholar) at Shanghai Institutions of Higher Learning (No. 2013-06), and the Innovation Program of Shanghai Municipal Education Commission (No. 2015ZZ007) (to D.Q.L.).
Conflict of Interest: The authors declare no potential conflict of interest.

REFERENCES

Acconcia, F., Barnes, C. J., Singh, R. R., Talukder, A. H., & Kumar, R. (2007). Phosphorylation-dependent regulation of nuclear localization and functions of integrin-linked kinase. *Proceedings of the National Academy of Sciences of the United States of America, 104,* 6782–6787.

Adam, L., Vadlamudi, R., Kondapaka, S. B., Chernoff, J., Mendelsohn, J., & Kumar, R. (1998). Heregulin regulates cytoskeletal reorganization and cell migration through the p21-activated kinase-1 via phosphatidylinositol-3 kinase. *The Journal of Biological Chemistry, 273,* 28238–28246.

Adam, L., Vadlamudi, R., Mandal, M., Chernoff, J., & Kumar, R. (2000). Regulation of microfilament reorganization and invasiveness of breast cancer cells by kinase dead p21-activated kinase-1. *The Journal of Biological Chemistry, 275,* 12041–12050.

Advani, S. J., Camargo, M. F., Seguin, L., Mielgo, A., Anand, S., Hicks, A. M., et al. (2015). Kinase-independent role for CRAF-driving tumour radioresistance via CHK2. *Nature Communications, 6,* 8154.

Ahmed, T., Shea, K., Masters, J. R., Jones, G. E., & Wells, C. M. (2008). A PAK4-LIMK1 pathway drives prostate cancer cell migration downstream of HGF. *Cellular Signalling, 20,* 1320–1328.

Ahn, H. K., Jang, J., Lee, J., Se Hoon, P., Park, J. O., Park, Y. S., et al. (2011). P21-activated kinase 4 overexpression in metastatic gastric cancer patients. *Translational Oncology, 4,* 345–349.

Akinmade, D., Talukder, A. H., Zhang, Y., Luo, W. M., Kumar, R., & Hamburger, A. W. (2008). Phosphorylation of the ErbB3 binding protein Ebp1 by p21-activated kinase 1 in breast cancer cells. *British Journal of Cancer, 98,* 1132–1140.

Al-Azayzih, A., Gao, F., & Somanath, P. R. (2015). P21 activated kinase-1 mediates transforming growth factor β1-induced prostate cancer cell epithelial to mesenchymal transition. *Biochimica et Biophysica Acta, 1853,* 1229–1239.

Aoki, H., Yokoyama, T., Fujiwara, K., Tari, A. M., Sawaya, R., Suki, D., et al. (2007). Phosphorylated Pak1 level in the cytoplasm correlates with shorter survival time in patients with glioblastoma. *Clinical Cancer Research, 13,* 6603–6609.

Arias-Romero, L. E., Villamar-Cruz, O., Huang, M., Hoeflich, K. P., & Chernoff, J. (2013). Pak1 kinase links ErbB2 to β-catenin in transformation of breast epithelial cells. *Cancer Research, 73,* 3671–3682.

Asthana, J., Kuchibhatla, A., Jana, S. C., Ray, K., & Panda, D. (2012). Dynein light chain 1 (LC8) association enhances microtubule stability and promotes microtubule bundling. *The Journal of Biological Chemistry, 287,* 40793–40805.

Bagheri-Yarmand, R., Mandal, M., Taludker, A. H., Wang, R. A., Vadlamudi, R. K., Kung, H. J., et al. (2001). Etk/Bmx tyrosine kinase activates Pak1 and regulates tumorigenicity of breast cancer cells. *The Journal of Biological Chemistry, 276,* 29403–29409.

Bagheri-Yarmand, R., Mazumdar, A., Sahin, A. A., & Kumar, R. (2006). LIM kinase 1 increases tumor metastasis of human breast cancer cells via regulation of the urokinase-type plasminogen activator system. *International Journal of Cancer, 118,* 2703–2710.

Bagheri-Yarmand, R., Vadlamudi, R. K., Wang, R. A., Mendelsohn, J., & Kumar, R. (2000). Vascular endothelial growth factor up-regulation via p21-activated kinase-1 signaling regulates heregulin-beta1-mediated angiogenesis. *The Journal of Biological Chemistry*, *275*, 39451–39457.

Bagrodia, S., Taylor, S. J., Creasy, C. L., Chernoff, J., & Cerione, R. A. (1995). Identification of a mouse p21Cdc42/Rac activated kinase. *The Journal of Biological Chemistry*, *270*, 22731–22737.

Balasenthil, S., Barnes, C. J., Rayala, S. K., & Kumar, R. (2004). Estrogen receptor activation at serine 305 is sufficient to upregulate cyclin D1 in breast cancer cells. *FEBS Letters*, *567*, 243–247.

Balasenthil, S., Sahin, A. A., Barnes, C. J., Wang, R. A., Pestell, R. G., Vadlamudi, R. K., et al. (2004). p21-Activated kinase-1 signaling mediates cyclin D1 expression in mammary epithelial and cancer cells. *The Journal of Biological Chemistry*, *279*, 1422–1428.

Banerjee, M., Worth, D., Prowse, D. M., & Nikolic, M. (2002). Pak1 phosphorylation on t212 affects microtubules in cells undergoing mitosis. *Current Biology*, *12*, 1233–1239.

Banko, M. R., Allen, J. J., Schaffer, B. E., Wilker, E. W., Tsou, P., White, J. L., et al. (2011). Chemical genetic screen for AMPKα2 substrates uncovers a network of proteins involved in mitosis. *Molecular Cell*, *44*, 878–892.

Barnes, C. J., Vadlamudi, R. K., Mishra, S. K., Jacobson, R. H., Li, F., & Kumar, R. (2003). Functional inactivation of a transcriptional corepressor by a signaling kinase. *Nature Structural Biology*, *10*, 622–628.

Barros, P., Lam, E. W., Jordan, P., & Matos, P. (2012). Rac1 signalling modulates a STAT5/BCL-6 transcriptional switch on cell-cycle-associated target gene promoters. *Nucleic Acids Research*, *40*, 7776–7787.

Bastea, L. I., Doppler, H., Pearce, S. E., Durand, N., Spratley, S. J., & Storz, P. (2013). Protein kinase D-mediated phosphorylation at Ser99 regulates localization of p21–activated kinase 4. *The Biochemical Journal*, *455*, 251–260.

Begum, A., Imoto, I., Kozaki, K., Tsuda, H., Suzuki, E., Amagasa, T., et al. (2009). Identification of PAK4 as a putative target gene for amplification within 19q13.12-q13.2 in oral squamous-cell carcinoma. *Cancer Science*, *100*, 1908–1916.

Bekri, S., Adelaide, J., Merscher, S., Grosgeorge, J., Caroli-Bosc, F., Perucca-Lostanlen, D., et al. (1997). Detailed map of a region commonly amplified at 11q13–>q14 in human breast carcinoma. *Cytogenetics and Cell Genetics*, *79*, 125–131.

Belletti, B., Nicoloso, M. S., Schiappacassi, M., Berton, S., Lovat, F., Wolf, K., et al. (2008). Stathmin activity influences sarcoma cell shape, motility, and metastatic potential. *Molecular Biology of the Cell*, *19*, 2003–2013.

Benton, B. K., Tinkelenberg, A., Gonzalez, I., & Cross, F. R. (1997). Cla4p, a Saccharomyces cerevisiae Cdc42p-activated kinase involved in cytokinesis, is activated at mitosis. *Molecular and Cellular Biology*, *17*, 5067–5076.

Berger, A., Hoelbl-Kovacic, A., Bourgeais, J., Hoefling, L., Warsch, W., Grundschober, E., et al. (2014). PAK-dependent STAT5 serine phosphorylation is required for BCR-ABL-induced leukemogenesis. *Leukemia*, *28*, 629–641.

Bokoch, G. M. (2003). Biology of the p21-activated kinases. *Annual Review of Biochemistry*, *72*, 743–781.

Bompard, G., Rabeharivelo, G., Cau, J., Abrieu, A., Delsert, C., & Morin, N. (2013). P21–activated kinase 4 (PAK4) is required for metaphase spindle positioning and anchoring. *Oncogene*, *32*, 910–919.

Bostner, J., Ahnstrom Waltersson, M., Fornander, T., Skoog, L., Nordenskjold, B., & Stal, O. (2007). Amplification of CCND1 and PAK1 as predictors of recurrence and tamoxifen resistance in postmenopausal breast cancer. *Oncogene*, *26*, 6997–7005.

Bostner, J., Skoog, L., Fornander, T., Nordenskjold, B., & Stal, O. (2010). Estrogen receptor-alpha phosphorylation at serine 305, nuclear p21-activated kinase 1 expression, and response to tamoxifen in postmenopausal breast cancer. *Clinical Cancer Research, 16*, 1624–1633.

Braun, A., Dang, K., Buslig, F., Baird, M. A., Davidson, M. W., Waterman, C. M., et al. (2014). Rac1 and Aurora A regulate MCAK to polarize microtubule growth in migrating endothelial cells. *The Journal of Cell Biology, 206*, 97–112.

Brown, L. A., Irving, J., Parker, R., Kim, H., Press, J. Z., Longacre, T. A., et al. (2006). Amplification of EMSY, a novel oncogene on 11q13, in high grade ovarian surface epithelial carcinomas. *Gynecologic Oncology, 100*, 264–270.

Brown, L. A., Kalloger, S. E., Miller, M. A., Shih Ie, M., McKinney, S. E., Santos, J. L., et al. (2008). Amplification of 11q13 in ovarian carcinoma. *Genes, Chromosomes & Cancer, 47*, 481–489.

Brunner, A. H., Hinterholzer, S., Riss, P., Heinze, G., Weiss, K., & Brustmann, H. (2011). Expression of γ-H2AX in endometrial carcinomas: An immunohistochemical study with p53. *Gynecologic Oncology, 121*, 206–211.

Brustmann, H., Hinterholzer, S., & Brunner, A. (2011). Expression of phosphorylated histone H2AX (γ-H2AX) in normal and neoplastic squamous epithelia of the uterine cervix: An immunohistochemical study with epidermal growth factor receptor. *International Journal of Gynecological Pathology, 30*, 76–83.

Buday, L., & Downward, J. (2007). Roles of cortactin in tumor pathogenesis. *Biochimica et Biophysica Acta, 1775*, 263–273.

Cai, S., Chen, R., Li, X., Cai, Y., Ye, Z., Li, S., et al. (2015). Downregulation of microRNA-23a suppresses prostate cancer metastasis by targeting the PAK6-LIMK1 signaling pathway. *Oncotarget, 6*, 3904–3917.

Cai, D., Iyer, A., Felekkis, K. N., Near, R. I., Luo, Z., Chernoff, J., et al. (2003). AND-34/BCAR3, a GDP exchange factor whose overexpression confers antiestrogen resistance, activates Rac, PAK1, and the cyclin D1 promoter. *Cancer Research, 63*, 6802–6808.

Cai, X. Z., Wang, J., Li, X. D., Wang, G. L., Liu, F. N., Cheng, M. S., et al. (2009). Curcumin suppresses proliferation and invasion in human gastric cancer cells by down-regulation of PAK1 activity and cyclin D1 expression. *Cancer Biology & Therapy, 8*, 1360–1368.

Cai, S., Ye, Z., Wang, X., Pan, Y., Weng, Y., Lao, S., et al. (2015). Overexpression of P21-activated kinase 4 is associated with poor prognosis in non-small cell lung cancer and promotes migration and invasion. *Journal of Experimental & Clinical Cancer Research, 34*, 48.

Callow, M. G., Clairvoyant, F., Zhu, S., Schryver, B., Whyte, D. B., Bischoff, J. R., et al. (2002). Requirement for PAK4 in the anchorage-independent growth of human cancer cell lines. *The Journal of Biological Chemistry, 277*, 550–558.

Carter, J. H., Douglass, L. E., Deddens, J. A., Colligan, B. M., Bhatt, T. R., Pemberton, J. O., et al. (2004). Pak-1 expression increases with progression of colorectal carcinomas to metastasis. *Clinical Cancer Research, 10*, 3448–3456.

Cau, J., Faure, S., Vigneron, S., Labbe, J. C., Delsert, C., & Morin, N. (2000). Regulation of Xenopus p21-activated kinase (X-PAK2) by Cdc42 and maturation-promoting factor controls Xenopus oocyte maturation. *The Journal of Biological Chemistry, 275*, 2367–2375.

Cerami, E., Gao, J., Dogrusoz, U., Gross, B. E., Sumer, S. O., Aksoy, B. A., et al. (2012). The cBio cancer genomics portal: An open platform for exploring multidimensional cancer genomics data. *Cancer Discovery, 2*, 401–404.

Chantaravisoot, N., Wongkongkathep, P., Loo, J. A., Mischel, P. S., & Tamanoi, F. (2015). Significance of filamin A in mTORC2 function in glioblastoma. *Molecular Cancer, 14*, 127.

Chatterjee, A., Ghosh, J., Ramdas, B., Mali, R. S., Martin, H., Kobayashi, M., et al. (2014). Regulation of Stat5 by FAK and PAK1 in oncogenic FLT3- and KIT-driven leukemogenesis. *Cell Reports, 9,* 1333–1348.

Chattopadhyay, I., Singh, A., Phukan, R., Purkayastha, J., Kataki, A., Mahanta, J., et al. (2010). Genome-wide analysis of chromosomal alterations in patients with esophageal squamous cell carcinoma exposed to tobacco and betel quid from high-risk area in India. *Mutation Research, 696,* 130–138.

Chen, S., Auletta, T., Dovirak, O., Hutter, C., Kuntz, K., El-ftesi, S., et al. (2008). Copy number alterations in pancreatic cancer identify recurrent PAK4 amplification. *Cancer Biology & Therapy, 7,* 1793–1802.

Chen, L., Liu, H., Liu, J., Zhu, Y., Xu, L., He, H., et al. (2013). Klotho endows hepatoma cells with resistance to anoikis via VEGFR2/PAK1 activation in hepatocellular carcinoma. *PloS One, 8,* e58413.

Chen, J., Lu, H., Yan, D., Cui, F., Wang, X., Yu, F., et al. (2015). PAK6 increase chemoresistance and is a prognostic marker for stage II and III colon cancer patients undergoing 5-FU based chemotherapy. *Oncotarget, 6,* 355–367.

Chen, H., Miao, J., Li, H., Wang, C., Li, J., Zhu, Y., et al. (2014). Expression and prognostic significance of p21-activated kinase 6 in hepatocellular carcinoma. *The Journal of Surgical Research, 189,* 81–88.

Cheung, P., Allis, C. D., & Sassone-Corsi, P. (2000). Signaling to chromatin through histone modifications. *Cell, 103,* 263–271.

Ching, Y. P., Leong, V. Y., Lee, M. F., Xu, H. T., Jin, D. Y., & Ng, I. O. (2007). P21-activated protein kinase is overexpressed in hepatocellular carcinoma and enhances cancer metastasis involving c-Jun NH2-terminal kinase activation and paxillin phosphorylation. *Cancer Research, 67,* 3601–3608.

Chinnadurai, G. (2009). The transcriptional corepressor CtBP: A foe of multiple tumor suppressors. *Cancer Research, 69,* 731–734.

Chow, H. Y., Jubb, A. M., Koch, J. N., Jaffer, Z. M., Stepanova, D., Campbell, D. A., et al. (2012). p21-Activated kinase 1 is required for efficient tumor formation and progression in a Ras-mediated skin cancer model. *Cancer Research, 72,* 5966–5975.

Cotteret, S., & Chernoff, J. (2005). Pak GITs to Aurora-A. *Developmental Cell, 9,* 573–574.

Cotteret, S., & Chernoff, J. (2006). Nucleocytoplasmic shuttling of Pak5 regulates its antiapoptotic properties. *Molecular and Cellular Biology, 26,* 3215–3230.

Cotteret, S., Jaffer, Z. M., Beeser, A., & Chernoff, J. (2003). p21-Activated kinase 5 (Pak5) localizes to mitochondria and inhibits apoptosis by phosphorylating BAD. *Molecular and Cellular Biology, 23,* 5526–5539.

Coussens, L. M., Zitvogel, L., & Palucka, A. K. (2013). Neutralizing tumor-promoting chronic inflammation: A magic bullet? *Science, 339,* 286–291.

Dadke, D., Fryer, B. H., Golemis, E. A., & Field, J. (2003). Activation of p21-activated kinase 1-nuclear factor kappaB signaling by Kaposi's sarcoma-associated herpes virus G protein-coupled receptor during cellular transformation. *Cancer Research, 63,* 8837–8847.

Dammann, K., Khare, V., & Gasche, C. (2014). Tracing PAKs from GI inflammation to cancer. *Gut, 63,* 1173–1184.

Dammann, K., Khare, V., Lang, M., Claudel, T., Harpain, F., Granofszky, N., et al. (2015). PAK1 modulates a PPARγ/NF-κB cascade in intestinal inflammation. *Biochimica et Biophysica Acta, 1853,* 2349–2360.

Daub, H., Gevaert, K., Vandekerckhove, J., Sobel, A., & Hall, A. (2001). Rac/Cdc42 and p65PAK regulate the microtubule-destabilizing protein stathmin through phosphorylation at serine 16. *The Journal of Biological Chemistry, 276,* 1677–1680.

Davis, S. J., Sheppard, K. E., Pearson, R. B., Campbell, I. G., Gorringe, K. L., & Simpson, K. J. (2013). Functional analysis of genes in regions commonly amplified in high-grade serous and endometrioid ovarian cancer. *Clinical Cancer Research, 19,* 1411–1421.

Deacon, S. W., Beeser, A., Fukui, J. A., Rennefahrt, U. E., Myers, C., Chernoff, J., et al. (2008). An isoform-selective, small-molecule inhibitor targets the autoregulatory mechanism of p21-activated kinase. *Chemistry & Biology*, *15*, 322–331.

Deguchi, A., Miyoshi, H., Kojima, Y., Okawa, K., Aoki, M., & Taketo, M. M. (2010). LKB1 suppresses p21-activated kinase-1 (PAK1) by phosphorylation of Thr109 in the p21-binding domain. *The Journal of Biological Chemistry*, *285*, 18283–18290.

den Hollander, P., & Kumar, R. (2006). Dynein light chain 1 contributes to cell cycle progression by increasing cyclin-dependent kinase 2 activity in estrogen-stimulated cells. *Cancer Research*, *66*, 5941–5949.

den Hollander, P., Rayala, S. K., Coverley, D., & Kumar, R. (2006). Ciz1, a novel DNA-binding coactivator of the estrogen receptor alpha, confers hypersensitivity to estrogen action. *Cancer Research*, *66*, 11021–11029.

Ding, Q., Xia, W., Liu, J. C., Yang, J. Y., Lee, D. F., Xia, J., et al. (2005). Erk associates with and primes GSK-3beta for its inactivation resulting in upregulation of beta-catenin. *Molecular Cell*, *19*, 159–170.

Edwards, D. C., Sanders, L. C., Bokoch, G. M., & Gill, G. N. (1999). Activation of LIM-kinase by Pak1 couples Rac/Cdc42 GTPase signalling to actin cytoskeletal dynamics. *Nature Cell Biology*, *1*, 253–259.

Eggers, C. M., Kline, E. R., Zhong, D., Zhou, W., & Marcus, A. I. (2012). STE20-related kinase adaptor protein α (STRADα) regulates cell polarity and invasion through PAK1 signaling in LKB1-null cells. *The Journal of Biological Chemistry*, *287*, 18758–18768.

Fang, Z. P., Jiang, B. G., Gu, X. F., Zhao, B., Ge, R. L., & Zhang, F. B. (2014). P21-activated kinase 5 plays essential roles in the proliferation and tumorigenicity of human hepatocellular carcinoma. *Acta Pharmacologica Sinica*, *35*, 82–88.

Faure, S., Vigneron, S., Doree, M., & Morin, N. (1997). A member of the Ste20/PAK family of protein kinases is involved in both arrest of Xenopus oocytes at G2/prophase of the first meiotic cell cycle and in prevention of apoptosis. *The EMBO Journal*, *16*, 5550–5561.

Faure, S., Vigneron, S., Galas, S., Brassac, T., Delsert, C., & Morin, N. (1999). Control of G2/M transition in Xenopus by a member of the p21-activated kinase (PAK) family: A link between protein kinase A and PAK signaling pathways? *The Journal of Biological Chemistry*, *274*, 3573–3579.

Fawdar, S., Trotter, E. W., Li, Y., Stephenson, N. L., Hanke, F., Marusiak, A. A., et al. (2013). Targeted genetic dependency screen facilitates identification of actionable mutations in FGFR4, MAP3K9, and PAK5 in lung cancer. *Proceedings of the National Academy of Sciences of the United States of America*, *110*, 12426–12431.

Fu, X., Feng, J., Zeng, D., Ding, Y., Yu, C., & Yang, B. (2014). PAK4 confers cisplatin resistance in gastric cancer cells via PI3K/Akt- and MEK/Erk-dependent pathways. *Bioscience Reports*. Epub ahead of print [PMID: 24471762].

Galisteo, M. L., Chernoff, J., Su, Y. C., Skolnik, E. Y., & Schlessinger, J. (1996). The adaptor protein Nck links receptor tyrosine kinases with the serine-threonine kinase Pak1. *The Journal of Biological Chemistry*, *271*, 20997–21000.

Gan, J., Zhang, Y., Ke, X., Tan, C., Ren, H., Dong, H., et al. (2015). Dysregulation of PAK1 is associated with DNA damage and is of prognostic importance in primary esophageal small cell carcinoma. *International Journal of Molecular Sciences*, *16*, 12035–12050.

Gao, J., Aksoy, B. A., Dogrusoz, U., Dresdner, G., Gross, B., Sumer, S. O., et al. (2013). Integrative analysis of complex cancer genomics and clinical profiles using the cBioPortal. *Science Signaling*, *6*, pl1.

Gao, C., Ma, T., Pang, L., & Xie, R. (2014). Activation of P21-activated protein kinase 2 is an independent prognostic predictor for patients with gastric cancer. *Diagnostic Pathology*, *9*, 55.

Gavard, J., & Gutkind, J. S. (2006). VEGF controls endothelial-cell permeability by promoting the beta-arrestin-dependent endocytosis of VE-cadherin. *Nature Cell Biology*, *8*, 1223–1234.

Goc, A., Al-Azayzih, A., Abdalla, M., Al-Husein, B., Kavuri, S., Lee, J., et al. (2013). P21 activated kinase-1 (Pak1) promotes prostate tumor growth and microinvasion via inhibition of transforming growth factor β expression and enhanced matrix metalloproteinase 9 secretion. *The Journal of Biological Chemistry*, *288*, 3025–3035.

Gong, W., An, Z., Wang, Y., Pan, X., Fang, W., Jiang, B., et al. (2009). P21-activated kinase 5 is overexpressed during colorectal cancer progression and regulates colorectal carcinoma cell adhesion and migration. *International Journal of Cancer*, *125*, 548–555.

Gonzalez-Villasana, V., Fuentes-Mattei, E., Ivan, C., Dalton, H. J., Rodriguez-Aguayo, C., Fernandez-de Thomas, R. J., et al. (2015). Rac1/Pak1/p38/MMP-2 axis regulates angiogenesis in ovarian cancer. *Clinical Cancer Research*, *21*, 2127–2137.

Goto, H., Tanabe, K., Manser, E., Lim, L., Yasui, Y., & Inagaki, M. (2002). Phosphorylation and reorganization of vimentin by p21-activated kinase (PAK). *Genes to Cells*, *7*, 91–97.

Gu, J., Li, K., Li, M., Wu, X., Zhang, L., Ding, Q., et al. (2013). A role for p21-activated kinase 7 in the development of gastric cancer. *The FEBS Journal*, *280*, 46–55.

Gu, X., Wang, C., Wang, X., Ma, G., Li, Y., Cui, L., et al. (2015). Efficient inhibition of human glioma development by RNA interference-mediated silencing of PAK5. *International Journal of Biological Sciences*, *11*, 230–237.

Guo, Q., Su, N., Zhang, J., Li, X., Miao, Z., Wang, G., et al. (2014). PAK4 kinase-mediated SCG10 phosphorylation involved in gastric cancer metastasis. *Oncogene*, *33*, 3277–3287.

Gururaj, A., Barnes, C. J., Vadlamudi, R. K., & Kumar, R. (2004). Regulation of phosphoglucomutase 1 phosphorylation and activity by a signaling kinase. *Oncogene*, *23*, 8118–8127.

Hammer, A., & Diakonova, M. (2015). Tyrosyl phosphorylated serine-threonine kinase PAK1 is a novel regulator of prolactin-dependent breast cancer cell motility and invasion. *Advances in Experimental Medicine and Biology*, *846*, 97–137.

Hammer, A., Rider, L., Oladimeji, P., Cook, L., Li, Q., Mattingly, R. R., et al. (2013). Tyrosyl phosphorylated PAK1 regulates breast cancer cell motility in response to prolactin through filamin A. *Molecular Endocrinology*, *27*, 455–465.

Han, K., Zhou, Y., Gan, Z. H., Qi, W. X., Zhang, J. J., Fen, T., et al. (2014). p21-Activated kinase 7 is an oncogene in human osteosarcoma. *Cell Biology International*, *38*, 1394–1402.

Hao, S., Luo, C., Abukiwan, A., Wang, G., He, J., Huang, L., et al. (2015). miR-137 inhibits proliferation of melanoma cells by targeting PAK2. *Experimental Dermatology*, *24*, 947–952. http://dx.doi.org/10.1111/exd.12812.

Haun, R. S., Fan, C. Y., Mackintosh, S. G., Zhao, H., & Tackett, A. J. (2014). CD109 overexpression in pancreatic cancer identified by cell-surface glycoprotein capture. *Journal of Proteomics and Bioinformatics*, Suppl 10, S10003.

He, S., Feng, M., Liu, M., Yang, S., Yan, S., Zhang, W., et al. (2014). P21-activated kinase 7 mediates cisplatin-resistance of esophageal squamous carcinoma cells with Aurora-A overexpression. *PloS One*, *9*, e113989.

He, H., Hirokawa, Y., Levitzki, A., & Maruta, H. (2000). An anti-Ras cancer potential of PP1, an inhibitor specific for Src family kinases: In vitro and in vivo studies. *Cancer Journal*, *6*, 243–248.

He, H., Levitzki, A., Zhu, H. J., Walker, F., Burgess, A., & Maruta, H. (2001). Platelet-derived growth factor requires epidermal growth factor receptor to activate p21-activated kinase family kinases. *The Journal of Biological Chemistry*, *276*, 26741–26744.

Hirokawa, Y., Levitzki, A., Lessene, G., Baell, J., Xiao, Y., Zhu, H., et al. (2007). Signal therapy of human pancreatic cancer and NF1-deficient breast cancer xenograft in mice by a combination of PP1 and GL-2003, anti-PAK1 drugs (Tyr-kinase inhibitors). *Cancer Letters*, *245*, 242–251.

Hirokawa, Y., Tikoo, A., Huynh, J., Utermark, T., Hanemann, C. O., Giovannini, M., et al. (2004). A clue to the therapy of neurofibromatosis type 2: NF2/merlin is a PAK1 inhibitor. *Cancer Journal, 10,* 20–26.

Ho, H., Aruri, J., Kapadia, R., Mehr, H., White, M. A., & Ganesan, A. K. (2012). RhoJ regulates melanoma chemoresistance by suppressing pathways that sense DNA damage. *Cancer Research, 72,* 5516–5528.

Holderness Parker, N., Donninger, H., Birrer, M. J., & Leaner, V. D. (2013). p21-activated kinase 3 (PAK3) is an AP-1 regulated gene contributing to actin organisation and migration of transformed fibroblasts. *PloS One, 8,* e66892.

Holm, C., Rayala, S., Jirstrom, K., Stal, O., Kumar, R., & Landberg, G. (2006). Association between Pak1 expression and subcellular localization and tamoxifen resistance in breast cancer patients. *Journal of the National Cancer Institute, 98,* 671–680.

Hoover, H., Li, J., Marchese, J., Rothwell, C., Borawoski, J., Jeffery, D. A., et al. (2015). Quantitative proteomic verification of membrane proteins as potential therapeutic targets located in the 11q13 amplicon in cancers. *Journal of Proteome Research, 14,* 3670–3679.

Hsu, E. C., Kulp, S. K., Huang, H. L., Tu, H. J., Salunke, S. B., Sullivan, N. J., et al. (2015). Function of integrin-linked Kinase in modulating the stemness of IL-6-abundant breast cancer cells by regulating γ-secretase-mediated Notch1 activation in caveolae. *Neoplasia, 17,* 497–508.

Hu, X., Guo, J., Zheng, L., Li, C., Zheng, T. M., Tanyi, J. L., et al. (2013). The heterochronic microRNA let-7 inhibits cell motility by regulating the genes in the actin cytoskeleton pathway in breast cancer. *Molecular Cancer Research, 11,* 240–250.

Huang, K., Chen, G., Luo, J., Zhang, Y., & Xu, G. (2015). Clinicopathological and cellular signature of PAK1 in human bladder cancer. *Tumour Biology, 36,* 2359–2368.

Huang, X., Gollin, S. M., Raja, S., & Godfrey, T. E. (2002). High-resolution mapping of the 11q13 amplicon and identification of a gene, TAOS1, that is amplified and overexpressed in oral cancer cells. *Proceedings of the National Academy of Sciences of the United States of America, 99,* 11369–11374.

Huang, Z., Traugh, J. A., & Bishop, J. M. (2004). Negative control of the Myc protein by the stress-responsive kinase Pak2. *Molecular and Cellular Biology, 24,* 1582–1594.

Ichigotani, Y., Yokozaki, S., Fukuda, Y., Hamaguchi, M., & Matsuda, S. (2002). Forced expression of NESH suppresses motility and metastatic dissemination of malignant cells. *Cancer Research, 62,* 2215–2219.

Ito, M., Nishiyama, H., Kawanishi, H., Matsui, S., Guilford, P., Reeve, A., et al. (2007). P21-activated kinase 1: A new molecular marker for intravesical recurrence after transurethral resection of bladder cancer. *The Journal of Urology, 178,* 1073–1079.

Iyer, S. C., Gopal, A., & Halagowder, D. (2015). Myricetin induces apoptosis by inhibiting P21 activated kinase 1 (PAK1) signaling cascade in hepatocellular carcinoma. *Molecular and Cellular Biochemistry, 407,* 223–237.

Jagadeeshan, S., Krishnamoorthy, Y. R., Singhal, M., Subramanian, A., Mavuluri, J., Lakshmi, A., et al. (2015). Transcriptional regulation of fibronectin by p21-activated kinase-1 modulates pancreatic tumorigenesis. *Oncogene, 34,* 455–464.

Jha, R. K., & Strauss, C. E. (2012). 3D structure analysis of PAKs: A clue to the rational design for affinity reagents and blockers. *Cellular Logistics, 2,* 69–77.

Jin, R., Liu, W., Menezes, S., Yue, F., Zheng, M., Kovacevic, Z., et al. (2014). The metastasis suppressor NDRG1 modulates the phosphorylation and nuclear translocation of β-catenin through mechanisms involving FRAT1 and PAK4. *Journal of Cell Science, 127,* 3116–3130.

Jung, I. D., Lee, J., Lee, K. B., Park, C. G., Kim, Y. K., Seo, D. W., et al. (2004). Activation of p21-activated kinase 1 is required for lysophosphatidic acid-induced focal adhesion kinase phosphorylation and cell motility in human melanoma A2058 cells. *European Journal of Biochemistry, 271,* 1557–1565.

Kamai, T., Shirataki, H., Nakanishi, K., Furuya, N., Kambara, T., Abe, H., et al. (2010). Increased Rac1 activity and Pak1 overexpression are associated with lymphovascular invasion and lymph node metastasis of upper urinary tract cancer. *BMC Cancer, 10*, 164. http://dx.doi.org/10.1186/1471-2407-10-164.

Kaneko, M., Saito, Y., Saito, H., Matsumoto, T., Matsuda, Y., Vaught, J. L., et al. (1997). Neurotrophic 3,9-bis[(alkylthio)methyl]-and-bis(alkoxymethyl)-K-252a derivatives. *Journal of Medicinal Chemistry, 40*, 1863–1869.

Kang, B., Pu, M., Hu, G., Wen, W., Dong, Z., Zhao, K., et al. (2011). Phosphorylation of H4 Ser 47 promotes HIRA-mediated nucleosome assembly. *Genes & Development, 25*, 1359–1364.

Karlsson, E., Waltersson, M. A., Bostner, J., Perez-Tenorio, G., Olsson, B., Hallbeck, A. L., et al. (2011). High-resolution genomic analysis of the 11q13 amplicon in breast cancers identifies synergy with 8p12 amplification, involving the mTOR targets S6K2 and 4EBP1. *Genes, Chromosomes & Cancer, 50*, 775–787.

Kaur, R., Liu, X., Gjoerup, O., Zhang, A., Yuan, X., Balk, S. P., et al. (2005). Activation of p21-activated kinase 6 by MAP kinase kinase 6 and p38 MAP kinase. *The Journal of Biological Chemistry, 280*, 3323–3330.

Kaur, R., Yuan, X., Lu, M. L., & Balk, S. P. (2008). Increased PAK6 expression in prostate cancer and identification of PAK6 associated proteins. *Prostate, 68*, 1510–1516.

Kesanakurti, D., Chetty, C., Rajasekhar Maddirela, D., Gujrati, M., & Rao, J. S. (2012). Functional cooperativity by direct interaction between PAK4 and MMP-2 in the regulation of anoikis resistance, migration and invasion in glioma. *Cell Death & Disease, 3*, e445.

Khare, V., Dammann, K., Asboth, M., Krnjic, A., Jambrich, M., & Gasche, C. (2015). Overexpression of PAK1 promotes cell survival in inflammatory bowel diseases and colitis-associated cancer. *Inflammatory Bowel Diseases, 21*, 287–296.

Khare, V., Lyakhovich, A., Dammann, K., Lang, M., Borgmann, M., Tichy, B., et al. (2013). Mesalamine modulates intercellular adhesion through inhibition of p-21 activated kinase-1. *Biochemical Pharmacology, 85*, 234–244.

Kim, T. W., Kang, Y. K., Park, Z. Y., Kim, Y. H., Hong, S. W., Oh, S. J., et al. (2014). SH3RF2 functions as an oncogene by mediating PAK4 protein stability. *Carcinogenesis, 35*, 624–634.

Kim, Y. B., Shin, Y. J., Roy, A., & Kim, J. H. (2015). The role of the pleckstrin homology domain-containing protein CKIP-1 in activation of p21-activated kinase 1 (PAK1). *The Journal of Biological Chemistry, 290*, 21076–21085.

Kim, E., Youn, H., Kwon, T., Son, B., Kang, J., Yang, H. J., et al. (2014). PAK1 tyrosine phosphorylation is required to induce epithelial-mesenchymal transition and radioresistance in lung cancer cells. *Cancer Research, 74*, 5520–5531.

Kimmelman, A. C., Hezel, A. F., Aguirre, A. J., Zheng, H., Paik, J. H., Ying, H., et al. (2008). Genomic alterations link Rho family of GTPases to the highly invasive phenotype of pancreas cancer. *Proceedings of the National Academy of Sciences of the United States of America, 105*, 19372–19377.

Kiosses, W. B., Hood, J., Yang, S., Gerritsen, M. E., Cheresh, D. A., Alderson, N., et al. (2002). A dominant-negative p65 PAK peptide inhibits angiogenesis. *Circulation Research, 90*, 697–702.

Kissil, J. L., Johnson, K. C., Eckman, M. S., & Jacks, T. (2002). Merlin phosphorylation by p21-activated kinase 2 and effects of phosphorylation on merlin localization. *The Journal of Biological Chemistry, 277*, 10394–10399.

Kissil, J. L., Wilker, E. W., Johnson, K. C., Eckman, M. S., Yaffe, M. B., & Jacks, T. (2003). Merlin, the product of the Nf2 tumor suppressor gene, is an inhibitor of the p21-activated kinase, Pak1. *Molecular Cell, 12*, 841–849.

Knaus, U. G., Morris, S., Dong, H. J., Chernoff, J., & Bokoch, G. M. (1995). Regulation of human leukocyte p21-activated kinases through G protein-coupled receptors. *Science, 269*, 221–223.

Kok, M., Zwart, W., Holm, C., Fles, R., Hauptmann, M., Van't Veer, L. J., et al. (2011). PKA-induced phosphorylation of ERα at serine 305 and high PAK1 levels is associated with sensitivity to tamoxifen in ER-positive breast cancer. *Breast Cancer Research and Treatment, 125*, 1–12.

Kou, B., Gao, Y., Du, C., Shi, Q., Xu, S., Wang, C. Q., et al. (2014). miR-145 inhibits invasion of bladder cancer cells by targeting PAK1. *Urologic Oncology, 32*, 846–854.

Kumagai, K., Nimura, Y., Mizota, A., Miyahara, N., Aoki, M., Furusawa, Y., et al. (2006). Arpc1b gene is a candidate prediction marker for choroidal malignant melanomas sensitive to radiotherapy. *Investigative Ophthalmology & Visual Science, 47*, 2300–2304.

Kumar, R., Gururaj, A. E., & Barnes, C. J. (2006). p21-Activated kinases in cancer. *Nature Reviews. Cancer, 6*, 459–471.

Kumar, R., & Hall, A. (2009). Cytoskeleton signaling in cancer. In R. Kumar & A. Hal (Eds.), *Cancer and metastasis reviews: 28 (1–2)*. 0167–7659.

Kumar, A., Molli, P. R., Pakala, S. B., Bui Nguyen, T. M., Rayala, S. K., & Kumar, R. (2009). PAK thread from amoeba to mammals. *Journal of Cellular Biochemistry, 107*, 579–585.

Lee, S. H., Kunz, J., Lin, S. H., & Yu-Lee, L. Y. (2007). 16-kDa prolactin inhibits endothelial cell migration by down-regulating the Ras-Tiam1-Rac1-Pak1 signaling pathway. *Cancer Research, 67*, 11045–11053.

Lee, S. R., Ramos, S. M., Ko, A., Masiello, D., Swanson, K. D., Lu, M. L., et al. (2002). AR and ER interaction with a p21-activated kinase (PAK6). *Molecular Endocrinology, 16*, 85–99.

Lee, J. H., Wittki, S., Brau, T., Dreyer, F. S., Kratzel, K., Dindorf, J., et al. (2013). HIV Nef, paxillin, and Pak1/2 regulate activation and secretion of TACE/ADAM10 proteases. *Molecular Cell, 49*, 668–679.

Li, F., Adam, L., Vadlamudi, R. K., Zhou, H., Sen, S., Chernoff, J., et al. (2002). p21-Activated kinase 1 interacts with and phosphorylates histone H3 in breast cancer cells. *EMBO Reports, 3*, 767–773.

Li, Y., Ke, Q., Shao, Y., Zhu, G., Geng, N., Jin, F., et al. (2015). GATA1 induces epithelial-mesenchymal transition in breast cancer cells through PAK5 oncogenic signaling. *Oncotarget, 6*, 4345–4356.

Li, L. H., Luo, Q., Zheng, M. H., Pan, C., Wu, G. Y., Lu, Y. Z., et al. (2012). P21-activated protein kinase 1 is overexpressed in gastric cancer and induces cancer metastasis. *Oncology Reports, 27*, 1435–1442.

Li, D. Q., Nair, S. S., Ohshiro, K., Kumar, A., Nair, V. S., Pakala, S. B., et al. (2012). MORC2 signaling integrates phosphorylation-dependent, ATPase-coupled chromatin remodeling during the DNA damage response. *Cell Reports, 2*, 1657–1669.

Li, Y., Shao, Y., Tong, Y., Shen, T., Zhang, J., Gu, H., et al. (2012). Nucleo-cytoplasmic shuttling of PAK4 modulates β-catenin intracellular translocation and signaling. *Biochimica et Biophysica Acta, 1823*, 465–475.

Li, Y., Wang, D., Zhang, H., Wang, C., Dai, W., Cheng, Z., et al. (2013). P21-activated kinase 4 regulates the cyclin-dependent kinase inhibitor p57(kip2) in human breast cancer. *Anatomical Record (Hoboken, N.J.: 2007), 296*, 1561–1567.

Li, X., Wen, W., Liu, K., Zhu, F., Malakhova, M., Peng, C., et al. (2011). Phosphorylation of caspase-7 by p21-activated protein kinase (PAK) 2 inhibits chemotherapeutic drug-induced apoptosis of breast cancer cell lines. *The Journal of Biological Chemistry, 286*, 22291–22299.

Li, D., Yao, X., & Zhang, P. (2013). The overexpression of P21-activated kinase 5 (PAK5) promotes paclitaxel-chemoresistance of epithelial ovarian cancer. *Molecular and Cellular Biochemistry, 383,* 191–199.

Li, Z., Zhang, H., Lundin, L., Thullberg, M., Liu, Y., Wang, Y., et al. (2010). p21-activated kinase 4 phosphorylation of integrin beta5 Ser-759 and Ser-762 regulates cell migration. *The Journal of Biological Chemistry, 285,* 23699–23710.

Li, T., Zhang, J., Zhu, F., Wen, W., Zykova, T., Li, X., et al. (2011). P21-activated protein kinase (PAK2)-mediated c-Jun phosphorylation at 5 threonine sites promotes cell transformation. *Carcinogenesis, 32,* 659–666.

Li, L. H., Zheng, M. H., Luo, Q., Ye, Q., Feng, B., Lu, A. G., et al. (2010). P21-activated protein kinase 1 induces colorectal cancer metastasis involving ERK activation and phosphorylation of FAK at Ser-910. *International Journal of Oncology, 37,* 951–962.

Li, Z., Zou, X., Xie, L., Chen, H., Chen, Y., Yeung, S. C., et al. (2015). Personalizing risk stratification by addition of PAK1 expression to TNM staging: Improving the accuracy of clinical decision for gastroesophageal junction adenocarcinoma. *International Journal of Cancer, 136,* 1636–1645.

Li, Z., Zou, X., Xie, L., Dong, H., Chen, Y., Liu, Q., et al. (2013). Prognostic importance and therapeutic implications of PAK1, a drugable protein kinase, in gastroesophageal junction adenocarcinoma. *PloS One, 8,* e80665.

Licciulli, S., Maksimoska, J., Zhou, C., Troutman, S., Kota, S., Liu, Q., et al. (2013). FRAX597, a small molecule inhibitor of the p21-activated kinases, inhibits tumorigenesis of neurofibromatosis type 2 (NF2)-associated Schwannomas. *The Journal of Biological Chemistry, 288,* 29105–29114.

Lin, S. L., Qi, S. T., Sun, S. C., Wang, Y. P., Schatten, H., & Sun, Q. Y. (2010). PAK1 regulates spindle microtubule organization during oocyte meiotic maturation. *Frontiers in Bioscience (Elite Edition), 2,* 1254–1264.

Liu, X., Busby, J., John, C., Wei, J., Yuan, X., & Lu, M. L. (2013). Direct interaction between AR and PAK6 in androgen-stimulated PAK6 activation. *PloS One, 8,* e77367.

Liu, J. S., Che, X. M., Chang, S., Qiu, G. L., He, S. C., Fan, L., et al. (2015). β-elemene enhances the radiosensitivity of gastric cancer cells by inhibiting Pak1 activation. *World Journal of Gastroenterology, 21,* 9945–9956.

Liu, T., Li, Y., Gu, H., Zhu, G., Li, J., Cao, L., et al. (2013). p21-Activated kinase 6 (PAK6) inhibits prostate cancer growth via phosphorylation of androgen receptor and tumorigenic E3 ligase murine double minute-2 (Mdm2). *The Journal of Biological Chemistry, 288,* 3359–3369.

Liu, F., Li, X., Wang, C., Cai, X., Du, Z., Xu, H., et al. (2009). Downregulation of p21-activated kinase-1 inhibits the growth of gastric cancer cells involving cyclin B1. *International Journal of Cancer, 125,* 2511–2519.

Liu, W., Liu, H., Liu, Y., Xu, L., Zhang, W., Zhu, Y., et al. (2014). Prognostic significance of p21-activated kinase 6 expression in patients with clear cell renal cell carcinoma. *Annals of Surgical Oncology, 21*(Suppl. 4), S575–S583.

Liu, W., Liu, Y., Liu, H., Zhang, W., Fu, Q., Xu, J., et al. (2015). Tumor suppressive function of p21-activated kinase 6 in hepatocellular carcinoma. *The Journal of Biological Chemistry, 290,* 28489–28501.

Liu, J., Liu, H., Zhang, W., Wu, Q., Liu, W., Liu, Y., et al. (2013). N-acetylglucosaminyltransferase V confers hepatoma cells with resistance to anoikis through EGFR/PAK1 activation. *Glycobiology, 23,* 1097–1109.

Liu, R. X., Wang, W. Q., Ye, L., Bi, Y. F., Fang, H., Cui, B., et al. (2010). p21-Activated kinase 3 is overexpressed in thymic neuroendocrine tumors (carcinoids) with ectopic ACTH syndrome and participates in cell migration. *Endocrine, 38,* 38–47.

Long, W., Yi, P., Amazit, L., LaMarca, H. L., Ashcroft, F., Kumar, R., et al. (2010). SRC-3Delta4 mediates the interaction of EGFR with FAK to promote cell migration. *Molecular Cell*, *37*, 321–332.

Lu, W., Qu, J. J., Li, B. L., Lu, C., Yan, Q., Wu, X. M., et al. (2013). Overexpression of p21-activated kinase 1 promotes endometrial cancer progression. *Oncology Reports*, *29*, 1547–1555.

Lu, W., Xia, Y. H., Qu, J. J., He, Y. Y., Li, B. L., Lu, C., et al. (2013). p21-Activated kinase 4 regulation of endometrial cancer cell migration and invasion involves the ERK1/2 pathway mediated MMP-2 secretion. *Neoplasma*, *60*, 493–503.

Luo, P., Fei, J., Zhou, J., & Zhang, W. (2015). microRNA-126 suppresses PAK4 expression in ovarian cancer SKOV3 cells. *Oncology Letters*, *9*, 2225–2229.

Mahlamaki, E. H., Kauraniemi, P., Monni, O., Wolf, M., Hautaniemi, S., & Kallioniemi, A. (2004). High-resolution genomic and expression profiling reveals 105 putative amplification target genes in pancreatic cancer. *Neoplasia*, *6*, 432–439.

Mak, G. W., Chan, M. M., Leong, V. Y., Lee, J. M., Yau, T. O., Ng, I. O., et al. (2011). Overexpression of a novel activator of PAK4, the CDK5 kinase-associated protein CDK5RAP3, promotes hepatocellular carcinoma metastasis. *Cancer Research*, *71*, 2949–2958.

Manavathi, B., Rayala, S. K., & Kumar, R. (2007). Phosphorylation-dependent regulation of stability and transforming potential of ETS transcriptional factor ESE-1 by p21-activated kinase 1. *The Journal of Biological Chemistry*, *282*, 19820–19830.

Manser, E., Leung, T., Salihuddin, H., Zhao, Z. S., & Lim, L. (1994). A brain serine/threonine protein kinase activated by Cdc42 and Rac1. *Nature*, *367*, 40–46.

Maroto, B., Ye, M. B., von Lohneysen, K., Schnelzer, A., & Knaus, U. G. (2008). P21-activated kinase is required for mitotic progression and regulates Plk1. *Oncogene*, *27*, 4900–4908.

Martin, G. A., Bollag, G., McCormick, F., & Abo, A. (1995). A novel serine kinase activated by rac1/CDC42Hs-dependent autophosphorylation is related to PAK65 and STE20. *The EMBO Journal*, *14*, 4385.

Maruta, H. (2011). Effective neurofibromatosis therapeutics blocking the oncogenic kinase PAK1. *Drug Discoveries & Therapeutics*, *5*, 266–278.

Maruta, H. (2014). Herbal therapeutics that block the oncogenic kinase PAK1: A practical approach towards PAK1-dependent diseases and longevity. *Phytotherapy Research*, *28*, 656–672.

Marx, J. (2004). Cancer research. Inflammation and cancer: The link grows stronger. *Science*, *306*, 966–968.

Master, Z., Jones, N., Tran, J., Jones, J., Kerbel, R. S., & Dumont, D. J. (2001). Dok-R plays a pivotal role in angiopoietin-1-dependent cell migration through recruitment and activation of Pak. *The EMBO Journal*, *20*, 5919–5928.

Matthaios, D., Foukas, P. G., Kefala, M., Hountis, P., Trypsianis, G., Panayiotides, I. G., et al. (2012). γ-H2AX expression detected by immunohistochemistry correlates with prognosis in early operable non-small cell lung cancer. *OncoTargets and Therapy*, *5*, 309–314.

Mazumdar, A., & Kumar, R. (2003). Estrogen regulation of Pak1 and FKHR pathways in breast cancer cells. *FEBS Letters*, *535*, 6–10.

McCarty, S. K., Saji, M., Zhang, X., Jarjoura, D., Fusco, A., Vasko, V. V., et al. (2010). Group I p21-activated kinases regulate thyroid cancer cell migration and are overexpressed and activated in thyroid cancer invasion. *Endocrine-Related Cancer*, *17*, 989–999.

McCarty, S. K., Saji, M., Zhang, X., Knippler, C. M., Kirschner, L. S., Fernandez, S., et al. (2014). BRAF activates and physically interacts with PAK to regulate cell motility. *Endocrine-Related Cancer*, *21*, 865–877.

McDonald, P. C., Fielding, A. B., & Dedhar, S. (2008). Integrin-linked kinase—Essential roles in physiology and cancer biology. *Journal of Cell Science, 121*, 3121–3132.

McFawn, P. K., Shen, L., Vincent, S. G., Mak, A., Van Eyk, J. E., & Fisher, J. T. (2003). Calcium-independent contraction and sensitization of airway smooth muscle by p21-activated protein kinase. *American Journal of Physiology. Lung Cellular and Molecular Physiology, 284*, L863–L870.

Meng, Q., Rayala, S. K., Gururaj, A. E., Talukder, A. H., O'Malley, B. W., & Kumar, R. (2007). Signaling-dependent and coordinated regulation of transcription, splicing, and translation resides in a single coregulator, PCBP1. *Proceedings of the National Academy of Sciences of the United States of America, 104*, 5866–5871.

Mira, J. P., Benard, V., Groffen, J., Sanders, L. C., & Knaus, U. G. (2000). Endogenous, hyperactive Rac3 controls proliferation of breast cancer cells by a p21-activated kinase-dependent pathway. *Proceedings of the National Academy of Sciences of the United States of America, 97*, 185–189.

Misra, U. K., Deedwania, R., & Pizzo, S. V. (2005). Binding of activated alpha2-macroglobulin to its cell surface receptor GRP78 in 1-LN prostate cancer cells regulates PAK-2-dependent activation of LIMK. *The Journal of Biological Chemistry, 280*, 26278–26286.

Molli, P. R., Li, D. Q., Bagheri-Yarmand, R., Pakala, S. B., Katayama, H., Sen, S., et al. (2010). Arpc1b, a centrosomal protein, is both an activator and substrate of Aurora A. *The Journal of Cell Biology, 190*, 101–114.

Moon, S. U., Kim, J. W., Sung, J. H., Kang, M. H., Kim, S. H., Chang, H., et al. (2015). p21-Activated kinase 4 (PAK4) as a predictive marker of gemcitabine sensitivity in pancreatic cancer cell lines. *Cancer Research and Treatment, 47*, 501–508.

Moshfegh, Y., Bravo-Cordero, J. J., Miskolci, V., Condeelis, J., & Hodgson, L. (2014). A Trio-Rac1-Pak1 signalling axis drives invadopodia disassembly. *Nature Cell Biology, 16*, 574–586.

Motwani, M., Li, D. Q., Horvath, A., & Kumar, R. (2013). Identification of novel gene targets and functions of p21-activated kinase 1 during DNA damage by gene expression profiling. *PloS One, 8*, e66585.

Murray, B. W., Guo, C., Piraino, J., Westwick, J. K., Zhang, C., Lamerdin, J., et al. (2010). Small-molecule p21-activated kinase inhibitor PF-3758309 is a potent inhibitor of oncogenic signaling and tumor growth. *Proceedings of the National Academy of Sciences of the United States of America, 107*, 9446–9451.

Nagelkerke, A., van Kuijk, S. J., Sweep, F. C., Nagtegaal, I. D., Hoogerbrugge, N., Martens, J. W., et al. (2011). Constitutive expression of γ-H2AX has prognostic relevance in triple negative breast cancer. *Radiotherapy and Oncology, 101*, 39–45.

Nazarian, R., Shi, H., Wang, Q., Kong, X., Koya, R. C., Lee, H., et al. (2010). Melanomas acquire resistance to B-RAF(V600E) inhibition by RTK or N-RAS upregulation. *Nature, 468*, 973–977.

Nekrasova, T., & Minden, A. (2011). PAK4 is required for regulation of the cell-cycle regulatory protein p21, and for control of cell-cycle progression. *Journal of Cellular Biochemistry, 112*, 1795–1806.

Neumann, M., Foryst-Ludwig, A., Klar, S., Schweitzer, K., & Naumann, M. (2006). The PAK1 autoregulatory domain is required for interaction with NIK in Helicobacter pylori-induced NF-kappaB activation. *Biological Chemistry, 387*, 79–86.

Nguyen, B. C., Be Tu, P. T., Tawata, S., & Maruta, H. (2015). Combination of immunoprecipitation (IP)-ATP_Glo kinase assay and melanogenesis for the assessment of potent and safe PAK1-blockers in cell culture. *Drug Discoveries & Therapeutics, 9*, 289–295.

Nguyen, B. C., Taira, N., & Tawata, S. (2014). Several herbal compounds in Okinawa plants directly inhibit the oncogenic/aging kinase PAK1. *Drug Discoveries & Therapeutics, 8*, 238–244.

Nheu, T. V., He, H., Hirokawa, Y., Tamaki, K., Florin, L., Schmitz, M. L., et al. (2002). The K252a derivatives, inhibitors for the PAK/MLK kinase family selectively block the growth of RAS transformants. *Cancer Journal, 8*, 328–336.

Nobes, C. D., & Hall, A. (1995). Rho, rac, and cdc42 GTPases regulate the assembly of multimolecular focal complexes associated with actin stress fibers, lamellipodia, and filopodia. *Cell, 81*, 53–62.

Ong, C. C., Gierke, S., Pitt, C., Sagolla, M., Cheng, C. K., Zhou, W., et al. (2015). Small molecule inhibition of group I p21-activated kinases in breast cancer induces apoptosis and potentiates the activity of microtubule stabilizing agents. *Breast Cancer Research, 17*, 59.

Ong, C. C., Jubb, A. M., Haverty, P. M., Zhou, W., Tran, V., Truong, T., et al. (2011). Targeting p21-activated kinase 1 (PAK1) to induce apoptosis of tumor cells. *Proceedings of the National Academy of Sciences of the United States of America, 108*, 7177–7182.

Ong, C. C., Jubb, A. M., Jakubiak, D., Zhou, W., Rudolph, J., Haverty, P. M., et al. (2013). P21-activated kinase 1 (PAK1) as a therapeutic target in BRAF wild-type melanoma. *Journal of the National Cancer Institute, 105*, 606–607.

O'Sullivan, G. C., Tangney, M., Casey, G., Ambrose, M., Houston, A., & Barry, O. P. (2007). Modulation of p21-activated kinase 1 alters the behavior of renal cell carcinoma. *International Journal of Cancer, 121*, 1930–1940.

Pakala, S. B., Nair, V. S., Reddy, S. D., & Kumar, R. (2012). Signaling-dependent phosphorylation of mitotic centromere-associated kinesin regulates microtubule depolymerization and its centrosomal localization. *The Journal of Biological Chemistry, 287*, 40560–40569.

Park, J., Kim, J. M., Park, J. K., Huang, S., Kwak, S. Y., Ryu, K. A., et al. (2015). Association of p21-activated kinase-1 activity with aggressive tumor behavior and poor prognosis of head and neck cancer. *Head & Neck, 37*, 953–963.

Park, M. H., Kim, D. J., You, S. T., Lee, C. S., Kim, H. K., Park, S. M., et al. (2012). Phosphorylation of β-catenin at serine 663 regulates its transcriptional activity. *Biochemical and Biophysical Research Communications, 419*, 543–549.

Park, M. H., Lee, H. S., Lee, C. S., You, S. T., Kim, D. J., Park, B. H., et al. (2013). p21-Activated kinase 4 promotes prostate cancer progression through CREB. *Oncogene, 32*, 2475–2482.

Pavey, S., Zuidervaart, W., van Nieuwpoort, F., Packer, L., Jager, M., Gruis, N., et al. (2006). Increased p21-activated kinase-1 expression is associated with invasive potential in uveal melanoma. *Melanoma Research, 16*, 285–296.

Pellegrino, L., Stebbing, J., Braga, V. M., Frampton, A. E., Jacob, J., Buluwela, L., et al. (2013). miR-23b regulates cytoskeletal remodeling, motility and metastasis by directly targeting multiple transcripts. *Nucleic Acids Research, 41*, 5400–5412.

Porchia, L. M., Guerra, M., Wang, Y. C., Zhang, Y., Espinosa, A. V., Shinohara, M., et al. (2007). 2-Amino-N-{4-[5-(2-phenanthrenyl)-3-(trifluoromethyl)-1H-pyrazol-1-yl]-phenyl} acetamide (OSU-03012), a celecoxib derivative, directly targets p21-activated kinase. *Molecular Pharmacology, 72*, 1124–1131.

Puto, L. A., Pestonjamasp, K., King, C. C., & Bokoch, G. M. (2003). p21-Activated kinase 1 (PAK1) interacts with the Grb2 adapter protein to couple to growth factor signaling. *The Journal of Biological Chemistry, 278*, 9388–9393.

Qian, Z., Zhu, G., Tang, L., Wang, M., Zhang, L., Fu, J., et al. (2014). Whole genome gene copy number profiling of gastric cancer identifies PAK1 and KRAS gene amplification as therapy targets. *Genes, Chromosomes & Cancer, 53*, 883–894.

Qing, H., Gong, W., Che, Y., Wang, X., Peng, L., Liang, Y., et al. (2012). PAK1-dependent MAPK pathway activation is required for colorectal cancer cell proliferation. *Tumour Biology, 33*, 985–994.

Qu, J., Cammarano, M. S., Shi, Q., Ha, K. C., de Lanerolle, P., & Minden, A. (2001). Activated PAK4 regulates cell adhesion and anchorage-independent growth. *Molecular and Cellular Biology, 21*, 3523–3533.

Radu, M., Lyle, K., Hoeflich, K. P., Villamar-Cruz, O., Koeppen, H., & Chernoff, J. (2015). p21-Activated kinase 2 regulates endothelial development and function through the Bmk1/Erk5 pathway. *Molecular and Cellular Biology, 35*, 3990–4005.

Radu, M., Semenova, G., Kosoff, R., & Chernoff, J. (2014). PAK signalling during the development and progression of cancer. *Nature Reviews. Cancer, 14*, 13–25.

Rane, C. K., & Minden, A. (2014). P21 activated kinases: Structure, regulation, and functions. *Small GTPases, 5*. pii: e28003.

Rayala, S. K., den Hollander, P., Balasenthil, S., Yang, Z., Broaddus, R. R., & Kumar, R. (2005). Functional regulation of oestrogen receptor pathway by the dynein light chain 1. *EMBO Reports, 6*, 538–544.

Rayala, S. K., Molli, P. R., & Kumar, R. (2006). Nuclear p21-activated kinase 1 in breast cancer packs off tamoxifen sensitivity. *Cancer Research, 66*, 5985–5988.

Rayala, S. K., Talukder, A. H., Balasenthil, S., Tharakan, R., Barnes, C. J., Wang, R. A., et al. (2006). P21-activated kinase 1 regulation of estrogen receptor-alpha activation involves serine 305 activation linked with serine 118 phosphorylation. *Cancer Research, 66*, 1694–1701.

Reddy, S. D., Ohshiro, K., Rayala, S. K., & Kumar, R. (2008). MicroRNA-7, a homeobox D10 target, inhibits p21-activated kinase 1 and regulates its functions. *Cancer Research, 68*, 8195–8200.

Reinardy, J. L., Corey, D. M., Golzio, C., Mueller, S. B., Katsanis, N., & Kontos, C. D. (2015). Phosphorylation of threonine 794 on Tie1 by Rac1/PAK1 reveals a novel angiogenesis regulatory pathway. *PloS One, 10*, e0139614.

Rettig, M., Trinidad, K., Pezeshkpour, G., Frost, P., Sharma, S., Moatamed, F., et al. (2012). PAK1 kinase promotes cell motility and invasiveness through CRK-II serine phosphorylation in non-small cell lung cancer cells. *PloS One, 7*, e42012.

Rider, L., Shatrova, A., Feener, E. P., Webb, L., & Diakonova, M. (2007). JAK2 tyrosine kinase phosphorylates PAK1 and regulates PAK1 activity and functions. *The Journal of Biological Chemistry, 282*, 30985–30996.

Roig, J., & Traugh, J. A. (1999). p21-Activated protein kinase gamma-PAK is activated by ionizing radiation and other DNA-damaging agents. Similarities and differences to alpha-PAK. *The Journal of Biological Chemistry, 274*, 31119–31122.

Rong, R., Surace, E. I., Haipek, C. A., Gutmann, D. H., & Ye, K. (2004). Serine 518 phosphorylation modulates merlin intramolecular association and binding to critical effectors important for NF2 growth suppression. *Oncogene, 23*, 8447–8454.

Ryu, B. J., Kim, S., Min, B., Kim, K. Y., Lee, J. S., Park, W. J., et al. (2014). Discovery and the structural basis of a novel p21-activated kinase 4 inhibitor. *Cancer Letters, 349*, 45–50.

Sanchez-Solana, B., Motwani, M., Li, D. Q., Eswaran, J., & Kumar, R. (2012). p21-Activated kinase-1 signaling regulates transcription of tissue factor and tissue factor pathway inhibitor. *The Journal of Biological Chemistry, 287*, 39291–39302.

Sato, M., Matsuda, Y., Wakai, T., Kubota, M., Osawa, M., Fujimaki, S., et al. (2013). P21-activated kinase-2 is a critical mediator of transforming growth factor-β-induced hepatoma cell migration. *Journal of Gastroenterology and Hepatology, 28*, 1047–1055.

Schraml, P., Schwerdtfeger, G., Burkhalter, F., Raggi, A., Schmidt, D., Ruffalo, T., et al. (2003). Combined array comparative genomic hybridization and tissue microarray analysis suggest PAK1 at 11q13.5–q14 as a critical oncogene target in ovarian carcinoma. *The American Journal of Pathology, 163*, 985–992.

Scott, R. W., Hooper, S., Crighton, D., Li, A., Konig, I., Munro, J., et al. (2010). LIM kinases are required for invasive path generation by tumor and tumor-associated stromal cells. *The Journal of Cell Biology, 191*, 169–185.

Sedelnikova, O. A., & Bonner, W. M. (2006). GammaH2AX in cancer cells: A potential biomarker for cancer diagnostics, prediction and recurrence. *Cell Cycle, 5*, 2909–2913.

Seguin, L., Kato, S., Franovic, A., Camargo, M. F., Lesperance, J., Elliott, K. C., et al. (2014). An integrin β3-KRAS-RalB complex drives tumour stemness and resistance to EGFR inhibition. *Nature Cell Biology, 16*, 457–468.

Serrano, I., McDonald, P. C., Lock, F., Muller, W. J., & Dedhar, S. (2013). Inactivation of the Hippo tumour suppressor pathway by integrin-linked kinase. *Nature Communications, 4*, 2976.

Shin, Y. J., Kim, Y. B., & Kim, J. H. (2013). Protein kinase CK2 phosphorylates and activates p21-activated kinase 1. *Molecular Biology of the Cell, 24*, 2990–2999.

Shrestha, Y., Schafer, E. J., Boehm, J. S., Thomas, S. R., He, F., Du, J., et al. (2012). PAK1 is a breast cancer oncogene that coordinately activates MAPK and MET signaling. *Oncogene, 31*, 3397–3408.

Shu, X. R., Wu, J., Sun, H., Chi, L. Q., & Wang, J. H. (2015). PAK4 confers the malignance of cervical cancers and contributes to the cisplatin-resistance in cervical cancer cells via PI3K/AKT pathway. *Diagnostic Pathology, 10*, 177.

Singh, R. R., Song, C., Yang, Z., & Kumar, R. (2005). Nuclear localization and chromatin targets of p21-activated kinase 1. *The Journal of Biological Chemistry, 280*, 18130–18137.

Siu, M. K., Chan, H. Y., Kong, D. S., Wong, E. S., Wong, O. G., Ngan, H. Y., et al. (2010). p21-Activated kinase 4 regulates ovarian cancer cell proliferation, migration, and invasion and contributes to poor prognosis in patients. *Proceedings of the National Academy of Sciences of the United States of America, 107*, 18622–18627.

Siu, M. K., Kong, D. S., Ngai, S. Y., Chan, H. Y., Jiang, L., Wong, E. S., et al. (2015). p21-Activated kinases 1, 2 and 4 in endometrial cancers: Effects on clinical outcomes and cell proliferation. *PloS One, 10*, e0133467.

Siu, M. K., Wong, E. S., Chan, H. Y., Kong, D. S., Woo, N. W., Tam, K. F., et al. (2010). Differential expression and phosphorylation of Pak1 and Pak2 in ovarian cancer: Effects on prognosis and cell invasion. *International Journal of Cancer, 127*, 21–31.

Siu, M. K., Yeung, M. C., Zhang, H., Kong, D. S., Ho, J. W., Ngan, H. Y., et al. (2010). p21-Activated kinase-1 promotes aggressive phenotype, cell proliferation, and invasion in gestational trophoblastic disease. *The American Journal of Pathology, 176*, 3015–3022.

Song, S., Li, X., Guo, J., Hao, C., Feng, Y., Guo, B., et al. (2015). Design, synthesis and biological evaluation of 1-phenanthryl-tetrahydroisoquinoline derivatives as novel p21-activated kinase 4 (PAK4) inhibitors. *Organic & Biomolecular Chemistry, 13*, 3803–3818.

Song, B., Wang, W., Zheng, Y., Yang, J., & Xu, Z. (2015). P21-activated kinase 1 and 4 were associated with colorectal cancer metastasis and infiltration. *The Journal of Surgical Research, 196*, 130–135.

Spratley, S. J., Bastea, L. I., Doppler, H., Mizuno, K., & Storz, P. (2011). Protein kinase D regulates cofilin activity through p21-activated kinase 4. *The Journal of Biological Chemistry, 286*, 34254–34261.

Strochlic, T. I., Viaud, J., Rennefahrt, U. E., Anastassiadis, T., & Peterson, J. R. (2010). Phosphoinositides are essential coactivators for p21-activated kinase 1. *Molecular Cell, 40*, 493–500.

Sun, G. G., Wei, C. D., Jing, S. W., & Hu, W. N. (2014). Interactions between filamin A and MMP-9 regulate proliferation and invasion in renal cell carcinoma. *Asian Pacific Journal of Cancer Prevention, 15*, 3789–3795.

Talukder, A. H., Li, D. Q., Manavathi, B., & Kumar, R. (2008). Serine 28 phosphorylation of NRIF3 confers its co-activator function for estrogen receptor-alpha transactivation. *Oncogene, 27*, 5233–5242.

Talukder, A. H., Meng, Q., & Kumar, R. (2006). CRIPak, a novel endogenous Pak1 inhibitor. *Oncogene, 25,* 1311–1319.

Tao, J., Li, H., Li, Q., & Yang, Y. (2014). CD109 is a potential target for triple-negative breast cancer. *Tumour Biology, 35,* 12083–12090.

Tao, J., Oladimeji, P., Rider, L., & Diakonova, M. (2011). PAK1-Nck regulates cyclin D1 promoter activity in response to prolactin. *Molecular Endocrinology, 25,* 1565–1578.

Tharakan, R., Lepont, P., Singleton, D., Kumar, R., & Khan, S. (2008). Phosphorylation of estrogen receptor alpha, serine residue 305 enhances activity. *Molecular and Cellular Endocrinology, 295,* 70–78.

Thiel, D. A., Reeder, M. K., Pfaff, A., Coleman, T. R., Sells, M. A., & Chernoff, J. (2002). Cell cycle-regulated phosphorylation of p21-activated kinase 1. *Current Biology, 12,* 1227–1232.

Thomas, J. L., Moncollin, V., Ravel-Chapuis, A., Valente, C., Corda, D., Mejat, A., et al. (2015). PAK1 and CtBP1 regulate the coupling of neuronal activity to muscle chromatin and gene expression. *Molecular and Cellular Biology, 35,* 4110–4120.

Tu, H. F., Chang, K. W., Chiang, W. F., Liu, C. J., Yu, E. H., Liu, S. T., et al. (2011). The frequent co-expression of the oncogenes PIK3CA and PAK1 in oral carcinomas. *Oral Oncology, 47,* 211–216.

Vadlamudi, R. K., Adam, L., Wang, R. A., Mandal, M., Nguyen, D., Sahin, A., et al. (2000). Regulatable expression of p21-activated kinase-1 promotes anchorage-independent growth and abnormal organization of mitotic spindles in human epithelial breast cancer cells. *The Journal of Biological Chemistry, 275,* 36238–36244.

Vadlamudi, R. K., Bagheri-Yarmand, R., Yang, Z., Balasenthil, S., Nguyen, D., Sahin, A. A., et al. (2004). Dynein light chain 1, a p21-activated kinase 1-interacting substrate, promotes cancerous phenotypes. *Cancer Cell, 5,* 575–585.

Vadlamudi, R. K., Barnes, C. J., Rayala, S., Li, F., Balasenthil, S., Marcus, S., et al. (2005). p21-Activated kinase 1 regulates microtubule dynamics by phosphorylating tubulin cofactor B. *Molecular and Cellular Biology, 25,* 3726–3736.

Vadlamudi, R. K., & Kumar, R. (2003). P21-activated kinases in human cancer. *Cancer Metastasis Reviews, 22,* 385–393.

Vadlamudi, R. K., Li, F., Adam, L., Nguyen, D., Ohta, Y., Stossel, T. P., et al. (2002). Filamin is essential in actin cytoskeletal assembly mediated by p21-activated kinase 1. *Nature Cell Biology, 4,* 681–690.

Vadlamudi, R. K., Li, F., Barnes, C. J., Bagheri-Yarmand, R., & Kumar, R. (2004). p41-Arc subunit of human Arp2/3 complex is a p21-activated kinase-1-interacting substrate. *EMBO Reports, 5,* 154–160.

Vadlamudi, R. K., Manavathi, B., Singh, R. R., Nguyen, D., Li, F., & Kumar, R. (2005). An essential role of Pak1 phosphorylation of SHARP in Notch signaling. *Oncogene, 24,* 4591–4596.

Van Tine, B. A., & Ellis, M. J. (2011). Understanding the estrogen receptor-positive breast cancer genome: Not even the end of the beginning. *Journal of the National Cancer Institute, 103,* 526–527.

Verde, F., Wiley, D. J., & Nurse, P. (1998). Fission yeast orb6, a ser/thr protein kinase related to mammalian rho kinase and myotonic dystrophy kinase, is required for maintenance of cell polarity and coordinates cell morphogenesis with the cell cycle. *Proceedings of the National Academy of Sciences of the United States of America, 95,* 7526–7531.

Viaud, J., & Peterson, J. R. (2009). An allosteric kinase inhibitor binds the p21-activated kinase autoregulatory domain covalently. *Molecular Cancer Therapeutics, 8,* 2559–2565.

Walsh, K., McKinney, M. S., Love, C., Liu, Q., Fan, A., Patel, A., et al. (2013). PAK1 mediates resistance to PI3K inhibition in lymphomas. *Clinical Cancer Research, 19,* 1106–1115.

Wang, X. X., Cheng, Q., Zhang, S. N., Qian, H. Y., Wu, J. X., Tian, H., et al. (2013). PAK5-Egr1-MMP2 signaling controls the migration and invasion in breast cancer cell. *Tumour Biology, 34*, 2721–2729.

Wang, X., Gong, W., Qing, H., Geng, Y., Zhang, Y., Peng, L., et al. (2010). p21-Activated kinase 5 inhibits camptothecin-induced apoptosis in colorectal carcinoma cells. *Tumour Biology, 31*, 575–582.

Wang, C., Li, Y., Zhang, H., Liu, F., Cheng, Z., Wang, D., et al. (2014). Oncogenic PAK4 regulates Smad2/3 axis involving gastric tumorigenesis. *Oncogene, 33*, 3473–3484.

Wang, R. A., Mazumdar, A., Vadlamudi, R. K., & Kumar, R. (2002). P21-activated kinase-1 phosphorylates and transactivates estrogen receptor-alpha and promotes hyperplasia in mammary epithelium. *The EMBO Journal, 21*, 5437–5447.

Wang, D., Sai, J., & Richmond, A. (2003). Cell surface heparan sulfate participates in CXCL1-induced signaling. *Biochemistry, 42*, 1071–1077.

Wang, S. E., Shin, I., Wu, F. Y., Friedman, D. B., & Arteaga, C. L. (2006). HER2/Neu (ErbB2) signaling to Rac1-Pak1 is temporally and spatially modulated by transforming growth factor beta. *Cancer Research, 66*, 9591–9600.

Wang, G., Song, Y., Liu, T., Wang, C., Zhang, Q., Liu, F., et al. (2015). PAK1-mediated MORC2 phosphorylation promotes gastric tumorigenesis. *Oncotarget, 6*, 9877–9886.

Wang, R. A., Vadlamudi, R. K., Bagheri-Yarmand, R., Beuvink, I., Hynes, N. E., & Kumar, R. (2003). Essential functions of p21-activated kinase 1 in morphogenesis and differentiation of mammary glands. *The Journal of Cell Biology, 161*, 583–592.

Wang, R. A., Zhang, H., Balasenthil, S., Medina, D., & Kumar, R. (2006). PAK1 hyperactivation is sufficient for mammary gland tumor formation. *Oncogene, 25*, 2931–2936.

Wang, Z., Zhang, X., Yang, Z., Du, H., Wu, Z., Gong, J., et al. (2012). MiR-145 regulates PAK4 via the MAPK pathway and exhibits an antitumor effect in human colon cells. *Biochemical and Biophysical Research Communications, 427*, 444–449.

Wang, J. X., Zhou, Y. N., Zou, S. J., Ren, T. W., & Zhang, Z. Y. (2010). Correlations of P21-activated kinase 1 expression to clinicopathological features of gastric carcinoma and patients' prognosis. *Chinese Journal of Cancer, 29*, 649–654.

Warters, R. L., Adamson, P. J., Pond, C. D., & Leachman, S. A. (2005). Melanoma cells express elevated levels of phosphorylated histone H2AX foci. *The Journal of Investigative Dermatology, 124*, 807–817.

Wary, K. K. (2003). Signaling through Raf-1 in the neovasculature and target validation by nanoparticles. *Molecular Cancer, 2*, 27.

Wasco, M. J., & Pu, R. T. (2008). Utility of antiphosphorylated H2AX antibody (gamma-H2AX) in diagnosing metastatic renal cell carcinoma. *Applied Immunohistochemistry & Molecular Morphology, 16*, 349–356.

Wells, C. M., Abo, A., & Ridley, A. J. (2002). PAK4 is activated via PI3K in HGF-stimulated epithelial cells. *Journal of Cell Science, 115*, 3947–3956.

Wen, X., Li, X., Liao, B., Liu, Y., Wu, J., Yuan, X., et al. (2009). Knockdown of p21-activated kinase 6 inhibits prostate cancer growth and enhances chemosensitivity to docetaxel. *Urology, 73*, 1407–1411.

Whale, A. D., Dart, A., Holt, M., Jones, G. E., & Wells, C. M. (2013). PAK4 kinase activity and somatic mutation promote carcinoma cell motility and influence inhibitor sensitivity. *Oncogene, 32*, 2114–2120.

Whalley, H. J., Porter, A. P., Diamantopoulou, Z., White, G. R., Castaneda-Saucedo, E., & Malliri, A. (2015). Cdk1 phosphorylates the Rac activator Tiam1 to activate centrosomal Pak and promote mitotic spindle formation. *Nature Communications, 6*, 7437.

Wilkerson, P. M., & Reis-Filho, J. S. (2013). The 11q13-q14 amplicon: Clinicopathological correlations and potential drivers. *Genes, Chromosomes & Cancer, 52*, 333–355.

Wilkes, M. C., Murphy, S. J., Garamszegi, N., & Leof, E. B. (2003). Cell-type-specific activation of PAK2 by transforming growth factor beta independent of Smad2 and Smad3. *Molecular and Cellular Biology, 23,* 8878–8889.

Wilson, T. R., Fridlyand, J., Yan, Y., Penuel, E., Burton, L., Chan, E., et al. (2012). Widespread potential for growth-factor-driven resistance to anticancer kinase inhibitors. *Nature, 487,* 505–509.

Wittmann, T., Bokoch, G. M., & Waterman-Storer, C. M. (2004). Regulation of microtubule destabilizing activity of Op18/stathmin downstream of Rac1. *The Journal of Biological Chemistry, 279,* 6196–6203.

Wong, L. E., Reynolds, A. B., Dissanayaka, N. T., & Minden, A. (2010). p120-catenin is a binding partner and substrate for Group B Pak kinases. *Journal of Cellular Biochemistry, 110,* 1244–1254.

Xia, C., Ma, W., Stafford, L. J., Marcus, S., Xiong, W. C., & Liu, M. (2001). Regulation of the p21-activated kinase (PAK) by a human Gbeta-like WD-repeat protein, hPIP1. *Proceedings of the National Academy of Sciences of the United States of America, 98,* 6174–6179.

Xiao, G. H., Beeser, A., Chernoff, J., & Testa, J. R. (2002). p21-Activated kinase links Rac/Cdc42 signaling to merlin. *The Journal of Biological Chemistry, 277,* 883–886.

Xu, J., Liu, H., Chen, L., Wang, S., Zhou, L., Yun, X., et al. (2012). Hepatitis B virus X protein confers resistance of hepatoma cells to anoikis by up-regulating and activating p21-activated kinase 1. *Gastroenterology, 143.* 199-212 e4.

Xue, J., Chen, L. Z., Li, Z. Z., Hu, Y. Y., Yan, S. P., & Liu, L. Y. (2015). MicroRNA-433 inhibits cell proliferation in hepatocellular carcinoma by targeting p21 activated kinase (PAK4). *Molecular and Cellular Biochemistry, 399,* 77–86.

Yang, F., Li, X., Sharma, M., Zarnegar, M., Lim, B., & Sun, Z. (2001). Androgen receptor specifically interacts with a novel p21-activated kinase, PAK6. *The Journal of Biological Chemistry, 276,* 15345–15353.

Yang, Z., Rayala, S., Nguyen, D., Vadlamudi, R. K., Chen, S., & Kumar, R. (2005). Pak1 phosphorylation of snail, a master regulator of epithelial-to-mesenchyme transition, modulates snail's subcellular localization and functions. *Cancer Research, 65,* 3179–3184.

Yang, Z., Vadlamudi, R. K., & Kumar, R. (2005). Dynein light chain 1 phosphorylation controls macropinocytosis. *The Journal of Biological Chemistry, 280,* 654–659.

Yang, H. J., Zheng, Y. B., Ji, T., Ding, X. F., Zhu, C., Yu, X. F., et al. (2013). Overexpression of ILK1 in breast cancer associates with poor prognosis. *Tumour Biology, 34,* 3933–3938.

Ye, D. Z., Jin, S., Zhuo, Y., & Field, J. (2011). p21-Activated kinase 1 (Pak1) phosphorylates BAD directly at serine 111 in vitro and indirectly through Raf-1 at serine 112. *PloS One, 6,* e27637.

Yeo, D., Huynh, N., Beutler, J. A., Christophi, C., Shulkes, A., Baldwin, G. S., et al. (2014). Glaucarubinone and gemcitabine synergistically reduce pancreatic cancer growth via down-regulation of P21-activated kinases. *Cancer Letters, 346,* 264–272.

Yi, C., Maksimoska, J., Marmorstein, R., & Kissil, J. L. (2010). Development of small-molecule inhibitors of the group I p21-activated kinases, emerging therapeutic targets in cancer. *Biochemical Pharmacology, 80,* 683–689.

Yoon, J. H., Mo, J. S., Ann, E. J., Ahn, J. S., Jo, E. H., Lee, H. J., et al. (2015). NOTCH1 intracellular domain negatively regulates PAK1 signaling pathway through direct interaction. *Biochimica et Biophysica Acta, 1863,* 179–188.

Yu, T., MacPhail, S. H., Banath, J. P., Klokov, D., & Olive, P. L. (2006). Endogenous expression of phosphorylated histone H2AX in tumors in relation to DNA double-strand breaks and genomic instability. *DNA Repair (Amst), 5,* 935–946.

Yuan, Z. Q., Kim, D., Kaneko, S., Sussman, M., Bokoch, G. M., Kruh, G. D., et al. (2005). ArgBP2gamma interacts with Akt and p21-activated kinase-1 and promotes cell survival. *The Journal of Biological Chemistry, 280,* 21483–21490.

Yuan, L., Santi, M., Rushing, E. J., Cornelison, R., & MacDonald, T. J. (2010). ERK activation of p21 activated kinase-1 (Pak1) is critical for medulloblastoma cell migration. *Clinical & Experimental Metastasis, 27*, 481–491.

Zhai, J., Qu, S., Li, X., Zhong, J., Chen, X., Qu, Z., et al. (2015). miR-129 suppresses tumor cell growth and invasion by targeting PAK5 in hepatocellular carcinoma. *Biochemical and Biophysical Research Communications, 464*, 161–167.

Zhang, X., Ems-McClung, S. C., & Walczak, C. E. (2008). Aurora A phosphorylates MCAK to control ran-dependent spindle bipolarity. *Molecular Biology of the Cell, 19*, 2752–2765.

Zhang, M., Siedow, M., Saia, G., & Chakravarti, A. (2010). Inhibition of p21-activated kinase 6 (PAK6) increases radiosensitivity of prostate cancer cells. *Prostate, 70*, 807–816.

Zhang, H. J., Siu, M. K., Yeung, M. C., Jiang, L. L., Mak, V. C., Ngan, H. Y., et al. (2011). Overexpressed PAK4 promotes proliferation, migration and invasion of choriocarcinoma. *Carcinogenesis, 32*, 765–771.

Zhang, D. G., Zhang, J., Mao, L. L., Wu, J. X., Cao, W. J., Zheng, J. N., et al. (2015). p21-Activated kinase 5 affects cisplatin-induced apoptosis and proliferation in hepatocellular carcinoma cells. *Tumour Biology, 36*, 3685–3691.

Zhang, K., Zhu, T., Gao, D., Zhang, Y., Zhao, Q., Liu, S., et al. (2014). Filamin A expression correlates with proliferation and invasive properties of human metastatic melanoma tumors: Implications for survival in patients. *Journal of Cancer Research and Clinical Oncology, 140*, 1913–1926.

Zhao, Z. S., Lim, J. P., Ng, Y. W., Lim, L., & Manser, E. (2005). The GIT-associated kinase PAK targets to the centrosome and regulates Aurora-A. *Molecular Cell, 20*, 237–249.

Zheng, M., Liu, J., Zhu, M., Yin, R., Dai, J., Sun, J., et al. (2015). Potentially functional polymorphisms in PAK1 are associated with risk of lung cancer in a Chinese population. *Cancer Medicine, 4*, 1781–1787.

Zhong, Z., Yeow, W. S., Zou, C., Wassell, R., Wang, C., Pestell, R. G., et al. (2010). Cyclin D1/cyclin-dependent kinase 4 interacts with filamin A and affects the migration and invasion potential of breast cancer cells. *Cancer Research, 70*, 2105–2114.

Zhou, W., Jubb, A. M., Lyle, K., Xiao, Q., Ong, C. C., Desai, R., et al. (2014). PAK1 mediates pancreatic cancer cell migration and resistance to MET inhibition. *The Journal of Pathology, 234*, 502–513.

Zhou, G. L., Zhuo, Y., King, C. C., Fryer, B. H., Bokoch, G. M., & Field, J. (2003). Akt phosphorylation of serine 21 on Pak1 modulates Nck binding and cell migration. *Molecular and Cellular Biology, 23*, 8058–8069.

Zhu, J., Huang, J. W., Tseng, P. H., Yang, Y. T., Fowble, J., Shiau, C. W., et al. (2004). From the cyclooxygenase-2 inhibitor celecoxib to a novel class of 3-phosphoinositide-dependent protein kinase-1 inhibitors. *Cancer Research, 64*, 4309–4318.

Zhu, G., Li, X., Guo, B., Ke, Q., Dong, M., & Li, F. (2015). PAK5-mediated E47 phosphorylation promotes epithelial-mesenchymal transition and metastasis of colon cancer. *Oncogene*. Epub ahead of print [PMID: 26212009].

Zhu, G., Wang, Y., Huang, B., Liang, J., Ding, Y., Xu, A., et al. (2012). A Rac1/PAK1 cascade controls β-catenin activation in colon cancer cells. *Oncogene, 31*, 1001–1012.

Ziegler-Heitbrock, H. W., & Ulevitch, R. J. (1993). CD14: Cell surface receptor and differentiation marker. *Immunology Today, 14*, 121–125.

Zucman-Rossi, J., Villanueva, A., Nault, J. C., & Llovet, J. M. (2015). Genetic landscape and biomarkers of hepatocellular carcinoma. *Gastroenterology, 149*. 1226–1239 e4.

CHAPTER FIVE

Sirtuins and the Estrogen Receptor as Regulators of the Mammalian Mitochondrial UPR in Cancer and Aging

D. Germain[1]

The Tisch Cancer Institute, Icahn School of Medicine at Mount Sinai, New York, NY, United States
[1]Corresponding author: e-mail address: doris.germain@mssm.edu

Contents

Advances in Cancer Research, Volume 130
ISSN 0065-230X
http://dx.doi.org/10.1016/bs.acr.2016.01.004

Abstract

By being both the source of ATP and the mediator of apoptosis, the mitochondria are key regulators of cellular life and death. Not surprisingly alterations in the biology of the mitochondria have implications in a wide array of diseases including cancer and age-related diseases such as neurodegeneration. To protect the mitochondria against damage the mitochondrial unfolded protein response (UPR^{mt}) orchestrates several pathways, including the protein quality controls, the antioxidant machinery, oxidative phosphorylation, mitophagy, and mitochondrial biogenesis. While several reports have implicated an array of transcription factors in the UPR^{mt}, most of the focus has been on studies of *Caenorhabditis elegans*, which led to the identification of ATFS-1, for which the mammalian homolog remains unknown. Meanwhile, there are studies which link the UPR^{mt} to sirtuins and transcription factors of the Foxo family in both *C. elegans* and mammalian cells but those have been largely overlooked. This review aims at emphasizing the potential importance of these studies by building on the large body of literature supporting the key role of the sirtuins in the maintenance of the integrity of the mitochondria in both cancer and aging. Further, the estrogen receptor alpha (ERα) and beta (ERβ) are known to confer protection against mitochondrial stress, and at least ERα has been linked to the UPR^{mt}. Considering the difference in gender longevity, this chapter also includes a discussion of the link between the ERα and ERβ and the mitochondria in cancer and aging.

1. INTRODUCTION

The study of the mitochondrial unfolded protein response (UPR^{mt}) is relatively recent. The Hoogenraad's group was the first to describe the transcriptional response activated by accumulation of misfolded proteins in the mitochondria (Zhao et al., 2002). Their work identified CHOP as the transcription factor necessary for the elevation in the transcription of hsp60, hsp10, and the protease ClpP (Zhao et al., 2002; Fig. 1). Subsequently, the Haynes's group extended the study of the UPR^{mt} using *Caenorhabditis elegans* as a model system (Benedetti, Haynes, Yang, Harding, & Ron, 2006; Haynes, Petrova, Benedetti, Yang, & Ron, 2007; Nargund, Fiorese, Pellegrino, Deng, & Haynes, 2015). In their work, the hsp6 and hsp60 promoters are used as the reporters for activation of the UPR^{mt}. Since then several studies have also used the hsp60 promoter as the unique reporter for the activation of the UPR^{mt}. The early study by Hoogenraad's group

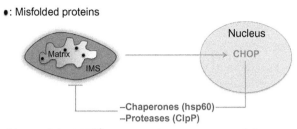

Fig. 1 The CHOP axis of the UPR^{mt} promotes the transcription of chaperones hsp60 and hsp10 as well as the protease ClpP. See text for further details. (See the color plate.)

therefore led to the generalized perception that activation of the transcription of chaperones defines the UPR^{mt}. For instance, as the retrograde response (RTG) that was described in yeast in response to decreased mitochondrial activity by Butow's group (Liu & Butow, 2006) does not lead to the transcription of chaperones, the RTG is considered distinct from the UPR^{mt} (Jovaisaite, Mouchiroud, & Auwerx, 2014). This limitation in the definition of the UPR^{mt} opens the risk of creating a fundamental misconception about the UPR^{mt}. Support for this concern is the observation that several siRNA clones identified in a genome-wide RNAi screen for negative regulators of the UPR^{mt} do not activate the hsp60 reporter (Bennett et al., 2014). Likewise, we found that the SIRT3 axis of the UPR^{mt}, which is one focus of this chapter, does not affect expression of hsp60, only the CHOP axis identified by the Hoogenraad's group (Papa & Germain, 2014). Therefore, as the field moves forward, it appears that an expansion of the current view of the UPR^{mt} should include the consideration that this process involves several axes, only one of which regulates hsp60, while others promote different cytoprotective outcomes.

Another intrinsic confusion in defining the UPR^{mt} is the origin of mitochondrial stress. Depletion of mitochondrial DNA, elevation in the production of reactive oxygen species (ROS) due to inhibition of the electron transport chain (ETC) complexes or accumulation of misfolded proteins have all been used to generate mitochondrial stress. However, no consensus has yet been formally stated as to whether or not the definition of the UPR^{mt} should be restricted to the response activated by accumulation of unfolded proteins as its name implies. The following section aims at addressing this issue.

1.1 The Mitochondrial UPR vs Mitochondrial Retrograde Signaling Pathway or ROS Defense Pathway

The first description of a UPR^{mt} came from the observation that proteins that fail to be properly folded in the lumen of the endoplasmic reticulum accumulate, leading to the swelling of the organelle and the transcriptional upregulation of the chaperone BiP. Since these early observations, the signaling cascades activated by the accumulation of misfolded proteins in the endoplasmic reticulum have been studied extensively. Three axes of the UPR^{ER} have been described, and they collectively lead to activation of a large transcriptional program that ultimately aims at reducing the proteotoxic stress in the lumen of the endoplasmic reticulum and restoring the integrity of the organelle. More recently, the signaling cascades activated upon accumulation of misfolded proteins in the lumen of the mitochondria has begun to be investigated and was named the UPR^{mt}. Therefore at least two UPR have been reported: the UPR^{ER} and the UPR^{mt}. While this chapter focuses on the UPR^{mt} it is important to clarify the role of the origin of mitochondrial stress relative to that of endoplasmic reticulum stress. As the first step of the secretory pathway, the lumen of the endoplasmic reticulum is exposed to a large volume of newly synthesized proteins destined for the endoplasmic reticulum itself, but also several other subcellular locations such as the Golgi, the plasma membrane, as well as the extracellular milieu. Considering the critical role of the endoplasmic reticulum in the secretory pathway, it is not surprising that this organelle contains a complex protein folding machinery. In a nut shell, the origin of the stress in the endoplasmic reticulum is clearly the result of accumulated misfolded proteins and, therefore, the name UPR^{mt} directly reflects proteotoxic stress.

In the mitochondria, the situation is more complex due to several factors. First, the function of the mitochondria is not primarily the folding of proteins. Second, the mitochondria have a genome that encodes 13 proteins involved in the ETC. The ETC complexes contain several subunits, most of which are encoded by the nuclear genome. Therefore, the proper stoichiometry of these complexes requires the coordination between the nuclear and mitochondrial genomes. Third, the mitochondria are the main source of ROS, which can lead to damage to DNA, proteins, and lipids. Therefore, unlike the endoplasmic reticulum, the accumulation of misfolded proteins in the mitochondria can arise from diverse sources. Direct sources include import of mutated mitochondrial proteins encoded by the nuclear genome, oxidation of mitochondrial proteins, and defect in the assembly of large ETC complexes leading to unassembled subunits that may, as a consequence, adopt an unfolded status. Indirect sources of accumulation of misfolded proteins in the mitochondria include mutation in mtDNA leading to mutated mitochondria proteins encoded by the mitochondria genome, misassembly of complexes due to deletion or insertion in the mtDNA, oxidation of lipids leading to defect in the assembly of ETC complexes and other transmembrane proteins and oxidation of chaperones and proteases leading indirectly to the accumulation of misfolded proteins.

Further, the effect of mutations in proteins of the ETC complexes can lead to more ROS, additional mutations in mtDNA and further misassembly. The various sources of mitochondrial stress have led to emergence of different terminology regarding signaling cascades activated upon mitochondrial stress: the retrograde signaling cascades, ROS defense pathway, and the UPR^{mt}. For instance, ROS is reported to activate the retrograde signaling cascades and ROS defense pathway but not the UPR^{mt}, again as defined by activation of the hsp60-reporter. Yet, a recent study reported that altering NAD$^+$ levels using poly(ADP-ribose) polymerase (PARP) inhibitors leads to a burst of ROS and activates both the UPR^{mt} and the ROS defense pathway (Mouchiroud et al., 2013) leading the authors to question how these two pathways are interconnected. Regardless if the origin of the mitochondrial stress is deletion of mtDNA, increased ROS, inhibition of the prohibitins, or chaperones or overexpression of misfolded proteins, ultimately all of these defects lead to the accumulation of misfolded proteins. Thus, it seems advisable not to make a distinction between UPR^{mt} and mitochondrial retrograde signaling. Rather, it should be considered that activation of hsp60 is only one aspect of the UPR^{mt} and that, since several transcription factors are implicated, the extent of the activation of the UPR^{mt} will vary depending on the strength and length of the stress so that, depending on the conditions, hsp60 may be activated or not.

2. THE SIRTUINS

Sirtuins are a family of seven proteins implicated in the regulation of several biological processes, notably in longevity, metabolism, and response to stress. They have been the focus of much attention due to the initial discovery that sirtuin-2 (sir-2) extends the life span of yeast (Kaeberlein, McVey, & Guarente, 1999). The biochemical characterization of sirtuins revealed that they have lysine deacetylase and ADP-ribosyltransferase activities, both of which require NAD$^+$ as a cofactor. Sirtuins show an array of subcellular localizations; SIRT1 is both nuclear and cytosolic; SIRT2 is cytoplasmic; SIRT3, 4, and 5 are found in the mitochondria; while SIRT6 and 7 are in the nucleus. For the purpose of this chapter only SIRT1 and SIRT3 will be discussed.

SIRT1 is the most studied of all sirtuins. It was originally described as a histone deacetylase but it was soon realized that SIRT1 deacetylases other proteins (Feige & Auwerx, 2008; Haigis & Sinclair, 2010; Houtkooper, Williams, & Auwerx, 2010; Lomb, Laurent, & Haigis, 2010). Among the substrates of SIRT1, peroxisome proliferator-activated receptor gamma coactivator (PCG1α) and forkhead transcription factors (FOXO) 3a are the most relevant to the UPR^{mt} and therefore, while other proteins are regulated by SIRT1 (Houtkooper, Pirinen, & Auwerx, 2012), only PCG1α and FOXO3a will be discussed here.

PGC1α is a major regulator of mitochondrial biogenesis and glycolysis. It forms complexes with either PPAR-alpha or estrogen-related receptor alpha (ERRα) and nuclear respiratory factor 1 (NRF1). The PGC1α–PPAR-alpha complex regulates lipid utilization, while the PGC1α–ERRα–NRF1 complex regulates mitochondrial biogenesis and decreases glycolysis (Houtkooper et al., 2012). The deacetylation of PGC1α by SIRT1 is required for formation of these complexes. The activity of SIRT1 is itself regulated by NAD$^+$ levels.

The transcription factor FOXO3a regulates several genes implicated in apoptosis, such as Bim, PUM, and FLIP. FOXO3a was also identified as a major regulator of Notch signaling in stem cell renewal. However, Foxo3a is also involved in the activation of the antioxidant enzyme such as catalase and manganese superoxide dismutase 2 (SOD2). The nuclear localization of FOXO3a is affected by its phosphorylation by Akt, which results in its nuclear export. In cancer, FOXO3a has been reported to have a role as an oncogene as well as a tumor suppressor (Myatt & Lam, 2007). The deacetylation of FOXO3a by SIRT1 has been proposed to not only affect its activity, but to direct FOXO3a to specific targets, therefore adding another level of regulation (Brunet et al., 2004; Motta et al., 2004).

Some of the substrates of SIRT3 have been characterized but it is likely that more substrates remain to be identified. Based on current knowledge, the only substrate of SIRT3 that is directly linked to the UPR^{mt} is the SOD2. The important finding of the regulation of SOD2 by SIRT3 arose from the observation that genetic ablation of the SIRT3 gene leads to an elevation in the levels of mitochondrial superoxide. Since SOD2 is required for the conversion of superoxide to hydrogen peroxide, this observation led the investigators to analyze SOD2 in the SIRT3 knockout mice. They found that in absence of SIRT3 SOD2 is hyperacetylated and they further established that SIRT3 is required for the deacetylation of SOD2 at lysine 122 (Tao et al., 2010).

3. UPR^{mt} IN CANCER: THE SIRTUINS AND THE UPR^{mt}

3.1 SIRT3 Is Downregulated in Cancer—Its Role as a Tumor Suppressor

The analysis of mouse embryonic fibroblasts (MEF) of the Sirt3 knockout mice showed a decrease in mitochondrial DNA integrity with age (Kim et al., 2010). As altered mitochondrial integrity is observed in several cancer types, the effect of Sirt3 deletion on immortalization capacity was investigated. It was found that Sirt3$^{-/-}$ MEF form a larger number of colonies in a colony formation assay. Further, while both Myc and Ras are required for the transformation of MEF, in the absence of Sirt3 either Myc or Ras was sufficient for immortalization (Kim et al., 2010). Moreover, the Sirt3$^{-/-}$ ras or Sirt3$^{-/-}$ myc MEF were found to have lower oxidative phosphorylation activity but significantly higher glycolysis (Kim et al., 2010). Further, infection of the Sirt3$^{-/-}$/Ras or myc MEF with a lentivirus expressing SOD2 inhibited their immortalization.

Importantly to the discussion of the UPR^{mt}, the authors also reported that the SOD2 promoter occupancy by the transcription factor FOXO3a was decreased in the Sirt3$^{-/-}$ MEF and that this was due to a decrease in the nuclear accumulation of FOXO3a. To further analyze the link between SIRT3 and FOXO3a, a dominant negative construct of SIRT3 was used and the level of FOXO3a found to be decreased. This observation suggests that SIRT3 somehow affects the nuclear accumulation of FOXO3a (Kim et al., 2010). This observation is also consistent with the findings by others (Sundaresan et al., 2009). Lastly, the investigators reported that the SIRT3 knockout mice develop mammary tumors, therefore supporting a tumor suppressor function of SIRT3 (Kim et al., 2010). Of particular interest was the observation that the mammary tumors in the Sirt3 knockout mice were exclusively estrogen receptor positive, which is rare in mice models of breast cancer. A potential explanation for the selection of ER-positive mammary tumor will be discussed in more details in the section on the role of the estrogen receptor in the UPR^{mt}.

Another key study in the establishment of SIRT3 as a tumor suppressor came from the Haigis laboratory (Finley, Carracedo, et al., 2011). As reported by Gius's group, they confirmed that Sirt3$^{-/-}$ MEF switch toward glycolysis and, they further showed, that this effect was associated with increased glucose usage as the Sirt3$^{-/-}$ cells showed lower intracellular glucose (Finley, Carracedo, et al., 2011). Since directing glucose away from the

TCA cycle is associated with increased proliferation in cancer cells, they also monitored the growth rate of the Sirt3$^{-/-}$ MEF and reported that these cells grow significantly more than their wild-type counterpart (Finley, Carracedo, et al., 2011). Further, the Sirt3$^{-/-}$ MEF were found to consume more glucose, suggesting that the upregulation of glycolysis is not simply a compensatory mechanism due to a reduction in mitochondria oxidative function, but rather it is the result of specific activation of the pathway. To further investigate this possibility, they analyzed the level of the HIF1α as it is a major driver of glycolysis. They reported that indeed HIF1α is upregulated in the Sirt3$^{-/-}$ cells and that the stabilization of HIFα was dependent on the increased superoxide accumulation resulting from the defect in SOD2 activity (Finley, Carracedo, et al., 2011). To validate the role of HIF1α in the tumor suppressor function of Sirt3, they inhibited the expression of HIF1α in Sirt3$^{-/-}$ ras MEF and found that inhibition of HIF rescues the increase in colony formation of the Sirt3$^{-/-}$ cells (Finley, Carracedo, et al., 2011). In addition, the level of Sirt3 was further analyzed in human primary cancers. They reported that at least one copy of the Sirt3 gene is deleted in 20% of all human cancers and in 40% of breast cancer (Finley, Carracedo, et al., 2011). Of importance to the discussion of the UPR^{mt}, the vast majority of SIRT3 deletions are heterozygous, suggesting that tumors select for the retention of the other allele. To further test the extent of the loss of SIRT3 in cancer, they then performed immunohistochemistry and found that in 87% of breast cancers, SIRT3 was either lower or undetectable (Finley, Carracedo, et al., 2011).

While these studies strongly support the tumor suppressor function of SIRT3, other studies suggest the opposite effect of SIRT3. Namely, SIRT3 is overexpressed in metabolically active tissues such as heart, and was found to prevent cell death by increasing the interaction between Ku70 and Bax (Sundaresan et al., 2009; Sundaresan, Samant, Pillai, Rajamohan, & Gupta, 2008). Indeed, this interaction was protective against cell death in an in vitro model of cervical cancer (Sundaresan et al., 2008). Also, SIRT3 is overexpressed in oral (Yang et al., 2007) and bladder (Li et al., 2010) cancers. Further, SIRT3 is overexpressed in lymph node-positive breast cancers, suggesting that SIRT3 is associated with advanced stage of the disease (Ashraf et al., 2006). Therefore, the apparent opposite reports regarding the role of SIRT3 in various cancers has complicated the interpretation of its role and it was suggested that perhaps the epigenetic landscape of particular tumor type may be at the origin of this dual effect. While this might be a potential explanation, another possibility is that SIRT3 is inducible at a later stage of the disease under stress conditions through the activation of the UPR^{mt}.

3.2 SIRT3 Is Upregulated by the UPR^{mt}

Our group has shown that SIRT3 is a key regulator of the UPR^{mt} (Papa & Germain, 2014). We reported that under mitochondrial proteotoxic stress, FOXO3a accumulates in the nucleus and is deacetylated. The transcriptional targets of FOXO3a, SOD2 and catalase, are also elevated. Since FOXO3a is a substrate of SIRT1, we analyzed SIRT1 levels but found no change. In contrast, SIRT3 was increased under these conditions both at the protein and transcript levels. Similarly to findings by other groups (Kim et al., 2010; Sundaresan et al., 2009) that SIRT3 regulates the nuclear translocation of FOXO3a, we reported that upon inhibition of SIRT3 by shRNA, the nuclear translocation of FOXO3a was abolished (Papa & Germain, 2014).

The induction of SOD2 and catalase under mitochondrial proteotoxic stress conditions was found to also be dependent on SIRT3. Since SIRT3 is in the mitochondria and FOXO3A in the cytoplasm, how SIRT3 can affect FOXO3A is unclear. The mitochondrial localization of FOXO3A and the cytoplasmic localization of SIRT3 have both been reported but are very controversial (Jacobs et al., 2008; Sundaresan et al., 2009). Therefore, whether SIRT3 affects FOXO3A directly or indirectly remains to be determined; however, the fact that several groups have made the same observation using entirely different experimental models demonstrates that indeed SIRT3 does regulate the nuclear accumulation of FOXO3a.

Because using the same mitochondrial proteotoxic stress model (Zhao et al., 2002) we used in our studies, Hoogenraad's group had previously reported that the transcription factor CHOP is implicated in the transcriptional upregulation of hsp60 and hsp10, we tested whether SIRT3 may act downstream of CHOP. If so, the activation of SOD2 and catalase would be predicted to be abolished when CHOP is inhibited, but neither was. However, their expression was abolished upon inhibition of SIRT3. Conversely, inhibition of SIRT3 had no effect on the level of LonP, hsp10, or hsp60 (Papa & Germain, 2014). This finding is significant as it was one of the first indications to suggest that the UPR^{mt} may have distinct, activated in parallel axes that promote the transcription of a distinct set of genes. More specifically, this finding suggests that the CHOP-dependent axis is responsible for promoting the expression of mitochondrial chaperones and proteases, while the SIRT3 axis stimulates the expression of the mitochondrial antioxidant machinery.

We also reported that mitophagy is observed in cells undergoing mito-chondrial proteotoxic stress (Papa & Germain, 2014). In agreement with this finding, several markers of mitophagy were found to be upregulated under these conditions. As for the expression of SOD2 and catalase, we found that mitophagy was dependent on SIRT3 but was independent of CHOP. We therefore concluded that the SIRT3 axis of the UPR^{mt} regulates both the antioxidant machinery and mitophagy. Based on these observations, we pro-posed that SIRT3 acts as mitochondrial checkpoint protein whereby mod-erately stressed mitochondrion may be repaired through an upregulation of the antioxidant machinery, while irreversibly damaged organelles would be selectively eliminated from the network by mitophagy. In agreement with this possibility using again the same mitochondrial proteotoxic stress model, Youle's group showed that accumulation of misfolded ornithine trans-carbamylase (OTCΔ) in the mitochondria leads to the accumulation of PINK and the translocation of the ubiquitin ligase PARK2 to the mitochon-dria offering therefore a potential mechanism of selection of the irreversibly damaged organelles (Jin & Youle, 2013).

In addition to the upregulation of the antioxidant SOD2 and mitophagy, we also reported that mitochondrial proteotoxic stress induces the expres-sion of the transcription factor NRF1 (Papa & Germain, 2011, 2014). As NRF1, along with PGC-1α, is a central regulator of the expression of genes involved in mitochondrial biogenesis, this finding highlights the fact that the UPR^{mt} orchestrates simultaneously the elimination of irreversibly damaged mitochondrion that is counterbalanced by the biogenesis of new organelles, as well as the repair of preexisting mitochondrion via the antioxidant machinery and the upregulation of oxidative phosphorylation. Given that the CHOP axis acts in parallel to upregulate the chaperone and the proteases for the monitoring of the protein quality control, these findings indicate that the UPR^{mt} represents a ballet of well-choreographed signaling pathways that collectively maintain the integrity of the entire network.

3.3 Reconciling the Up- and Downregulation of SIRT3 in Breast Cancer

The undeniable evidence generated by the Haigis and Gius groups, showing that SIRT3 acts as a tumor suppressor, is hard to reconcile with the reports from several groups that SIRT3 is upregulated, notably in lymph node-positive breast cancer, and with our own work that SIRT3 regulates at least one axis of the UPR^{mt}. We propose a model whereby SIRT3 serves as a rheostat of ROS in cancer cells (Fig. 2). In this model, a decrease in SIRT3

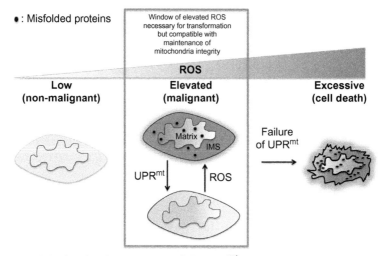

Fig. 2 Model whereby the activation of the UPR^{mt} may be necessary to protect the integrity of the mitochondrial network under increased oxidative stress conditions as well as acting as a rheostat of ROS to maintain ROS levels within the elevated range. (See the color plate.)

is necessary during transformation to elevate ROS levels and to promote the shift to glycolysis. However, in cells in which ROS reach excessive levels, UPR^{mt} may induce SIRT3 allowing ROS to decrease to levels that are sufficient to be utilized as signaling molecules in cancer cells, yet within a range of concentrations that is compatible with the viability of the organelle. In addition, the inducible expression of SIRT3 in these cells would allow the elimination of irreversibly damaged mitochondrion from the mitochondrial network and for the restoration of a healthier and uniform network (Fig. 2). Importantly, the upregulation of NRF1 by the UPR^{mt} acts to increase mitochondrial biogenesis and oxidative phosphorylation. This model is compatible with the observation that only one allele of SIRT3 is lost in cancer, preserving SIRT3 ability to be expressed.

3.4 The SIRT1/FOXO Axis of the UPR^{mt} in C. elegans

Auwerx's group initiated a study aimed at investigating the link between metabolism and longevity through the modulation of NAD$^+$ levels. The activity of the sirtuins is strictly dependent on NAD$^+$. In addition to the sirtuins, PARP proteins PARP1 and 2 are the main consumer of NAD$^+$. As such, when PARP is inhibited, NAD$^+$ levels rise and can activate the Sirtuins. This group first reported that in aged mice the levels of NAD$^+$ are low and correlated with the hyperacetylation of the substrate of SIRT1,

PCG1α (Mouchiroud et al., 2013). This group then turned to *C. elegans* to further investigate the effect of NAD$^+$ on the life span. They found that feeding worms with PARP inhibitors extended their life span by 15–23% and that this effect was associated with increased oxidative phosphorylation and increased ATP levels (Mouchiroud et al., 2013). To investigate the signaling pathway implicated in the increased longevity phenotype observed when NAD$^+$ was increased, they then turned their attention to two pathways, the UPR^{mt} and the so-called ROS defense pathway. The distinction between these two pathways arises from the observation that ROS does not activate the UPR^{mt} (Durieux, Wolff, & Dillin, 2011), which is again defined by the activation of the hsp60 or 6 promoter reporters in *C. elegans*. The ROS defense pathway, on the other hand, is characterized by the nuclear translocation of FOXO transcription factor daf-16 (Berdichevsky, Viswanathan, Horvitz, & Guarente, 2006) leading to the activation of the antioxidant machinery (Honda & Honda, 1999). As stated by the authors: *"it is unclear whether and if so these two pathways are activated by NAD$^+$ and how they are intertwined."* One potential explanation is that the definition of the UPR^{mt} should not be restricted to the activation of hsp6 and 60 reporters and that the ROS defense pathway is simply another axis of the UPR^{mt}. In support of this possibility they found that both hsp6 reporter and translocation of FOXO and transcription of Sod-3 (the equivalent of FOXO3a and SOD2 in mammalian cells) are activated by PARP inhibitors (Mouchiroud et al., 2013). Further, they found that in their experimental conditions SIRT1 is the sirtuin implicated in the deacetylation of FOXO3a (Mouchiroud et al., 2013). To reconcile their findings, the authors referred to the NAD$^+$/SIRT1/UPR^{mt}/SOD signaling axis. They further went on to validate these findings in mammalian cells (Mouchiroud et al., 2013).

Clearly, the pathway described by the Auwerx's group is highly reminiscent to the SIRT/FOXO3a/SOD2 axis of the UPR^{mt} we reported (Papa & Germain, 2014). Considering the intimate interconnection between SIRT1 and SIRT3, these pathways are very likely to be similar. This possibility is further discussed in the following section.

3.5 The Sirtuins Axis of the UPR^{mt}: A Unifying Model

On one hand, the pathway described by Auwerx's group implicates the activation of SIRT1 by an elevation of NAD$^+$ leading to the deacetylation and activation of FOXO3a, which then promotes the transcription of SOD2.

On the other hand, the pathway we have described implicates SIRT3 in the regulation of FOXO3a and the transcription of SOD2. While we and others have reported now the SIRT3-dependent nuclear localization of FOXO3a, the mechanism that is responsible for a matrix deacetylase regulating FOXO3a in the cytoplasm poses a conceptual difficulty. Simone's group has reported an AMPK-dependent FOXO3a–SIRT3 complex in the mitochondria (Peserico et al., 2013). While this complex may offer a direct explanation for the regulation of FOXO3a by SIRT3, the mitochondrial localization of FOXO3a remains controversial.

Other studies have implicated a direct regulation of FOXO3a by AMPK. Namely, AMPK has been reported to phosphorylate FOXO3a at several sites; phosphorylation of FOXO3a on serine 413 was reported to be essential for the formation of an active transcriptional complex in the nucleus (Greer et al., 2007). Since AMPK activation results in an increase in NAD^+, and the activation of SIRT1 and that SIRT1 deacetylates FOXO3a, these studies raise the possibility that both phosphorylation and deacetylation affect FOXO3a and that the net outcome on the transcriptional activity of FOXO3a may be context dependent. In this regard, the AMPK–FOXO3a pathway of oxidative stress was independent of AMP level (Colombo & Moncada, 2009).

A direct link between SIRT1 and SIRT3 is provided by the finding that PGC1α regulates the transcription of SIRT3 (Kong et al., 2010). Chang's group reported that adenovirus-mediated overexpression of PGC1α stimulated the transcription of SIRT3, while it had no effect on any of the other Sirtuins (Kong et al., 2010). Conversely, inhibition of PCG1α by siRNA reduced the expression of SIRT3. They further demonstrated that PGC1α binds to the promoter of SIRT3 through estrogen-receptor related binding sites and mapped this binding site to position −407 to −399 of the SIRT3 promoter (Kong et al., 2010). Deletion of this site abolished the upregulation of SIRT3 by PGC1α overexpression. Importantly, they found that SIRT3 was required for the upregulation of genes implicated in mitochondrial biogenesis by PGC1α. Namely, inhibition of SIRT3 by shRNA abolished the regulation of ATP synthase, cytochrome *c*, and SOD2 by PGC1α (Kong et al., 2010). Further, while PGC1α overexpression leads to an increase in mitochondrial DNA copy number, this effect of PGC1α was also abolished in absence of SIRT3. This study therefore defines SIRT3 as a novel transcriptional target of PGC1α and suggests that SIRT3 is at least in part necessary for the effect of PGC1α on the mitochondria. Therefore, since SIRT1 regulates PGC1α and PGC1α regulates SIRT3, and because SIRT3 and SIRT1 both regulate FOXO3a, the finding of the SIRT1/SOD axis by the Auwerx's group and our finding of the SIRT3/SOD axis are likely to be intimately linked.

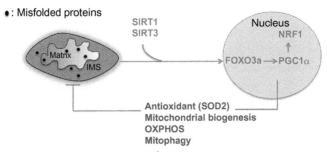

Fig. 3 The SIRT/FOXO3a axis of the UPR^mt promotes the activation of a complex transcriptional program involving FOXO3a, PGC1α, and NRF1 leading to the transcription of antioxidant genes such as SOD2, increased mitochondrial biogenesis, oxidative phosphorylation, and mitophagy. See text for further details. (See the color plate.)

The implication of the SIRT1 and SIRT3 cross talk is not limited to SOD2, however. PGC1α acts directly to increase the transcription of genes implicated in oxidative phosphorylation. SIRT3 has been reported to directly bind to complexes regulating oxidative phosphorylation (Ahn et al., 2008; Cimen et al., 2010; Finley, Haas, et al., 2011; Hirschey et al., 2010). Further several reports support a direct regulation of oxidative phosphorylation by SIRT3. In SIRT3 knockout cells, the activities of complexes I and III are reduced (Cimen et al., 2010; Kim et al., 2010), ROS levels are elevated (Bell, Emerling, Ricoult, & Guarente, 2011), and ATP production is reduced (Ahn et al., 2008). Therefore, both PGC1α and SIRT3 regulate oxidative phosphorylation.

The third aspect of the SIRT3 axis of the UPR^mt we have reported is the induction of autophagy (Papa & Germain, 2014). Considering that several studies have reported a role for SIRT1 in regulating autophagy (Jeong, Moon, Lee, Seol, & Park, 2013; Lee et al., 2008; Morselli et al., 2010a), the cross talk between SIRT1 and SIRT3 covers all aspects of this axis of the UPR^mt.

Finally, overexpression of SIRT3 has been also reported to promote the expression of PGC1α (Shi, Wang, Stieren, & Tong, 2005). These findings suggested a tightly intertwined network between SIRT1, SIRT3, FOXO3a, and PGC1α leading to increased mitochondrial biogenesis, upregulation of SOD2 and autophagy (Fig. 3).

3.6 Evidences Supporting the Activation of UPR^mt in Mouse Models of Cancer

A number of mouse models of recurrent cancers as well as circulating cancer cells support the possibility that the UPR^mt may be required for cancer cells survival.

The Kalluri's group has recently reported that PGC1α is essential for the metastatic potential of circulating cancer cells (LeBleu et al., 2014). Injection of 4T1 mammary epithelial cells in the fat pad of mice is a reliable model of lung metastasis as 100% of mice develop metastasis. Using this model, they isolated circulating cancer cells and performed transcriptome analysis. This analysis revealed that oxidative phosphorylation is the most differentially upregulated pathway in these cells compared to the parental cells (LeBleu et al., 2014). Among the genes that were associated with this phenotype, they reported PGC1α, PCG1β, NRF1, and ERRα. Subsequently they found that PGC1α is upregulated not only in the 4T1 model but also in a variety of metastatic models such as MDA-MB231 breast cancer cells, B16F10 mouse melanoma cells, and 786-O renal carcinoma cells (LeBleu et al., 2014). Their analysis revealed that circulating cells exhibited increased mitochondrial DNA and elevated ATP production suggesting that the enhanced oxidative phosphorylation is associated with increased mitochondrial biogenesis. Modulation of PGC1α modulated the expression of mitochondrial biogenesis genes; PGC1α overexpression enhanced invasion capacity. However, inhibition of PGC1α had no effect on the growth of primary tumors. Further, inhibition of PGC1α reduced the number of metastases to the lung (LeBleu et al., 2014). While it would be interesting to know whether inhibition of NRF1 and ERRα also leads to similar inhibition of metastasis, the results presented in this study are sufficient to support the notion that increased mitochondrial biogenesis is necessary for survival of cells under stress conditions.

Draetta's group reached a similar conclusion using a model of recurrent pancreatic cancer. In their model, inducible ras was used to drive the growth of these tumors and inhibition of ras led to their complete regression. However, a small residual population survived in absence of ras and upon reactivation of ras these cells rapidly generated recurrent tumors. They performed mutational profiles of these lesions and found no significant differences between the primary and the recurrent tumors. However, transcriptome analysis revealed enrichment in several metabolic pathways, autophagy, and oxidative phosphorylation (Viale et al., 2014). Their studies confirmed that oxidative phosphorylation and mitochondrial biogenesis are specifically upregulated in these recurrent lesions.

Similarly, DePinho's group found an upregulation of mitochondrial biogenesis and oxidative phosphorylation in a model of T-cell lymphoma that activate the ALT pathway in order to survive telomere shortening crisis (Hu et al., 2012). Of particular interest in terms of the potential link to the UPR^{mt} is the fact that in their model, SOD2 was essential for the survival of these recurrent cancers, which were found to be very sensitive to SOD2 inhibition.

More examples of cancer models where oxidative phosphorylation is upregulated include a report of lymphoma cells undergoing "therapy-induced senescence" or TIS. In this Eµ-myc driven lymphoma model of TIS, cells were made resistant to apoptosis by the overexpression of BCL-2. The authors found that these cells utilize a hybrid form of energy metabolism using both glycolysis but also oxidative phosphorylation. Proteomic analysis of these cells showed a drastic elevation in the proteins of ETC suggesting a potential elevation in NRF1 or PGC1α, but this was not reported in this study (Dorr et al., 2013). The same upregulation of oxidative phosphorylation was also observed in drug-selected melanomas (Roesch et al., 2010).

Yet another example of a tumor model where the Sirtuin axis of the UPR^{mt} is likely to be upregulated came from Kranenburg's group (Vellinga et al., 2015). In this study gene a expression profile was performed on 119 liver metastases, of which 64 arose from patients that had been treated with chemotherapy. This analysis revealed that oxidative phosphorylation was the most upregulated pathway in chemotherapy-treated tumors. Since mitochondria biogenesis and ETC complexes were upregulated, this finding suggested that chemotherapy induces a change in metabolism. While the authors did not considered this possibility, one alternative explanation is that the oxidative stress generated by chemotherapy imposes a selective pressure on cells causing them to combat excessive ROS and do so by activating the UPR^{mt}. To directly test their hypothesis, the investigators established colonospheres from primary colon cancers, as well as liver metastases, and exposed these primary cultures to chemotherapy. They found that chemotherapy selectively induces an increase in mitochondrial mass and an upregulation in oxidative phosphorylation (Vellinga et al., 2015). Most importantly for the discussion of the UPR^{mt}, they found that SIRT1 expression was selectively upregulated and was within the top 5% of upregulated genes. To test whether SIRT1 plays an important role in the mitochondrial phenotype they observed, they inhibited SIRT1 using nicotinamide (NAM). They found that NAM inhibited not only the increase in oxidative phosphorylation but also the elevation in mitochondrial mass (Vellinga et al., 2015). Further, SIRT1 knockdown, using two different shRNAs against SIRT1, also abolished the effect of chemotherapy on mitochondrial mass (Vellinga et al., 2015). Because SIRT1 regulates PCG1α, they then turned their attention to the role of PGC1α. In agreement with the direct regulation of PGC1α by SIRT1, they found that inhibition of PGC1α by shRNA also leads to the suppression of the effect of chemotherapy on the mitochondria. Lastly, the authors then investigated whether inhibition of SIRT1 or PGC1α affects the viability of the colonospheres after chemotherapy. They found that inhibition of either SIRT1 or PGC1α leads to a twofold increase in cell death following chemotherapy (Vellinga et al., 2015). To further substantiate this observation, they also performed a xenograft experiment using colon cancer cells with and without knockdown of SIRT1 and treated mice with chemotherapy. They observed that tumors in which the expression of SIRT1 is inhibited were more sensitive to chemotherapy then tumors expressing SIRT1 (Vellinga et al., 2015).

Therefore, while a formal demonstration that the UPR^{mt} is activated and essential for the survival of circulating cells, recurrent tumors, and metastases is not yet established, the collective finding of an upregulation of mitochondrial biogenesis by multiple investigators certainly suggest that this analysis should be undertaken.

4. UPR^{mt} IN CANCER: THE ESTROGEN RECEPTORS AND THE UPR^{mt}

4.1 The Discovery of the Estrogen Receptor Arm of the UPR^{mt}

The estrogen receptor alpha (ERα) acts as a transcription factor and is the major therapeutic target against breast cancer. The recent genome-wide analysis of the binding of the ERα revealed the extraordinary extent of its transcriptional targets (Carroll et al., 2006; Mohammed et al., 2015). In addition we are only beginning to understand how the multiple layers of post-translational (Bhat-Nakshatri et al., 2008) and epigenetic regulation affect the pattern of binding of the ERα across the genome and the tissue specificity of such pattern (Franco, Nagari, & Kraus, 2015; Gertz et al., 2013). Our discovery of a role of the estrogen receptor in the UPR^{mt} originally arose from the investigation of the role of the intermembrane space (IMS) in the UPR^{mt}. While the accumulation of misfolded proteins in the mitochondrial matrix has been explored by the Hoogenraad's group, the effect of the accumulation of misfolded proteins in the mitochondrial IMS has never been addressed. Considering that ROS is produced on both sides of the inner-membrane and therefore can lead to oxidation and misfolding of proteins in both the matrix and the IMS, but the IMS has much lower protein quality control (proteases and chaperones) as well as

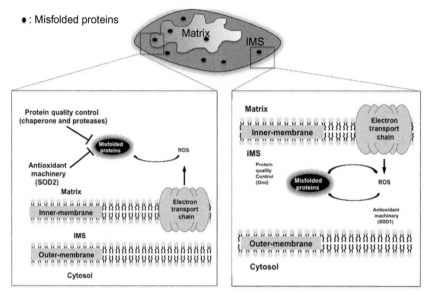

Fig. 4 The antioxidant and the protein quality control capacity of the matrix are superior than those of the intermembrane space. (See the color plate.)

antioxidant capacity than the matrix (Fig. 4), investigating how cells respond to proteotoxic stress in this important subcompartment of the mitochondria appeared to be a critical gap in our knowledge of the UPR^{mt}.

Therefore, we aimed at examining the effects of proteotoxic stress in the IMS using the expression of a mutant form of endonuclease G, which as we previously reported, forms aggregates in the IMS (Radke et al., 2008). Hoogenraad's group used accumulation of the misfolded matrix protein OTCΔ (Martinus et al., 1996; Zhao et al., 2002). They reported the activation of hsp60, hsp10, and ClpP through activation of the transcription factor CHOP (Martinus et al., 1996; Zhao et al., 2002). While we confirmed the activation of CHOP by inducing matrix stress, we found that IMS stress did not (Papa & Germain, 2011), suggesting that IMS stress and matrix stress do not trigger the same response. Further, we confirmed that, as with matrix stress, IMS stress does not activate the UPR of the endoplasmic reticulum. As ERα had been shown to localize in the mitochondria and estrogen is implicated in the regulation of mitochondrial functions (Pedram, Razandi, Wallace, & Levin, 2006), we investigated whether ERα is affected by IMS stress. We found that IMS stress, but not matrix stress, activated ERα (Papa & Germain, 2011). Two estrogen receptors exist, ERα and ERβ. We reported that ERα, but not ERβ, was activated upon IMS stress.

To investigate the mechanism by which the ERα is activated, we tested the phosphorylation of the ERα on serine 167, which is known to activate ERα even in absence of estrogen (Lannigan, 2003). We found that IMS stress leads to the phosphorylation of ERα and further confirmed that AKT was mediating this phosphorylation.

To explore the mechanism leading to the phosphorylation of ERα by AKT, given that ROS activates AKT (Campbell et al., 2001; Sun et al., 2001; Vilgelm et al., 2006), we tested the phosphorylation of AKT following IMS stress in presence or absence of NAC. We found that NAC abolished both the phosphorylation of AKT as well as phosphorylation of the ERα (Papa & Germain, 2011). We also found that IMS stress did not affect cellular viability, suggesting that activation of the ERα may promote the transcription of genes that protect the mitochondria against such insult. Given that Klinge's group had reported that the ERα regulates the transcription of NRF1 (Mattingly et al., 2008), we tested whether IMS stress induces the expression of NRF1 and found that indeed NRF1 is activated and dependent on the expression of the ERα (Papa & Germain, 2011). A summary of the ERα axis of the UPR^{mt} is shown in Fig. 5. Since NRF1, along with PGC1α, is a major transcription factor mediating increased oxidative phosphorylation and mitochondrial biogenesis, this finding suggests that the ERα/NRF1 axis of the UPR^{mt} has a redundant function with the SIRT/FOXO3 axis.

Importantly, the regulation of the NRF1 by the estrogen receptor has more recently been confirmed in vivo (Ivanova et al., 2013). Klinge's group showed that estrogen increases the expression of NRF1 in both the mammary gland and uterus of mice. However, the transcriptional targets of NRF1, such as the mitochondrial transcription factor (TFAM), were elevated in the mammary gland but not the uterus. This is because in the uterus,

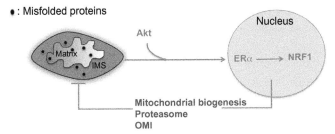

Fig. 5 The ERα axis of the UPR^{mt} promotes the transcription of NRF1, the protease OMI, and increases the activity of the proteasome. See text for further details. (See the color plate.)

estrogen inhibits the expression of the coactivators of NRF1 (Ivanova et al., 2013). Further, they reported that estrogen also stimulated the nuclear accumulation of NRF1 and PGC1α in the mammary gland but PGC1α was actually reduced in the uterus. Therefore, this study indicates that the regulation of the expression of NRF1 by the estrogen receptor is tissue specific (Ivanova et al., 2013). In terms of the UPR^{mt}, the latter finding suggests another level of complexity as in our model the induction of NRF1 transcription was affected through phosphorylation by AKT (activation) of the ERα, a process independent of estrogen. Since AKT and estrogen synergize in the activation of the ERα, and phosphorylation of the ERα by AKT was reported to have drastic effects on the genome-wide binding of ERα, the implication is that the regulation of the ERα/NRF1 axis of the UPR^{mt} is not only tissue-specific but affected by the levels of estrogen. The contribution of estrogen may explain some gender difference in life span and will be discussed in further details later in this chapter.

In addition to NRF1, we reported that IMS stress activates IMS-specific aspects of the UPR^{mt}, notably the protease OMI, as well as the activity of the 26S proteasome, which we had previously reported play important roles in limiting the accumulation of misfolded proteins in the IMS (Radke et al., 2008). Lastly, we found that inhibition of the proteasome reduced the viability of cells under IMS stress conditions. We concluded that the ERα/NRF1/proteasome axis of the UPR^{mt} is a cytoprotective response that contributes to the maintenance of the integrity of the mitochondria.

4.2 The IMS of the Mitochondria as a Sensitive Trigger of the UPR^{mt}?

Compared to the intensive studies of the inner-membrane (ETC), outer-membrane (permeabilization during apoptosis), and matrix (Krebs cycle, glycolysis, etc.), the IMS has largely been overlooked. The general view is that the IMS is a passive subcompartment, which acts mainly as a storage space for a few pro-apoptotic proteins. In reality, however, the IMS contains over 100 proteins (Herrmann & Riemer, 2010). Collectively, the various functions of these proteins indicate that the IMS acts as a logistic hub that orchestrates metabolic processes, import of proteins, oxidative folding, protein degradation, transport of metabolites, lipids and metals ions, export of ferrous precursors, assembly of the respiratory chain, detoxification of ROS, and ROS-mediated signaling (Herrmann & Riemer, 2010).

Oxidative protein folding in the IMS is of particular interest since IMS is only one of the two cellular compartments in which this process takes place; the other is the endoplasmic reticulum. Each cycle of folding generates one molecule of ROS. Oxidation of cysteines leads to the formation of disulfide bonds, which, if inappropriate, will lead to misfolding and protein aggregation. While ROS generated by oxidative folding is the only source of ROS in the endoplasmic reticulum, the activity of the ETC is an important additional source of ROS in the IMS. Therefore, the IMS is considered one of the most oxidative cellular compartments, implying that IMS proteins are at higher risk of misfolding (Herrmann & Riemer, 2010). This fact highlights the crucial importance of detecting and signaling to the nucleus the presence of misfolded proteins in the IMS.

The IMS has also an important role in the assembly of the ETC complexes. The inner-membrane is considered the most protein-enriched membrane of the cell, with up to 42 subunits per complex, including some soluble subunits facing the IMS. Several mutations in the various subunits of these complexes have been reported in cancer (Lemarie & Grimm, 2011). Since these mutations affect the efficacy of the electron transport across the inner-membrane and generate more ROS, this observation is consistent with the notion that cancer cells suffer from chronic oxidative stress in the IMS.

Therefore, contrary to the general perception, the IMS represents an important logistic hub that orchestrates essential mitochondrial functions. In term of accumulation of misfolded proteins, the fact that the IMS contains (1) no heat shock proteins, (2) limited proteases and antioxidant enzymes compared to the matrix, and (3) one of the subcellular compartments with most elevated levels of ROS, all converge to argue that the IMS may be a very sensitive sensor of misfolded proteins. Importantly, accumulation of misfolded proteins in the IMS in cells expressing the ERα did not activate CHOP and hsp60. However, in cells that do not express the ERα, both IMS stress and matrix stress led to the activation of hsp60. Since ERα is expressed in several tissues, one interpretation of these findings is that in these tissues all three axes, the ERα, CHOP, and SIRT3 axis of the UPR^{mt}, may be activated while in ERα-negative tissues only the CHOP and SIRT3 axes are. The potential implication of this differential in gene expression profile of the UPR^{mt} among tissues is not trivial since Dillin's group reported that activation of the UPR^{mt} in some tissues, but not others, is linked to longevity (Durieux et al., 2011). A detailed discussion of this study is the topic of a section later in this chapter.

4.3 Lyn Kinase, the New Kid on the Block of the ERα Axis of the UPR^{mt}?

Support for the importance of the IMS as a critical sensor of accumulation of oxidized and misfolded proteins came from the recent study by Lodish's group. They reported that ROS generated by the ETC activates a series of hierarchical signaling events involving the Lyn kinase upstream of the Syk kinase-mediated activation of AKT (Patterson et al., 2015). Gene profile of this response activated genes implicated in transcription, translation, protein folding, metabolism, cell cycle regulation, and tumor suppression (Patterson et al., 2015). Importantly for the discussion of the ERα axis of the UPR^{mt}, they found that a pool of Lyn and Syk localizes to the IMS of the mitochondria. They further obtained evidence that this pathway may be highly conserved through evolution as orthologues of Syk were found in every vertebrate but not in yeast, plants, or bacteria (Patterson et al., 2015). They proposed a critical role of ROS in signaling across species and suggested that this pathway was activated in several tissues and might represent an ancient pathway. Considering that we discovered the ERα axis of the UPR^{mt} as response to stress emanating specifically from the IMS and that we found ROS and AKT are essential upstream activators of ERα, it is tempting to speculate that Lyn and Syk represent the missing links between ROS and activation of AKT in this axis of the UPR^{mt}. This possibility will be tested in the future.

4.4 The Intramitochondrial ERα and ERβ: Link to the UPR^{mt}?

While our study of the estrogen receptor in the UPR^{mt} has focused on ERα and more specifically the nuclear fraction of the ERα, we, like others, have found the ERα and ERβ to be localized in the mitochondria. In fact our original hypothesis to explain the activation of the ERα by IMS stress was that IMS stress may promote the translocation of ERα from the mitochondria to the nucleus. While we found no evidence for such translocation and focused on the nuclear form of the ERα, a role for the intramitochondrial form of the ERα and possibly also ERβ cannot be ruled out. Therefore, while evidence linking the intramitochondrial ERs to the UPR^{mt} has not yet been obtained, the mounting number of reports supporting an important role of mitochondrial ER in the integrity of the organelle imposes a discussion.

4.5 Mitochondrial ER Protects Against Apoptosis via Upregulation of SOD2 Activity

It is more than 10 years ago that the localization of the ERα and ERβ in the mitochondria was reported (Chen, Delannoy, Cooke, & Yager, 2004). Levin's group subsequently reported that in a breast cancer cell line,

MCF-7, approximately 85% of the ER localized to the nucleus, 5% to the plasma membrane, and 10% to the mitochondria (Pedram et al., 2006). Further, they were the first to report that while the ERβ is much less abundant than ERα in these cells, ERβ was the most concentrated in the mitochondria. They then investigated whether estrogen can protect against apoptosis using UV irradiation-mediated cytochrome c release as a model system. They found that addition of estrogen blocked the release of cytochrome c under these conditions and that the presence of the ER was necessary for the effect of estrogen (Pedram et al., 2006). Interestingly, as expression of the ligand-binding domain of the ER only was able to recapitulate the protective effect of estrogen in ER-negative cell lines, this result suggests that the protective effect of the ER in the mitochondria is independent of it transcriptional function since the DNA-binding domain is dispensable. In agreement with this possibility they found that estrogen led to an increase in SOD2 enzymatic activity within 20 min after the addition of estrogen, a time frame that is indeed incompatible with a transcriptional effect of the ER (Pedram et al., 2006). Further, they found that treatment with the antioxidant NAC abolished the UV-induced translocation of cytochrome c to the cytoplasm. They concluded that the upregulation of SOD2 activity is the main mechanism by which estrogen protects against apoptosis. Since the same group has pioneered the nongenomic action of the ER at the plasma membrane, they suggested that much like the reported mechanism of action of the ER at the plasma membrane, the ER in the mitochondria may associate with kinase to mediate the phosphorylation and activation of SOD2. This interesting possibility remains to be demonstrated.

This study by Levin's group was followed by another aimed at testing the role of mitochondrial ER in resistance to the antiestrogen drug tamoxifen. Tamoxifen was the first antiestrogen drug to be developed for the treatment of ERα-positive breast cancer. However, resistance is frequently observed and while many mechanisms have been proposed, the role of the mitochondria in this setting was never investigated. Levin's group first showed that while treatment with tamoxifen leads to an increase in ROS production in MCF-7 cells that are sensitive to such treatment, in a clone of MCF-7 that are resistant to tamoxifen (MCF7-TR), tamoxifen failed to stimulate ROS production (Razandi, Pedram, Jordan, Fuqua, & Levin, 2013). To test the role of ROS in cell death induced by tamoxifen, they used rotenone to inhibit complex I and found that pretreatment with rotenone impaired by 68% the ability of tamoxifen to induce ROS. To ensure that the source of ROS was mitochondrial in nature, they measured ROS using staining with

Mito-SOX. They found that tamoxifen increased mitochondrial ROS by threefold and that this effect was inhibited by cotreatment with estrogen. Since the mitochondria express both ERα and ERβ, they then tried to identify which of the ER is implicated in this effect of tamoxifen. Following a successful inhibition of ERα and ERβ by siRNA, they reported that inhibition of ERβ, but not ERα, affected the production of ROS and cell death induced by tamoxifen (Razandi et al., 2013). As they had previously reported that estrogen stimulates the activity of SOD2, they logically tested whether tamoxifen blocks the activation of SOD2. They found that SOD2 activity but not its protein level was inhibited by tamoxifen and that ERβ was necessary for this effect to occur (Razandi et al., 2013). To link the effect of tamoxifen on SOD2 activity and resistance to tamoxifen, SOD2 was knocked down by siRNA in tamoxifen resistant cells. Reduction in SOD2 increased apoptosis by 15-fold upon treatment with tamoxifen. To validate this result in vivo, they then performed a xenograft experiment were tumors where injected with either control lentivirus or lentivirus expressing siRNA against SOD2. In agreement with the in vitro data, they observed a substantial reduction in tumor volumes in those tumors in which SOD2 expression was inhibited. Characterization of the tumors at the end of this experiment confirmed the link between inhibition of SOD2 and increased apoptosis. Therefore, these results indicate that inhibition of SOD2 can restore sensitivity to tamoxifen (Razandi et al., 2013).

The cytoplasmic fraction of ERβ has also been validated clinically in several studies. In advanced ovarian cancer, breast cancer, and lung cancer, cytoplasmic staining of ERβ is associated with worst outcomes (Ciucci et al., 2014; De Stefano et al., 2011; Mah et al., 2011; Shaaban et al., 2008; Zhang et al., 2009). Therefore, the available data strongly support an important role of the mitochondrial ER in cancer, namely drug resistance via its ability to regulate at the posttranslational level the activity of SOD2, a marker of the UPR^{mt}.

Adding to the role of the ER in the mitochondria are the reports of the regulation of 17β-hydroxysteroid dehydrogenase 10 (HSD17B10) by the ERα (Yang, He, & Schulz, 2005). HSD17B10 is an enzyme that converts estrogen into estrone in the mitochondria in a NAD$^+$-dependent fashion. Colocalization as well as direct interaction of the ERα and HSD17B10 has been shown and the authors of this study proposed that the levels of estrogen regulate this interaction. At high concentrations of estrogen, the interaction was disrupted, allowing the conversion of estrogen to estrone, while at low concentrations, estrogen stimulated the interaction and inhibited HSD17B10 (Jazbutyte, Kehl, Neyses, & Pelzer, 2009). A more recent study suggested an additional role for the interaction of ERα and HSD17B10 in the regulation of mitochondria-encoded genes. This finding arose from the fact that HSD17B10 is one of the three proteins composing the RNase P complex, which is required for the processing of the 5' end of mitochondrial tRNA and therefore affecting translation of mitochondria-encoded transcripts. The authors reported that estrogen leads to a significant elevation in mitochondrial protein translation (Sanchez et al., 2015). While intriguing, these results appear contradictory to the results reported in the Jazbutyte study. Since this latter study was performed in cardiomyocytes, while the study from Sanchez was conducted in MCF7 breast cancer cells, perhaps this discrepancy reflects a tissue specificity of the interaction between the ERα and HSD17B10. Nevertheless, the potential impact of the ERs on mitochondrial protein translation represents a very novel and interesting possibility that should be further explored in the future.

The effects of estrogen receptors on the mitochondria therefore appear to act at both nuclear genome level as well as the mitochondria level. In terms of its action on nuclear-encoded genes that modulate the mitochondria, we and others have reported the effect of the ER on the proteasome, Omi and the NRF1 (Ivanova et al., 2013; Papa & Germain, 2011). However, an effect on several other genes regulating glycolytic enzymes, TCA cycle, and ATP synthase has been reported (Kostanyan & Nazaryan, 1992; Nilsen, Irwin, Gallaher, & Brinton, 2007). Further, estrogen has been reported to also drastically affect the transcription of genes encoded by the mitochondrial genome. For instance estrogen is reported to increase by 16-fold the expression of cytochrome c oxidase subunit II (Van Itallie & Dannies, 1988), as well as all three subunits of complex IV and subunits 6 and 8 of ATP synthase (Chen et al., 2003; Chen, Gokhale, Li, Trush, & Yager, 1998). In strong support of an especially important role of ERβ in this setting, most of the genes modified by the knockdown of ERβ in mice are mitochondrial structural proteins (O'Lone et al., 2007).

5. SUMMARY OF THE ROLES OF SIRTUINS AND THE ESTROGEN RECEPTORS IN THE UPR^mt IN CANCER

Hoogenraad's group has pioneered the study of the UPR^{mt} using expression of mutant OTC in the matrix as a direct means to induce accumulation of misfolded proteins. Using this system they discovered that the transcription factor CHOP promotes the expression of the mitochondrial chaperones hsp10 and hsp60 as well as the matrix protease ClpP. Subsequent work on the UPR^{mt} in *C. elegans* has been restricted to the induction of hsp60 or 6 promoters driving a reporter to monitor the activation of the UPR^{mt}. Haynes's group has generated undeniably important advances in our understanding of the UPR^{mt}. However, restricting the definition of the UPR^{mt} to the activation of a single reporter has created an unfortunate oversimplification of this pathway. We and others have reported that other axes of the UPR^{mt} are activated by mitochondrial proteotoxic stress that does not affect the expression of hsp60. In addition, Kaeberlein's group also reported that not all RNAi clones identified in their screen activate hsp60 but only hsp6, which led this group to propose substantial differences in the regulation of individual targets of the UPR^{mt}. In this chapter, we have focused on the role of SIRT3 and SIRT1, which both regulate, either directly or indirectly, PGC1α and FOXO3A leading to the expression of SOD2. In addition, PGC1α regulates genes involved in mitochondrial biogenesis as well as in oxidative phosphorylation. Further, both SIRT1 and SIRT3 are linked to the induction of autophagy. We specifically showed that SIRT3 is required for the induction of mitophagy in response to mitochondrial proteotoxic stress. SIRT3 was, however, dispensable for the induction of hsp60 and therefore, using the current approach in *C. elegans*, genetic screens designed to identify regulators of the UPR^{mt} would fail to identify SIRT3 as an inducer of the UPR^{mt}.

In addition to the sirtuins, we also reported the role of the ERα, which directly promotes the expression of NRF1. As NRF1 can form a complex with PGC1α, NRF1 can mediate a cross talk between the sirtuins and ERα axis of the UPR^{mt}. While the role of ERα and ERβ in the mitochondria has not yet been formally linked to the UPR^{mt}, the finding that mitochondrial ER can regulate the activity of SOD2 offers a potential link. Lastly, while preliminary, the interaction of ERβ with 17β-hydroxysteroid dehydrogenase and the role of this enzyme in the regulation of mitochondrial tRNA processing open the interesting possibility that estrogen and the ER can affect the rate of mitochondrial protein translation. In support of a role of the regulation of mitochondrial translation in the UPR^{mt}, attenuation of mitochondrial translation has been linked to the UPR^{mt} in the context of longevity. The following sections focus on the role of the UPR^{mt} in aging.

6. UPR^{mt} IN AGING

6.1 Inhibition of Mitochondrial Protein Translation Activates the UPR^{mt} and Promotes Longevity

The mitochondria have been identified as a major regulator of longevity. The mitochondrion has over a thousand proteins. Of those only 13 are encoded by the mitochondrial genome; however, these mitochondria-encoded proteins are all implicated in respiratory chain complexes indicating an important role in the regulation of oxidative phosphorylation. Since each of the electron chain complexes contains several proteins, their assembly requires a stoichiometric balance between the subunits encoded by the nuclear genome and those encoded by the mitochondrial genome. Further, translation of the mitochondria-encoded proteins requires separate translation machinery, including mitochondrial ribosomal proteins.

Auwerx's group identified the mitochondria ribosomal protein S5 (Mrps5) in a screen for longevity genes in mice (Houtkooper et al., 2013). Their screen consisted of exploiting the BXD family of mice, in which life span among strains varies from 365 to 900 days. Having identified Mrps5 as a longevity gene in mice, they then turned to *C. elegans* to validate their findings using the worm homologue. The first evidence linking Mrps5 to life span came from the observation that Mrp expression declines with age. Further, linkage analysis revealed that not only Mrps5, but also several Mrp family members, were associated with longevity. Further, looking at the gene set that covary with Mrps5, they found that genes implicated in oxidative phosphorylation, which are known to be linked to longevity, were those that covary with Mrps5 (Houtkooper et al., 2010). To further test the role of Mrps5 in longevity, they inhibited its expression by RNAi and found that it is sufficient to extend life span (Houtkooper et al., 2013). This phenotype was associated with decreased mitochondrial activity and ATP production.

Pathways regulating longevity are the insulin/IGF signaling, calorie restriction, and mitochondrial dysfunction. Using genetic approach they found that neither IGF signaling nor calorie restriction was required for the effect of Mrps5 on longevity (Houtkooper et al., 2013). They therefore turned their attention to mitochondrial dysfunction and the UPR^{mt} and found that inhibition of Mrps5 induces the hsp60 and 6 reporters activity. Further, to confirm the activation of the UPR^{mt} by Mrsp5 (Houtkooper et al., 2013), they used two markers of the UPR^{mt} in *C. elegans*, HAF1 and UBL5, which are necessary for the transcription of these chaperones.

As mitochondrial protein translation is inhibited by antibiotics, rather than using depletion of Mrsp5, they used treatment with the antibiotic doxycycline or rapamycin to inhibit mitochondrial protein translation and found that such treatment also leads to extension in life span (Houtkooper et al., 2013). Doxycycline also activated the hsp60 reporter. They then used the observation that treatment with antibiotics activates the UPR^{mt} to validate the activation of the UPR^{mt} by inhibition of mitochondrial translation in mice. As they observed in worms, treatment with rapamycin in mice also activated the UPR^{mt}. They concluded that extension of life span due to inhibition of mitochondrial protein translation is due to the activation of the UPR^{mt}.

Interestingly, another study by the Nystrom's group had also reported a role of mitochondrial protein translation in longevity in the yeast *Saccharomyces cerevisiae*. In *S. cerevisiae*, the pathway regulating the communication between the mitochondria and nucleus is referred as the RTG retrograde signaling, a pathway identified by Butow's group. The RTG was identified using yeast lacking mitochondrial DNA and this group found that the CIT2 gene is potently activated by the absence of mtDNA (Chelstowska & Butow, 1995). Therefore, in their study, the Nystrom's group tested whether defects in mitochondrial protein translation affected the expression of CIT2. As they found no effect on the expression of CIT2, they concluded that the RTG is not implicated. While this study did not investigate the potential link to the UPR^{mt}, they reported that defect in mitochondrial protein translation activated the yeast equivalent of SIRT1 and that SIRT1 was essential for the effect on longevity they observed (Caballero et al., 2011). It would therefore be interesting to test whether the activation of the substrates of SIRT1 such as FOXO3a and PGCα is observed in this model as well.

6.2 Defect in the ETC Complexes Activates the UPR^{mt} and Promotes Longevity

One of the most innovative findings regarding the UPR^{mt} came from Dillin's group who addressed a central question regarding the aging process. Notably they asked how the changes in physiology that are observed in aging occur in multiple organs simultaneously. Further, they listed several reports that indicate that signals emerging from specific tissues are driving aging in the entire organism (Durieux et al., 2011). To address the role of specific tissue in aging, they used transgenic worms expressing shRNA against the nuclear-encoded cytochrome *c* oxidase-1 subunit Vb/COX4 (cco-1) to induce ETC defects. They performed knockdown in three-specific tissues: intestine, neurons, and muscles and found that inhibition of cco-1 in muscles had no effect on life span; however, it significantly increased longevity when inhibited in both intestine and neuronal tissues. Then, because defect in the ETC was reported to induce the UPR^{mt}, again as defined by induction of the hsp60 reporter in worms, they investigated the role of the UPR^{mt}. They found that defect in cco-1 is a potent inducer of the UPR^{mt} (Durieux et al., 2011) and that inhibition of ubl-5, which is required for the transcription of hsp60 in worms, is essential in the increased longevity conferred by inhibition of cco-1. Interestingly, the timing of the inhibition of cco-1 on longevity was found to be critical since inhibition after the L4 larval stage did not affect longevity. This finding suggested that inactivation during the larval stage of development is sufficient to maintain the activation of the UPR^{mt} in the adult animals. Based on these findings they then hypothesized that the induction of the UPR^{mt} in one tissue may lead to the induction of the UPR^{mt} in another tissue. In agreement with this possibility they found that the inhibition of cco-1 in the neurons led to the activation of the UPR^{mt} in the intestine (Durieux et al., 2011). Based on these findings they proposed a model whereby cells experiencing ETC defect can produce a signal that activates the UPR^{mt}, these cells then send an extracellular signal they named a mitokine that migrates through the circulation to reach another tissue and induce the UPR^{mt} (Durieux et al., 2011).

Clearly the UPR^{mt} activated in muscles cannot be the same as the UPR^{mt} activated in the neurons and intestine, despite the fact that in all cases hsp60 is activated. Since neurons and intestine, but not muscles, express the estrogen receptor, it is tempting to speculate that expression of the $ER\alpha$ axis of the UPR^{mt} may be what distinguish the UPR^{mt} in these tissues. Further support to this possibility arises from the well-known extended longevity of females. This aspect will be discussed later in this chapter.

The conclusion of Dillin's group study was, however, challenged by Kaeberlein's group who reported that UPR^{mt} is not required for longevity (Bennett et al., 2014). This group performed an RNAi screen for genes that induce the UPR^{mt} using the hsp6-reporter and identified 95 inducers, 39 of which were genes targeting the ETC and 22 targeted the mitochondrial ribosomal subunits. Of the 95 clones, 29 had been previously reported and 66 new. In their study, the authors focused on 34 clones that were validated by sequence and found that of those 34, only half were able to also activate the hsp60 reporter. They also found that while some clones increased life span, others significantly reduced it (Bennett et al., 2014). Further, they reported that deletion of atfs-1, while able to abolish the activation of hsp6 and 60 reporters, fails to affect life span. In their discussion, they highlighted the point that their results are actually consistent with the observation that deletion of mitochondrial prohibitin 2, while a potent activator of the UPR^{mt}, actually also reduces life span. Therefore, they authors raised the point that UPR^{mt} is still poorly characterized and imprecisely defined and that their results point to a perhaps more complex picture where ATFS-1 may regulate the expression of only a subset of UPR^{mt} targets. This interpretation is consistent with our work showing that the expression of hsp60 is regulated by the CHOP axis of the UPR^{mt} but is unaffected by the sirtuins axis. Conversely, targets of the sirtuins axis are not affected by CHOP (Papa & Germain, 2014).

Further, another important point raised by Kaeberlein's group is that the differences observed in the regulation of particular targets may also reflect the degree of mitochondrial stress used in individual studies. In this scenario, some stress conditions may lead to the activation of broader range of targets while others only a subset of genes. This situation is supported by the fact that it is precisely what is observed in cells undergoing stress in the endoplasmic reticulum. The three axes of this pathway ATF-6, IRE, and PERK can be either activated together or sequentially, depending on the level of stress experienced (Rutkowski & Kaufman, 2004).

One important point to add is the type of stress. Currently, several different sources of mitochondrial stress are being used, including ROS, misfolded proteins, depletion of mtDNA, inhibition of prohibitins, reduced mitochondrial protein translation, modulation of the NAD$^+$ levels, and defect in the ETC. Adding to the confusion are the conflicting results showing for instance that ROS does not activate the UPR^{mt}, based on activation of the hsp60 reporter, while ROS does activate SIRT1 (Houtkooper et al., 2013), while drugs able to increase NAD$^+$ levels promote both SIRT1 and hsp60 and boost ROS. Therefore, it appears that as the field moves forward, a better distinction needs to be made regarding the activation of the UPR^{mt} and the type and level of stress being applied.

The link between the UPR^{mt} and longevity has been largely dominated by the analysis of the hsp60 axis, with the exception of the study by Auwerx's group involving SIRT1, FOXO3A, and SOD2 (Mouchiroud et al., 2013). Considering this study and our work on the sirtuins in the UPR^{mt}, the following sections aim at summarizing the link between the sirtuins and longevity.

6.3 SIRT1 and Aging

The role of sirtuins in longevity has been a topic of major interest based on the impact of the sirtuins on mitochondrial biogenesis and the regulation of oxidative stress. As most longevity studies use model organisms, such as yeast and *C. elegans*, which express Sir-2, the homologue of SIRT1 in mammalian cells, the focus has been on the role of SIRT1 in aging. However, other sirtuins, namely, SIRT3 is also implicated in life span extension and will be discussed in the following section.

While originally described in yeast, the role of Sir2 on life span extension in yeast has been extended to *C. elegans* and *Drosophila* (Kaeberlein et al., 1999; Tissenbaum & Guarente, 2001; Whitaker et al., 2013). Sir2 was found to extend life span induced by calorie restriction in yeast by increasing oxidative phosphorylation (Lin et al., 2002). However, it is important to note that other pathways may also play a role, since other studies have reported sir2-independent effect of calorie restriction (Kaeberlein, Kirkland, Fields, & Kennedy, 2004; Lamming et al., 2005). In *C. elegans*, SIR2-mediated life span extension has also been linked to the activation of FOXO transcription factor and the induction of autophagy (Lin, Hsin, Libina, & Kenyon, 2001; Morselli et al., 2010b). Reduction in the $NAD^+/NADH$ ratio has been associated with aging and thought to be responsible for the increase in mitochondrial ROS.

A study by Sinclair's group has reported that the decline in NAD^+ during aging leads to a reduction in the activity of SIRT1. One of the most innovative aspects of this study is the finding that SIRT1 is able to regulate mitochondria through a PGC1α-independent pathway (Gomes et al., 2013). They reported that SIRT1 stabilizes HIF1α via the ubiquitin ligase VHL and that the resulting elevation in HIF1α modulates the ability of Myc to activate the TFAM (Gomes et al., 2013). Further, AMPK was found to act as a switch between the PGC1α-dependent and -independent pathways driven by SIRT1. They therefore referred to the activation of HIF1α by this pathway as a pseudohypoxic state, induced by the decline in NAD^+ (Gomes et al., 2013). Further, they demonstrated that restoring NAD^+ levels in old mice was able to restore mitochondrial function, indicating that this process is reversible. Interestingly, decline in SIRT3 has also been reported to lead to the stabilization of HIF1α (Finley, Carracedo, et al., 2011), therefore raising the possibility that loss of function of SIRT1 and 3 during aging, at least in part, leads to mitochondrial dysfunction by the activation of HIF1α driven pathways.

6.4 SIRT3 and Aging

The discovery of single nucleotide polymorphisms (SNP) in the SIRT3 gene in centenarians has generated great interest in linking SIRT3 function and aging (Bellizzi et al., 2005; Hurst, Williams, & Pal, 2002; Rose et al., 2003). Strangely, the G477T transversion in exon 3 of SIRT3 does not lead to a change in an amino acid, but humans carrying this SNP live beyond the average age. How this SNP increases longevity is not known (Rose et al., 2003).

However, since the SIRT3 gene maps to a region of the genome where other genes involved in longevity are found, one possibility is that this SNP interacts with other regions within this cluster. The SNP discovered in intron 5 of SIRT3, however, leads to improved enhancer activity and increases the expression of SIRT3 (Bellizzi et al., 2005).

The third SNP in the SIRT3 gene has the opposite effect to the other two SNP; it increases the risk of age-related metabolic syndrome. In agreement with the loss of function of SIRT3, this SNP does lead to a change in amino acid that reduces the deacetylase activity of SIRT3 (Hirschey et al., 2011).

In agreement with the correlative link between SIRT3 and longevity in humans, while the SIRT3 knockout mice do not show any severe phenotypes, they are prone to age-related diseases such as cardiac failure, cancer, and metabolic syndrome (Hirschey et al., 2011). Further, these mice show hyperacetylation of mitochondrial proteins and mitochondrial defect, an effect that is not shared by the other mitochondrial sirtuins, SIRT4 and 5 (Lombard et al., 2007).

Aging has been linked to increased oxidative stress, which can lead to increased rate of mitochondrial DNA mutations. Mice that are deficient in polymerase gamma (PolG), also known as the mutator mice, show premature aging linked to increased rate of mutation in their mtDNA (Trifunovic et al., 2004). However, exercise was found to abolish completely the premature aging phenotype of these mice and further, mutations in mtDNA were also abolished (Safdar et al., 2011). One possible explanation for this observation raised by Kincaid and Bossy-Wetzel (2013) is that exercise activates PGC1α and SIRT3 leading to expression of SOD2 and a reduction in ROS-mediated mtDNA mutation. Another possibility is that because SIRT3 was reported to deacetylate 8-oxoguanine-DNA glycosylase (OGC1), which localizes to the nucleus but also to the mitochondria, it can increase the DNA repair capacity. It would therefore be of interest to test whether SIRT3 is essential for the protective effect of exercise in the PolG mice.

6.5 SOD2 and Aging

A link between the levels and activity of SOD2 and longevity has also been established. Using transgenic flies designed to have inducible expression of SOD2, it was shown that induction of SOD2 increases the mean life span by 16%, but in some transgenic lines the increase in life span was as high as 33%

(Sun, Folk, Bradley, & Tower, 2002). The variability of the effect of SOD2 expression in different transgenic lines was shown to directly correlate with the level of activity of SOD2.

In support of this finding, inhibition of SOD2 in flies showed acceleration of age-related phenotypes. Using P-element insertion screen, a fly line in which the expression of SOD2 is lost was generated. Analysis of this line showed that life spans were reduced by 20–40% and that the effect on life span was directly related to the level of inhibition since flies with 50% and 75% reduction showed reduction in life span of 38% and 43%, respectively (Paul et al., 2007). All flies with reduced SOD2 expression had an age-related mortality therefore indicating that SOD2 plays a role in determining the rate of demographic aging. Phenotypical characterization of these flies established that neuronal cell death was accelerated in flies lacking SOD2 expression, suggesting that maintenance of neurons is especially sensitive to levels of SOD2. Further, olfactory capacity, which is known to decline with age, was found to be reduced in absence of SOD2. These two complementary studies therefore suggest that SOD2 is a longevity gene. A further support to this observation, the overexpression of SOD2 in yeast is also linked to a 30% life span extension (Fabrizio et al., 2003). Lastly, a more recent study showed that the life extension properties of cranberry supplement require the expression of SOD2 (Sun, Yolitz, Alberico, Sun, & Zou, 2014).

6.6 FOXO3a and Aging

The link between FOXO3a and aging has also been the topic of intensive research. The first study to report FOXO3a as a longevity gene was performed using a baseline analysis of longevity cases identified between 1991 and 1993 as those who had survived by 2007 to the age of 95 years or more. All participants who died before the age of 81 were grouped as the average-lived controls cases. Five genes were analyzed in this study but only FOXO3a showed an association with longevity (Willcox et al., 2008). Five loci of two SNP within each allele were tested in this study. The association between FOXO3a SNP and age-related diseases, such as coronary heart disease, stroke, and cancer, was also analyzed. The authors reported a significant protective effect of homozygosity of a selected SNP with regard to coronary heart disease and a borderline relation with cancer. This study therefore established a strong association between FOXO3a and longevity. As a result several other studies followed in various ethnic populations, namely, in the southern Italian centenarian study (Anselmi et al., 2009; Flachsbart et al., 2009; Li et al., 2009), in a German centenarians population and in the Han Chinese population. All of these studies confirmed the original study and established a link between FOXO3a and longevity.

The correlation between FOXO3a polymorphisms and longevity in humans was further analyzed in a recent meta-analysis. In this study a total of 5241 cases and 5724 controls from different ethnic groups were analyzed. The results revealed a significant association between specific alleles and longevity but only in males.

7. SUMMARY OF THE LINK BETWEEN THE SIRT3/FOXO3a/SOD2 AXIS OF THE UPR^{mt} AND AGING

While evidence linking SIRT1 and SOD2 to longevity has been generated in experimental models, strong epidemiologic data have been obtained in humans to link both SIRT3 and FOXO3a. Collectively, these results raise the distinct possibility that the common denominator of the effect of these individual genes on longevity is that they all lead to alterations in the UPR^{mt}. This implies that the SIRT/FOXO3a/SOD2 axis of the UPR^{mt} is a key node within the complex signaling pathways that is activated upon mitochondrial stress. This possibility represents an important question to be address in the future.

Of note is the interesting gender difference observed in the longevity phenotype associated with SNP in the *FOXO3a* gene. The selective benefit of these alleles in males suggests that females may have alternative ways to achieve longevity. One obvious possibility is that by having higher levels of estrogen, females also activate more strongly the ER-dependent axis of the UPR^{mt}. Since the ER has been shown to regulate the activity of SOD2 in the mitochondria, this regulation may allow an alternative mechanism to maintain elevated levels of SOD2, even in absence of FOXO3a, therefore leading to a lack of selection for these SNP in females.

Another important observation supporting the possibility that the ER axis and the SIRT3 axis of the UPR^{mt} may compensate for each other is that the SIRT3 knockout mice develop specifically estrogen receptor-positive mammary tumors (Kim et al., 2010). This observation is remarkable since while most breast cancers are ER positive in humans, in the vast majority of mouse models of breast cancers, mammary tumors are ER negative. The fact that SIRT3 knockout mice select specifically ER-positive cells supports the model that in the absence of the SIRT3 axis of the UPR^{mt}, the maintenance of the integrity of the mitochondria becomes dependent on the expression of the ER. This possibility is also supported by the fact that SIRT3 is reduced with age and that most breast cancers in postmenopausal women are ER positive.

Lastly, the observation that the activation of the UPR^{mt} early in life confers protection against mitochondrial stress over the entire adulthood raises the intriguing possibility that exposure to estrogen in premenopausal females may be sufficient to confer protection through activation of the ER axis of the UPR^{mt} even after the estrogen levels drop after menopause. While purely speculative at this stage, testing this possibility will be important in the future. This latter possibility raises the issue of the role of the estrogen receptors in longevity, which is the focus of the next section.

8. THE ESTROGEN RECEPTORS IN AGING

It is well established that in many species, including humans, females live longer than males, although this observation is not universal. Life style and environmental conditions are likely to impact gender differences and, therefore, experimental models whereby these factors can be differentiated from the biological factors of the gender difference are needed to address this question.

One of the most used models of longevity is the Wistar rat. In this species, females live about 10% longer than males. This difference has been attributed to estrogen since the life span of ovariectomized females was reduced compared to untreated females (Borras et al., 2003; Fox et al., 2006; Maklakov, Fricke, & Arnqvist, 2007). Further, transplantation of young ovaries to old females extended their life span (Paganini-Hill, Corrada, & Kawas, 2006). This observation is well in line with the fact that estrogen replacement therapy can increase life expectancy in humans (Ettinger, Friedman, Bush, & Quesenberry, 1996). In some strains of mice, such as the C57BL6, however, the males live longer than females, but in a variant of this strain, the C57BL6J, this difference is not observed and both males and females have the same life expectancy (Sanz et al., 2007). These differences offer the opportunity to conduct comparative aging studies. The general conclusion from such studies is that estrogen promotes a lower production of mitochondrial ROS, specifically in strains where females live longer. In contrast, in strains where the life expectancy of males and females is the same, the production of ROS is the same between genders, and in strains where males live longer than females, mitochondrial ROS is lower in males. Therefore, a direct correlation exists between life expectancy and mitochondrial ROS at least among mouse strains (Sanz et al., 2007; Vina & Borras, 2010). Considering the ER axis of the UPR^{mt}, and the role of both ERα and ERβ in the mitochondria and their direct action on SOD2, discussed in the earlier sections, the observation that the role of estrogen in longevity is linked to mitochondrial ROS production is in perfect agreement with the possibility that the ER axis of the UPR^{mt} contributes to the gender difference in life expectancy.

9. SIRTUINS AND CIRCADIAN RHYTHM IN CANCER AND AGING

Considering that dysregulation of the circadian rhythm has been linked to both cancer and aging, and that sirtuins as well as the estrogen-receptor related, a key coactivator PGC1α, are regulated by circadian rhythm, a discussion of this topic appeared essential for the completion of this chapter, although a detailed discussion of the machinery of the circadian rhythm is outside the scope of this review.

In relation to the UPR^{mt} both SIRT1 and SIRT3 have been identified as regulators of circadian rhythm. SIRT1 deacetylates PER2, promoting its degradation and allowing rhythmicity of the circadian rhythm (Asher et al., 2008). In addition, SIRT1 also deacetylates BMAL1, which then forms a transcriptional complex with CLOCK and the regulation of expression of circadian rhythm genes. Of note, the activity of SIRT1, rather than its levels, was found to be important in the context of circadian rhythm regulation (Nakahata et al., 2008). The circadian clock is regulated by the central pacemaker located in the suprachiasmatic nucleus, a region of the hypothalamus. SIRT1 has been implicated in this central clock and is linked to aging, a topic that was reviewed extensively (Giblin, Skinner, & Lombard, 2014; Verdin, 2014). These studies therefore link SIRT1 to both the central and peripheral clocks.

The circadian rhythm has been linked to mitochondrial function since the levels of metabolites show circadian oscillation (Dallmann, Viola, Tarokh, Cajochen, & Brown, 2012; Eckel-Mahan et al., 2012; Minami et al., 2009). SIRT3 was recently identified as a potential explanation of these observations. Bass's group reported that embryonic fibroblasts of bam1 knockout mice show decreased levels of oxygen consumption. Further, they found that NAD^{+} levels were lowered in the mitochondria of these mice and that this observation was linked to an increase in the acetylation of mitochondrial proteins and inhibition of SIRT3 activity (Peek et al., 2013).

A key coactivator of PGC1α is the ERRα. Rhythmical expression of several nuclear receptors in metabolically active tissues has been reported (Yang et al., 2006). More specifically ERRα expression profile shows a diurnal rhythm in several tissues (Yang et al., 2006). More recently direct evidence of the regulation of circadian rhythm by ERRα was demonstrated using a genome-wide ChIP on chip analysis of ERRα binding. This study revealed that ERRα is present on the promoters of several clock genes, including Bma1 and Clock (Charest-Marcotte et al., 2010). Further, the same group also showed that ERRα knockout mice have disturbed diurnal rhythms of the clock genes, Bma1 and Clock, as well as others (Dufour et al., 2011). These studies therefore offer a direct link between ERRα/PCG1α and the regulation of circadian rhythm.

10. CONCLUDING REMARKS

The UPR^{mt} is a young field and currently there is no consensus on its precise definition. Most focus on the UPR^{mt} has been using hsp60 reporter as readout of its activation and the finding that in *C. elegans*, ATFS-1 is the transcription factor necessary for the expression of hsp60 in response to a variety of mitochondrial stresses. As the homolog of ATFS-1 in mammalian cells is pending, some in the field have begun to question whether the UPR^{mt} exists in mammalian cells. This is despite the fact that activation of hsp60 was originally described in mammalian cells by Hoogenraad's group and found to involve the transcription factor CHOP. But the contribution of CHOP in this response has been largely ignored since.

The contribution of Sirtuins has also been overlooked despite the observation by Auwerx's group that the Sirtuin/FOXO/SOD2 axis is conserved from *C. elegans* to mammalian cells. As with the Hoogenraad's group, our work used accumulation of misfolding in the mitochondria as a source of stress and led to the discovery of an overlapping pathway involving a SIRT3/FOXO3a/SOD2 axis. This pathway offers a direct link between proteotoxic stress in the mitochondria and the transcriptional machinery able to promote mitochondrial biogenesis, oxidative phosphorylation, and mitophagy. In addition, the estrogen receptor has long been known to have protective effect on the mitochondria and we described a role of the ERα in the UPR^{mt}. In light of these findings, the uncertainty of the existence of the

UPR^{mt} in mammalian cells appears unfounded. In contrast, our knowledge of the UPR^{mt} in mammalian cells is much better advanced than the current portrait.

One factor that has contributed to the poor definition of the UPR^{mt} is the fact that unlike the endoplasmic reticulum, the origin of the stress leading to the accumulation of misfolded proteins can be direct or indirect in the mitochondria. This has led to a diverse nomenclature to define the signaling pathways between the mitochondria and the nucleus, such as retrograde signaling and ROS defense pathway.

Another contributing factor to the current confusion regarding the definition of the UPR^{mt} is the restriction of its activation to the hsp60 reporter. As highlighted by Kaeberlein's group several genes able to activate the hsp6 reporter do not activate the hsp60 reporter. As the field evolves, it seems mandatory that this arbitrary restriction to define the UPR^{mt} is reconsidered and that activation of hsp60 and/or hsp6 be seen as only one aspect of this complex signaling pathway.

Importantly, while the aim of this review was to focus on the sirtuins and the estrogen receptors, important contributions to the UPR^{mt} have been reported by several groups. Notably, Altieri's group has reported the tumor-specific elevation in hsp90 in the mitochondria in mice and human cells (Siegelin et al., 2011). The role of PGC1α in the retrograde mitochondria-nucleus signaling has been described and reviewed recently (Jones, Yao, Vicencio, Karkucinska-Wieckowska, & Szabadkai, 2012). The link between mitophagy and accumulation of misfolded proteins in the mitochondria has been studied in *Drosophila* (Pimenta de Castro et al., 2012). Genetic screens for genes activated by ROS-mediated UPR^{mt} have been performed (Runkel, Liu, Baumeister, & Schulze, 2013). Protoetoxic stress induced by the deletion of mortalin was shown to be rescued by increased mitophagy (Burbulla et al., 2014). Considering the increased interest in the UPR^{mt} it will be important in the future to integrate these findings as to create a more comprehensive picture of this pathway.

The finding from Dillin's group that activation of the UPR^{mt} varies among tissues argues that the genomic and epigenetic landscape of various tissues will affect the array of genes activated upon mitochondrial stress. In this setting, it appears that the role of the ERα axis of the UPR^{mt} is favorably placed to explain at least some of these tissue specificities.

The contribution of the IMS also needs to be considered more closely. Our work has pioneered the notion that this subcompartment may act as a very sensitive sensor of accumulation of misfolded proteins in the mitochondria. The recent study by the Lodish's group indicating that the IMS activates an ancient signaling cascade in response to oxidative stress-generated from defect in the ETC strongly supports an important role for the IMS (Patterson et al., 2015).

In conclusion, the mammalian UPR^{mt} represents an exciting new field of mitochondrial biology that is likely to impact several diseases and may provide the missing link between aging, circadian rhythm, life style, and gender difference observed in several of these diseases. Much remains to be done and exciting findings will certainly emerge from the study of the UPR^{mt}.

REFERENCES

Ahn, B. H., Kim, H. S., Song, S., Lee, I. H., Liu, J., Vassilopoulos, A., et al. (2008). A role for the mitochondrial deacetylase Sirt3 in regulating energy homeostasis. *Proceedings of the National Academy of Sciences of the United States of America, 105*, 14447–14452.

Anselmi, C. V., Malovini, A., Roncarati, R., Novelli, V., Villa, F., Condorelli, G., et al. (2009). Association of the FOXO3A locus with extreme longevity in a southern Italian centenarian study. *Rejuvenation Research, 12*, 95–104.

Asher, G., Gatfield, D., Stratmann, M., Reinke, H., Dibner, C., Kreppel, F., et al. (2008). SIRT1 regulates circadian clock gene expression through PER2 deacetylation. *Cell, 134*, 317–328.

Ashraf, N., Zino, S., Macintyre, A., Kingsmore, D., Payne, A. P., George, W. D., et al. (2006). Altered sirtuin expression is associated with node-positive breast cancer. *British Journal of Cancer, 95*, 1056–1061.

Bell, E. L., Emerling, B. M., Ricoult, S. J., & Guarente, L. (2011). SirT3 suppresses hypoxia inducible factor 1alpha and tumor growth by inhibiting mitochondrial ROS production. *Oncogene, 30*, 2986–2996.

Bellizzi, D., Rose, G., Cavalcante, P., Covello, G., Dato, S., De Rango, F., et al. (2005). A novel VNTR enhancer within the SIRT3 gene, a human homologue of SIR2, is associated with survival at oldest ages. *Genomics, 85*, 258–263.

Benedetti, C., Haynes, C. M., Yang, Y., Harding, H. P., & Ron, D. (2006). Ubiquitin-like protein 5 positively regulates chaperone gene expression in the mitochondrial unfolded protein response. *Genetics, 174*, 229–239.

Bennett, C. F., Vander Wende, H., Simko, M., Klum, S., Barfield, S., Choi, H., et al. (2014). Activation of the mitochondrial unfolded protein response does not predict longevity in *Caenorhabditis elegans*. *Nature Communications, 5*, 3483.

Berdichevsky, A., Viswanathan, M., Horvitz, H. R., & Guarente, L. (2006). C. elegans SIR-2.1 interacts with 14-3-3 proteins to activate DAF-16 and extend life span. *Cell, 125*, 1165–1177.

Bhat-Nakshatri, P., Wang, G., Appaiah, H., Luktuke, N., Carroll, J. S., Geistlinger, T. R., et al. (2008). AKT alters genome-wide estrogen receptor alpha binding and impacts estrogen signaling in breast cancer. *Molecular and Cellular Biology, 28*, 7487–7503.

Borras, C., Sastre, J., Garcia-Sala, D., Lloret, A., Pallardo, F. V., & Vina, J. (2003). Mitochondria from females exhibit higher antioxidant gene expression and lower oxidative damage than males. *Free Radical Biology & Medicine, 34*, 546–552.

Brunet, A., Sweeney, L. B., Sturgill, J. F., Chua, K. F., Greer, P. L., Lin, Y., et al. (2004). Stress-dependent regulation of FOXO transcription factors by the SIRT1 deacetylase. *Science, 303*, 2011–2015.

Burbulla, L. F., Fitzgerald, J. C., Stegen, K., Westermeier, J., Thost, A. K., Kato, H., et al. (2014). Mitochondrial proteolytic stress induced by loss of mortalin function is rescued by Parkin and PINK1. *Cell Death & Disease*, *5*, e1180.

Caballero, A., Ugidos, A., Liu, B., Oling, D., Kvint, K., Hao, X., et al. (2011). Absence of mitochondrial translation control proteins extends life span by activating sirtuin-dependent silencing. *Molecular Cell*, *42*, 390–400.

Campbell, R. A., Bhat-Nakshatri, P., Patel, N. M., Constantinidou, D., Ali, S., & Nakshatri, H. (2001). Phosphatidylinositol 3-kinase/AKT-mediated activation of estrogen receptor alpha: A new model for anti-estrogen resistance. *The Journal of Biological Chemistry*, *276*, 9817–9824.

Carroll, J. S., Meyer, C. A., Song, J., Li, W., Geistlinger, T. R., Eeckhoute, J., et al. (2006). Genome-wide analysis of estrogen receptor binding sites. *Nature Genetics*, *38*, 1289–1297.

Charest-Marcotte, A., Dufour, C. R., Wilson, B. J., Tremblay, A. M., Eichner, L. J., Arlow, D. H., et al. (2010). The homeobox protein Prox1 is a negative modulator of ERRα/PGC-1α bioenergetic functions. *Genes & Development*, *24*, 537–542.

Chelstowska, A., & Butow, R. A. (1995). RTG genes in yeast that function in communication between mitochondria and the nucleus are also required for expression of genes encoding peroxisomal proteins. *The Journal of Biological Chemistry*, *270*, 18141–18146.

Chen, J. Q., Delannoy, M., Cooke, C., & Yager, J. D. (2004). Mitochondrial localization of ERalpha and ERbeta in human MCF7 cells. *American Journal of Physiology. Endocrinology and Metabolism*, *286*, E1011–E1022.

Chen, J., Delannoy, M., Odwin, S., He, P., Trush, M. A., & Yager, J. D. (2003). Enhanced mitochondrial gene transcript, ATP, bcl-2 protein levels, and altered glutathione distribution in ethinyl estradiol-treated cultured female rat hepatocytes. *Toxicological Sciences: An Official Journal of the Society of Toxicology*, *75*, 271–278.

Chen, J., Gokhale, M., Li, Y., Trush, M. A., & Yager, J. D. (1998). Enhanced levels of several mitochondrial mRNA transcripts and mitochondrial superoxide production during ethinyl estradiol-induced hepatocarcinogenesis and after estrogen treatment of HepG2 cells. *Carcinogenesis*, *19*, 2187–2193.

Cimen, H., Han, M. J., Yang, Y., Tong, Q., Koc, H., & Koc, E. C. (2010). Regulation of succinate dehydrogenase activity by SIRT3 in mammalian mitochondria. *Biochemistry*, *49*, 304–311.

Ciucci, A., Zannoni, G. F., Travaglia, D., Petrillo, M., Scambia, G., & Gallo, D. (2014). Prognostic significance of the estrogen receptor beta (ERbeta) isoforms ERbeta1, ERbeta2, and ERbeta5 in advanced serous ovarian cancer. *Gynecologic Oncology*, *132*, 351–359.

Colombo, S. L., & Moncada, S. (2009). AMPKalpha1 regulates the antioxidant status of vascular endothelial cells. *The Biochemical Journal*, *421*, 163–169.

Dallmann, R., Viola, A. U., Tarokh, L., Cajochen, C., & Brown, S. A. (2012). The human circadian metabolome. *Proceedings of the National Academy of Sciences of the United States of America*, *109*, 2625–2629.

De Stefano, I., Zannoni, G. F., Prisco, M. G., Fagotti, A., Tortorella, L., Vizzielli, G., et al. (2011). Cytoplasmic expression of estrogen receptor beta (ERbeta) predicts poor clinical outcome in advanced serous ovarian cancer. *Gynecologic Oncology*, *122*, 573–579.

Dorr, J. R., Yu, Y., Milanovic, M., Beuster, G., Zasada, C., Dabritz, J. H., et al. (2013). Synthetic lethal metabolic targeting of cellular senescence in cancer therapy. *Nature*, *501*, 421–425.

Dufour, C. R., Levasseur, M. P., Pham, N. H., Eichner, L. J., Wilson, B. J., Charest-Marcotte, A., et al. (2011). Genomic convergence among ERRalpha, PROX1, and BMAL1 in the control of metabolic clock outputs. *PLoS Genetics*, *7*, e1002143.

Durieux, J., Wolff, S., & Dillin, A. (2011). The cell-non-autonomous nature of electron transport chain-mediated longevity. *Cell, 144*, 79–91.

Eckel-Mahan, K. L., Patel, V. R., Mohney, R. P., Vignola, K. S., Baldi, P., & Sassone-Corsi, P. (2012). Coordination of the transcriptome and metabolome by the circadian clock. *Proceedings of the National Academy of Sciences of the United States of America, 109*, 5541–5546.

Ettinger, B., Friedman, G. D., Bush, T., & Quesenberry, C. P., Jr. (1996). Reduced mortality associated with long-term postmenopausal estrogen therapy. *Obstetrics and Gynecology, 87*, 6–12.

Fabrizio, P., Liou, L. L., Moy, V. N., Diaspro, A., Valentine, J. S., Gralla, E. B., et al. (2003). SOD2 functions downstream of Sch9 to extend longevity in yeast. *Genetics, 163*, 35–46.

Feige, J. N., & Auwerx, J. (2008). Transcriptional targets of sirtuins in the coordination of mammalian physiology. *Current Opinion in Cell Biology, 20*, 303–309.

Finley, L. W., Carracedo, A., Lee, J., Souza, A., Egia, A., Zhang, J., et al. (2011). SIRT3 opposes reprogramming of cancer cell metabolism through HIF1alpha destabilization. *Cancer Cell, 19*, 416–428.

Finley, L. W., Haas, W., Desquiret-Dumas, V., Wallace, D. C., Procaccio, V., Gygi, S. P., et al. (2011). Succinate dehydrogenase is a direct target of sirtuin 3 deacetylase activity. *PLoS One, 6*, e23295.

Flachsbart, F., Caliebe, A., Kleindorp, R., Blanche, H., von Eller-Eberstein, H., Nikolaus, S., et al. (2009). Association of FOXO3A variation with human longevity confirmed in German centenarians. *Proceedings of the National Academy of Sciences of the United States of America, 106*, 2700–2705.

Fox, C. W., Scheibly, K. L., Wallin, W. G., Hitchcock, L. J., Stillwell, R. C., & Smith, B. P. (2006). The genetic architecture of life span and mortality rates: Gender and species differences in inbreeding load of two seed-feeding beetles. *Genetics, 174*, 763–773.

Franco, H. L., Nagari, A., & Kraus, W. L. (2015). TNFalpha signaling exposes latent estrogen receptor binding sites to alter the breast cancer cell transcriptome. *Molecular Cell, 58*, 21–34.

Gertz, J., Savic, D., Varley, K. E., Partridge, E. C., Safi, A., Jain, P., et al. (2013). Distinct properties of cell-type-specific and shared transcription factor binding sites. *Molecular Cell, 52*, 25–36.

Giblin, W., Skinner, M. E., & Lombard, D. B. (2014). Sirtuins: Guardians of mammalian healthspan. *Trends in Genetics, 30*, 271–286.

Gomes, A. P., Price, N. L., Ling, A. J., Moslehi, J. J., Montgomery, M. K., Rajman, L., et al. (2013). Declining NAD(+) induces a pseudohypoxic state disrupting nuclear-mitochondrial communication during aging. *Cell, 155*, 1624–1638.

Greer, E. L., Oskoui, P. R., Banko, M. R., Maniar, J. M., Gygi, M. P., Gygi, S. P., et al. (2007). The energy sensor AMP-activated protein kinase directly regulates the mammalian FOXO3 transcription factor. *The Journal of Biological Chemistry, 282*, 30107–30119.

Haigis, M. C., & Sinclair, D. A. (2010). Mammalian sirtuins: Biological insights and disease relevance. *Annual Review of Pathology, 5*, 253–295.

Haynes, C. M., Petrova, K., Benedetti, C., Yang, Y., & Ron, D. (2007). ClpP mediates activation of a mitochondrial unfolded protein response in C. elegans. *Developmental Cell, 13*, 467–480.

Herrmann, J. M., & Riemer, J. (2010). The intermembrane space of mitochondria. *Antioxidants & Redox Signaling, 13*, 1341–1358.

Hirschey, M. D., Shimazu, T., Goetzman, E., Jing, E., Schwer, B., Lombard, D. B., et al. (2010). SIRT3 regulates mitochondrial fatty-acid oxidation by reversible enzyme deacetylation. *Nature, 464*, 121–125.

Hirschey, M. D., Shimazu, T., Jing, E., Grueter, C. A., Collins, A. M., Aouizerat, B., et al. (2011). SIRT3 deficiency and mitochondrial protein hyperacetylation accelerate the development of the metabolic syndrome. *Molecular Cell, 44*, 177–190.

Honda, Y., & Honda, S. (1999). The daf-2 gene network for longevity regulates oxidative stress resistance and Mn-superoxide dismutase gene expression in *Caenorhabditis elegans*. *The FASEB Journal, 13*, 1385–1393.

Houtkooper, R. H., Mouchiroud, L., Ryu, D., Moullan, N., Katsyuba, E., Knott, G., et al. (2013). Mitonuclear protein imbalance as a conserved longevity mechanism. *Nature, 497*, 451–457.

Houtkooper, R. H., Pirinen, E., & Auwerx, J. (2012). Sirtuins as regulators of metabolism and healthspan. *Nature Reviews. Molecular Cell Biology, 13*, 225–238.

Houtkooper, R. H., Williams, R. W., & Auwerx, J. (2010). Metabolic networks of longevity. *Cell, 142*, 9–14.

Hu, J., Hwang, S. S., Liesa, M., Gan, B., Sahin, E., Jaskelioff, M., et al. (2012). Anti-telomerase therapy provokes ALT and mitochondrial adaptive mechanisms in cancer. *Cell, 148*, 651–663.

Hurst, L. D., Williams, E. J., & Pal, C. (2002). Natural selection promotes the conservation of linkage of co-expressed genes. *Trends in Genetics, 18*, 604–606.

Ivanova, M. M., Radde, B. N., Son, J., Mehta, F. F., Chung, S. H., & Klinge, C. M. (2013). Estradiol and tamoxifen regulate NRF-1 and mitochondrial function in mouse mammary gland and uterus. *Journal of Molecular Endocrinology, 51*, 233–246.

Jacobs, K. M., Pennington, J. D., Bisht, K. S., Aykin-Burns, N., Kim, H. S., Mishra, M., et al. (2008). SIRT3 interacts with the daf-16 homolog FOXO3a in the mitochondria, as well as increases FOXO3a dependent gene expression. *International Journal of Biological Sciences, 4*, 291–299.

Jazbutyte, V., Kehl, F., Neyses, L., & Pelzer, T. (2009). Estrogen receptor alpha interacts with 17beta-hydroxysteroid dehydrogenase type 10 in mitochondria. *Biochemical and Biophysical Research Communications, 384*, 450–454.

Jeong, J. K., Moon, M. H., Lee, Y. J., Seol, J. W., & Park, S. Y. (2013). Autophagy induced by the class III histone deacetylase Sirt1 prevents prion peptide neurotoxicity. *Neurobiology of Aging, 34*, 146–156.

Jin, S. M., & Youle, R. J. (2013). The accumulation of misfolded proteins in the mitochondrial matrix is sensed by PINK1 to induce PARK2/Parkin-mediated mitophagy of polarized mitochondria. *Autophagy, 9*, 1750–1757.

Jones, A. W., Yao, Z., Vicencio, J. M., Karkucinska-Wieckowska, A., & Szabadkai, G. (2012). PGC-1 family coactivators and cell fate: Roles in cancer, neurodegeneration, cardiovascular disease and retrograde mitochondria-nucleus signalling. *Mitochondrion, 12*, 86–99.

Jovaisaite, V., Mouchiroud, L., & Auwerx, J. (2014). The mitochondrial unfolded protein response, a conserved stress response pathway with implications in health and disease. *The Journal of Experimental Biology, 217*, 137–143.

Kaeberlein, M., Kirkland, K. T., Fields, S., & Kennedy, B. K. (2004). Sir2-independent life span extension by calorie restriction in yeast. *PLoS Biology, 2*, E296.

Kaeberlein, M., McVey, M., & Guarente, L. (1999). The SIR2/3/4 complex and SIR2 alone promote longevity in *Saccharomyces cerevisiae* by two different mechanisms. *Genes & Development, 13*, 2570–2580.

Kim, H. S., Patel, K., Muldoon-Jacobs, K., Bisht, K. S., Aykin-Burns, N., Pennington, J. D., et al. (2010). SIRT3 is a mitochondria-localized tumor suppressor required for maintenance of mitochondrial integrity and metabolism during stress. *Cancer Cell, 17*, 41–52.

Kincaid, B., & Bossy-Wetzel, E. (2013). Forever young: SIRT3 a shield against mitochondrial meltdown, aging, and neurodegeneration. *Frontiers in Aging Neuroscience, 5*, 48.

Kong, X., Wang, R., Xue, Y., Liu, X., Zhang, H., Chen, Y., et al. (2010). Sirtuin 3, a new target of PGC-1alpha, plays an important role in the suppression of ROS and mitochondrial biogenesis. *PLoS One, 5,* e11707.

Kostanyan, A., & Nazaryan, K. (1992). Rat brain glycolysis regulation by estradiol-17 beta. *Biochimica et Biophysica Acta, 1133,* 301–306.

Lamming, D. W., Latorre-Esteves, M., Medvedik, O., Wong, S. N., Tsang, F. A., Wang, C., et al. (2005). HST2 mediates SIR2-independent life-span extension by calorie restriction. *Science, 309,* 1861–1864.

Lannigan, D. A. (2003). Estrogen receptor phosphorylation. *Steroids, 68,* 1–9.

LeBleu, V. S., O'Connell, J. T., Gonzalez Herrera, K. N., Wikman, H., Pantel, K., Haigis, M. C., et al. (2014). PGC-1alpha mediates mitochondrial biogenesis and oxidative phosphorylation in cancer cells to promote metastasis. *Nature Cell Biology, 16,* 992–1003. 1001–1015.

Lee, I. H., Cao, L., Mostoslavsky, R., Lombard, D. B., Liu, J., Bruns, N. E., et al. (2008). A role for the NAD-dependent deacetylase Sirt1 in the regulation of autophagy. *Proceedings of the National Academy of Sciences of the United States of America, 105,* 3374–3379.

Lemarie, A., & Grimm, S. (2011). Mitochondrial respiratory chain complexes: Apoptosis sensors mutated in cancer? *Oncogene, 30,* 3985–4003.

Li, S., Banck, M., Mujtaba, S., Zhou, M. M., Sugrue, M. M., & Walsh, M. J. (2010). p53-induced growth arrest is regulated by the mitochondrial SirT3 deacetylase. *PLoS One, 5,* e10486.

Li, Y., Wang, W. J., Cao, H., Lu, J., Wu, C., Hu, F. Y., et al. (2009). Genetic association of FOXO1A and FOXO3A with longevity trait in Han Chinese populations. *Human Molecular Genetics, 18,* 4897–4904.

Lin, K., Hsin, H., Libina, N., & Kenyon, C. (2001). Regulation of the *Caenorhabditis elegans* longevity protein DAF-16 by insulin/IGF-1 and germline signaling. *Nature Genetics, 28,* 139–145.

Lin, S. J., Kaeberlein, M., Andalis, A. A., Sturtz, L. A., Defossez, P. A., Culotta, V. C., et al. (2002). Calorie restriction extends *Saccharomyces cerevisiae* lifespan by increasing respiration. *Nature, 418,* 344–348.

Liu, Z., & Butow, R. A. (2006). Mitochondrial retrograde signaling. *Annual Review of Genetics, 40,* 159–185.

Lomb, D. J., Laurent, G., & Haigis, M. C. (2010). Sirtuins regulate key aspects of lipid metabolism. *Biochimica et Biophysica Acta, 1804,* 1652–1657.

Lombard, D. B., Alt, F. W., Cheng, H. L., Bunkenborg, J., Streeper, R. S., Mostoslavsky, R., et al. (2007). Mammalian Sir2 homolog SIRT3 regulates global mitochondrial lysine acetylation. *Molecular and Cellular Biology, 27,* 8807–8814.

Mah, V., Marquez, D., Alavi, M., Maresh, E. L., Zhang, L., Yoon, N., et al. (2011). Expression levels of estrogen receptor beta in conjunction with aromatase predict survival in non-small cell lung cancer. *Lung Cancer, 74,* 318–325.

Maklakov, A. A., Fricke, C., & Arnqvist, G. (2007). Sexual selection affects lifespan and aging in the seed beetle. *Aging Cell, 6,* 739–744.

Martinus, R. D., Garth, G. P., Webster, T. L., Cartwright, P., Naylor, D. J., Hoj, P. B., et al. (1996). Selective induction of mitochondrial chaperones in response to loss of the mitochondrial genome. *European Journal of Biochemistry, 240,* 98–103.

Mattingly, K. A., Ivanova, M. M., Riggs, K. A., Wickramasinghe, N. S., Barch, M. J., & Klinge, C. M. (2008). Estradiol stimulates transcription of nuclear respiratory factor-1 and increases mitochondrial biogenesis. *Molecular Endocrinology, 22,* 609–622.

Minami, Y., Kasukawa, T., Kakazu, Y., Iigo, M., Sugimoto, M., Ikeda, S., et al. (2009). Measurement of internal body time by blood metabolomics. *Proceedings of the National Academy of Sciences of the United States of America, 106,* 9890–9895.

Mohammed, H., Russell, I. A., Stark, R., Rueda, O. M., Hickey, T. E., Tarulli, G. A., et al. (2015). Progesterone receptor modulates ERalpha action in breast cancer. *Nature, 523*, 313–317.

Morselli, E., Maiuri, M. C., Markaki, M., Megalou, E., Pasparaki, A., Palikaras, K., et al. (2010a). Caloric restriction and resveratrol promote longevity through the Sirtuin-1-dependent induction of autophagy. *Cell Death & Disease, 1*, e10.

Morselli, E., Maiuri, M. C., Markaki, M., Megalou, E., Pasparaki, A., Palikaras, K., et al. (2010b). The life span-prolonging effect of sirtuin-1 is mediated by autophagy. *Autophagy, 6*, 186–188.

Motta, M. C., Divecha, N., Lemieux, M., Kamel, C., Chen, D., Gu, W., et al. (2004). Mammalian SIRT1 represses forkhead transcription factors. *Cell, 116*, 551–563.

Mouchiroud, L., Houtkooper, R. H., Moullan, N., Katsyuba, E., Ryu, D., Canto, C., et al. (2013). The NAD(+)/sirtuin pathway modulates longevity through activation of mitochondrial UPR and FOXO signaling. *Cell, 154*, 430–441.

Myatt, S. S., & Lam, E. W. (2007). The emerging roles of forkhead box (Fox) proteins in cancer. *Nature Reviews. Cancer, 7*, 847–859.

Nakahata, Y., Kaluzova, M., Grimaldi, B., Sahar, S., Hirayama, J., Chen, D., et al. (2008). The NAD+-dependent deacetylase SIRT1 modulates CLOCK-mediated chromatin remodeling and circadian control. *Cell, 134*, 329–340.

Nargund, A. M., Fiorese, C. J., Pellegrino, M. W., Deng, P., & Haynes, C. M. (2015). Mitochondrial and nuclear accumulation of the transcription factor ATFS-1 promotes OXPHOS recovery during the UPR(mt). *Molecular Cell, 58*, 123–133.

Nilsen, J., Irwin, R. W., Gallaher, T. K., & Brinton, R. D. (2007). Estradiol in vivo regulation of brain mitochondrial proteome. *The Journal of Neuroscience, 27*, 14069–14077.

O'Lone, R., Knorr, K., Jaffe, I. Z., Schaffer, M. E., Martini, P. G., Karas, R. H., et al. (2007). Estrogen receptors alpha and beta mediate distinct pathways of vascular gene expression, including genes involved in mitochondrial electron transport and generation of reactive oxygen species. *Molecular Endocrinology, 21*, 1281–1296.

Paganini-Hill, A., Corrada, M. M., & Kawas, C. H. (2006). Increased longevity in older users of postmenopausal estrogen therapy: The Leisure World Cohort Study. *Menopause, 13*, 12–18.

Papa, L., & Germain, D. (2011). Estrogen receptor mediates a distinct mitochondrial unfolded protein response. *Journal of Cell Science, 124*, 1396–1402.

Papa, L., & Germain, D. (2014). SirT3 regulates the mitochondrial unfolded protein response. *Molecular and Cellular Biology, 34*, 699–710.

Patterson, H. C., Gerbeth, C., Thiru, P., Vogtle, N. F., Knoll, M., Shahsafaei, A., et al. (2015). A respiratory chain controlled signal transduction cascade in the mitochondrial intermembrane space mediates hydrogen peroxide signaling. *Proceedings of the National Academy of Sciences of the United States of America, 112*, E5679–E5688.

Paul, A., Belton, A., Nag, S., Martin, I., Grotewiel, M. S., & Duttaroy, A. (2007). Reduced mitochondrial SOD displays mortality characteristics reminiscent of natural aging. *Mechanisms of Ageing and Development, 128*, 706–716.

Pedram, A., Razandi, M., Wallace, D. C., & Levin, E. R. (2006). Functional estrogen receptors in the mitochondria of breast cancer cells. *Molecular Biology of the Cell, 17*, 2125–2137.

Peek, C. B., Affinati, A. H., Ramsey, K. M., Kuo, H. Y., Yu, W., Sena, L. A., et al. (2013). Circadian clock NAD+ cycle drives mitochondrial oxidative metabolism in mice. *Science, 342*, 1243417.

Peserico, A., Chiacchiera, F., Grossi, V., Matrone, A., Latorre, D., Simonatto, M., et al. (2013). A novel AMPK-dependent FoxO3A-SIRT3 intramitochondrial complex sensing glucose levels. *Cellular and Molecular Life Sciences, 70*, 2015–2029.

Pimenta de Castro, I., Costa, A. C., Lam, D., Tufi, R., Fedele, V., Moisoi, N., et al. (2012). Genetic analysis of mitochondrial protein misfolding in *Drosophila melanogaster*. *Cell Death and Differentiation*, *19*, 1308–1316.

Radke, S., Chander, H., Schafer, P., Meiss, G., Kruger, R., Schulz, J. B., et al. (2008). Mitochondrial protein quality control by the proteasome involves ubiquitination and the protease Omi. *The Journal of Biological Chemistry*, *283*, 12681–12685.

Razandi, M., Pedram, A., Jordan, V. C., Fuqua, S., & Levin, E. R. (2013). Tamoxifen regulates cell fate through mitochondrial estrogen receptor beta in breast cancer. *Oncogene*, *32*, 3274–3285.

Roesch, A., Fukunaga-Kalabis, M., Schmidt, E. C., Zabierowski, S. E., Brafford, P. A., Vultur, A., et al. (2010). A temporarily distinct subpopulation of slow-cycling melanoma cells is required for continuous tumor growth. *Cell*, *141*, 583–594.

Rose, G., Dato, S., Altomare, K., Bellizzi, D., Garasto, S., Greco, V., et al. (2003). Variability of the SIRT3 gene, human silent information regulator Sir2 homologue, and survivorship in the elderly. *Experimental Gerontology*, *38*, 1065–1070.

Runkel, E. D., Liu, S., Baumeister, R., & Schulze, E. (2013). Surveillance-activated defenses block the ROS-induced mitochondrial unfolded protein response. *PLoS Genetics*, *9*, e1003346.

Rutkowski, D. T., & Kaufman, R. J. (2004). A trip to the ER: Coping with stress. *Trends in Cell Biology*, *14*, 20–28.

Safdar, A., Bourgeois, J. M., Ogborn, D. I., Little, J. P., Hettinga, B. P., Akhtar, M., et al. (2011). Endurance exercise rescues progeroid aging and induces systemic mitochondrial rejuvenation in mtDNA mutator mice. *Proceedings of the National Academy of Sciences of the United States of America*, *108*, 4135–4140.

Sanchez, M. I., Shearwood, A. M., Chia, T., Davies, S. M., Rackham, O., & Filipovska, A. (2015). Estrogen-mediated regulation of mitochondrial gene expression. *Molecular Endocrinology*, *29*, 14–27.

Sanz, A., Hiona, A., Kujoth, G. C., Seo, A. Y., Hofer, T., Kouwenhoven, E., et al. (2007). Evaluation of sex differences on mitochondrial bioenergetics and apoptosis in mice. *Experimental Gerontology*, *42*, 173–182.

Shaaban, A. M., Green, A. R., Karthik, S., Alizadeh, Y., Hughes, T. A., Harkins, L., et al. (2008). Nuclear and cytoplasmic expression of ERbeta1, ERbeta2, and ERbeta5 identifies distinct prognostic outcome for breast cancer patients. *Clinical Cancer Research*, *14*, 5228–5235.

Shi, T., Wang, F., Stieren, E., & Tong, Q. (2005). SIRT3, a mitochondrial sirtuin deacetylase, regulates mitochondrial function and thermogenesis in brown adipocytes. *The Journal of Biological Chemistry*, *280*, 13560–13567.

Siegelin, M. D., Dohi, T., Raskett, C. M., Orlowski, G. M., Powers, C. M., Gilbert, C. A., et al. (2011). Exploiting the mitochondrial unfolded protein response for cancer therapy in mice and human cells. *The Journal of Clinical Investigation*, *121*, 1349–1360.

Sun, J., Folk, D., Bradley, T. J., & Tower, J. (2002). Induced overexpression of mitochondrial Mn-superoxide dismutase extends the life span of adult *Drosophila melanogaster*. *Genetics*, *161*, 661–672.

Sun, M., Paciga, J. E., Feldman, R. I., Yuan, Z., Coppola, D., Lu, Y. Y., et al. (2001). Phosphatidylinositol-3-OH Kinase (PI3K)/AKT2, activated in breast cancer, regulates and is induced by estrogen receptor alpha (ERalpha) via interaction between ERalpha and PI3K. *Cancer Research*, *61*, 5985–5991.

Sun, Y., Yolitz, J., Alberico, T., Sun, X., & Zou, S. (2014). Lifespan extension by cranberry supplementation partially requires SOD2 and is life stage independent. *Experimental Gerontology*, *50*, 57–63.

Sundaresan, N. R., Gupta, M., Kim, G., Rajamohan, S. B., Isbatan, A., & Gupta, M. P. (2009). Sirt3 blocks the cardiac hypertrophic response by augmenting Foxo3a-dependent antioxidant defense mechanisms in mice. *The Journal of Clinical Investigation, 119,* 2758–2771.

Sundaresan, N. R., Samant, S. A., Pillai, V. B., Rajamohan, S. B., & Gupta, M. P. (2008). SIRT3 is a stress-responsive deacetylase in cardiomyocytes that protects cells from stress-mediated cell death by deacetylation of Ku70. *Molecular and Cellular Biology, 28,* 6384–6401.

Tao, R., Coleman, M. C., Pennington, J. D., Ozden, O., Park, S. H., Jiang, H., et al. (2010). Sirt3-mediated deacetylation of evolutionarily conserved lysine 122 regulates MnSOD activity in response to stress. *Molecular Cell, 40,* 893–904.

Tissenbaum, H. A., & Guarente, L. (2001). Increased dosage of a sir-2 gene extends lifespan in *Caenorhabditis elegans. Nature, 410,* 227–230.

Trifunovic, A., Wredenberg, A., Falkenberg, M., Spelbrink, J. N., Rovio, A. T., Bruder, C. E., et al. (2004). Premature ageing in mice expressing defective mitochondrial DNA polymerase. *Nature, 429,* 417–423.

Van Itallie, C. M., & Dannies, P. S. (1988). Estrogen induces accumulation of the mitochondrial ribonucleic acid for subunit II of cytochrome oxidase in pituitary tumor cells. *Molecular Endocrinology, 2,* 332–337.

Vellinga, T. T., Borovski, T., de Boer, V. C., Fatrai, S., van Schelven, S., Trumpi, K., et al. (2015). SIRT1/PGC1alpha-dependent increase in oxidative phosphorylation supports chemotherapy resistance of colon cancer. *Clinical Cancer Research, 21,* 2870–2879.

Verdin, E. (2014). The many faces of sirtuins: Coupling of NAD metabolism, sirtuins and lifespan. *Nature Medicine, 20,* 25–27.

Viale, A., Pettazzoni, P., Lyssiotis, C. A., Ying, H., Sanchez, N., Marchesini, M., et al. (2014). Oncogene ablation-resistant pancreatic cancer cells depend on mitochondrial function. *Nature, 514,* 628–632.

Vilgelm, A., Lian, Z., Wang, H., Beauparlant, S. L., Klein-Szanto, A., Ellenson, L. H., et al. (2006). Akt-mediated phosphorylation and activation of estrogen receptor alpha is required for endometrial neoplastic transformation in Pten+/− mice. *Cancer Research, 66,* 3375–3380.

Vina, J., & Borras, C. (2010). Women live longer than men: Understanding molecular mechanisms offers opportunities to intervene by using estrogenic compounds. *Antioxidants & Redox Signaling, 13,* 269–278.

Whitaker, R., Faulkner, S., Miyokawa, R., Burhenn, L., Henriksen, M., Wood, J. G., et al. (2013). Increased expression of Drosophila Sir2 extends life span in a dose-dependent manner. *Aging, 5,* 682–691.

Willcox, B. J., Donlon, T. A., He, Q., Chen, R., Grove, J. S., Yano, K., et al. (2008). FOXO3A genotype is strongly associated with human longevity. *Proceedings of the National Academy of Sciences of the United States of America, 105,* 13987–13992.

Yang, X., Downes, M., Yu, R. T., Bookout, A. L., He, W., Straume, M., et al. (2006). Nuclear receptor expression links the circadian clock to metabolism. *Cell, 126,* 801–810.

Yang, S. Y., He, X. Y., & Schulz, H. (2005). Multiple functions of type 10 17beta-hydroxysteroid dehydrogenase. *Trends in Endocrinology and Metabolism: TEM, 16,* 167–175.

Yang, H., Yang, T., Baur, J. A., Perez, E., Matsui, T., Carmona, J. J., et al. (2007). Nutrient-sensitive mitochondrial NAD+ levels dictate cell survival. *Cell, 130,* 1095–1107.

Zhang, G., Liu, X., Farkas, A. M., Parwani, A. V., Lathrop, K. L., Lenzner, D., et al. (2009). Estrogen receptor beta functions through nongenomic mechanisms in lung cancer cells. *Molecular Endocrinology, 23,* 146–156.

Zhao, Q., Wang, J., Levichkin, I. V., Stasinopoulos, S., Ryan, M. T., & Hoogenraad, N. J. (2002). A mitochondrial specific stress response in mammalian cells. *The EMBO Journal, 21,* 4411–4419.

CHAPTER SIX

Keratinocyte Carcinoma as a Marker of a High Cancer-Risk Phenotype

J. Small, V. Barton, B. Peterson, A.J. Alberg[1]
Medical University of South Carolina, Charleston, SC, United States
[1]Corresponding author: e-mail address: alberg@musc.edu

Contents

Abstract

Keratinocyte carcinoma (KC) (also referred to as nonmelanoma skin cancer) is by far the most common form of human cancer. A personal history of KC is well established to be associated with increased risk of recurrent KC and malignant melanoma, a less common yet more fatal form of skin cancer. More surprising is that a substantial body of epidemiologic evidence now indicates that a personal history of KC is significantly associated with an overall elevated risk of noncutaneous malignancies. This association is not limited to one or a few types of cancer but applies across many different types of malignancy. This association has been consistently observed in prospective studies across genders for both major histologic types of KC, basal cell carcinoma and squamous cell carcinoma. The risk of other cancers has been even stronger in those with younger compared with older age of onset of KC.

Advances in Cancer Research, Volume 130
ISSN 0065-230X
http://dx.doi.org/10.1016/bs.acr.2016.01.003

A robust body of evidence lends support to the notion that KC may be a marker of a high cancer-risk phenotype. The underlying mechanisms for this association remain to be elucidated, but the cross-cutting nature of this association across numerous malignancies suggests that research to uncover these mechanisms is a promising line of inquiry that could potentially yield valuable insight into human carcinogenesis.

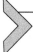

1. INTRODUCTION

Keratinocyte carcinoma (KC) (also referred to as nonmelanoma skin cancer (NMSC)) is by far the most common form of human cancer. A personal history of KC is well established to be associated with increased risk of recurrent KC (American Cancer Society, 2007). Based on shared risk factors and susceptibility profiles it is not surprising that a personal history of KC is also associated with a markedly increased risk of malignant melanoma, another form of cutaneous carcinoma that is far more lethal but less common than KC. More surprising is that a substantial body of epidemiologic evidence now indicates that a personal history of KC is consistently associated with an overall elevated risk of noncutaneous malignancies. In the later sections, after providing background on the occurrence of KC in populations and factors associated with KC risk, this evidence is characterized and evaluated. Evidence is also summarized from studies that have examined KC in relation to increased risk of fatal outcomes such as survival after a diagnosis with a noncutaneous malignancy, cancer-specific mortality, and all-cause mortality.

2. BACKGROUND AND DESCRIPTIVE EPIDEMIOLOGY OF KC

Skin cancer is classified based on whether melanocytes, the melanin-producing cells of the epidermis, are involved in its genesis. Malignant melanoma is skin cancer that begins in the melanocytes, whereas KC (or NMSC) encompasses all skin cancers not originating in the melanocytes. The predominant histologic subtypes of KC are basal cell carcinoma (BCC) and squamous cell carcinoma (SCC). With respect to its occurrence in populations, KC differs importantly from malignant melanoma. KC has a considerably higher incidence rate but a much lower mortality rate than malignant melanoma. The mortality rate for KC is approximately one-fourth of that for melanoma (0.7 vs 2.7 per 100,000 per year) (CDC, 2015; Lewis & Weinstock, 2007). Malignant melanoma accounts for the vast majority of skin cancer deaths because it is much more invasive and therefore more likely to metastasize than KC (Scotto, Fears, Kraemer, & Fraumeni, 1996).

The risk of developing KC is largely determined by a combination of skin type and exposure to solar ultraviolet radiation (UVR) (Karagas, Weinstock, & Nelson, 2006). Those with photosensitive skin types are typically fair skinned and have a propensity to sunburn, blister, and/or freckle when exposed to UVR and therefore have a greater susceptibility to the damaging effects of UVR on the skin than those with less sun-sensitive phenotypes (Karagas et al., 2006). The risk of KC associated with UVR is dose-dependent, with risk increasing the greater the duration and intensity of exposure.

2.1 KC Incidence and Mortality

KC is the single most common form of cancer, accounting for 33–50% of all new cancer diagnoses each year. Up to 3.5 million new cases are diagnosed annually in the United States, with approximately 2.8 million of those diagnoses being BCC and 700,000 being SCC (Rogers et al., 2010).

KC has a particularly high incidence rate in Australia. In 2008, there were a reported 434,000 new cases of KC, four times greater than all other cancers combined (Australian Institute of Health and Welfare and Cancer Australia, 2008). The estimated prevalence of KC is 2% in Australia, with the highest prevalence found among men (Perera, Gnaneswaran, Staines, Win, & Sinclair, 2015).

Despite being so common, KC is only rarely fatal. KC is estimated to cause more than 3000 deaths annually in the United States, primarily among the elderly (Karia, Han, & Schmults, 2013; Rogers et al., 2010). The mortality rate for KC is only 0.7 deaths per 100,000 people per year (Lewis & Weinstock, 2007). The low mortality rate is consistent with the fact that KC tends not to invade surrounding tissues or metastasize. Subtype-specific mortality rates indicate that SCC is the more fatal form of KC due to its greater metastatic potential, with as many as 2% of squamous cell diagnoses resulting in death. BCC, while more commonly diagnosed, is rarely fatal (Karia et al., 2013).

2.2 Primary Histological Types of KC

In many research studies BCC and SCC are collectively referred to as KC, but these two histologic types of KC are clinically and epidemiologically distinct. As summarized in Table 1, BCC and SCC have unique features

Table 1 A Comparison of Clinical and Epidemiologic Characteristics of the Two Major Forms of Keratinocyte Carcinoma, Basal Cell Carcinoma of the Skin (BCC) and Squamous Cell Carcinoma of the Skin (SCC)

Characteristic	Basal Cell Carcinoma	Squamous Cell Carcinoma
Originating cells	Basal skin cells	Squamous skin cells
Premalignant forms	None	Bowen's disease, actinic keratosis
Percent of KC	65–80%	~20%
Incidence rate (per 100,000)		
Males	309.9	97.2
Females	165.5	32.4
Probability of metastasis	0.0028–0.55%	~3%
Host susceptibility factors	Sun-sensitive skin phenotype Male sex Older age Immunosuppression Major inherited predisposition (e.g., xeroderma pigmentosum)	Sun-sensitive skin phenotype Male sex Older age Immunosuppression Major inherited predisposition (e.g., xeroderma pigmentosum)
Major environmental risk factor	Ultraviolet radiation exposure	Ultraviolet radiation exposure
Other risk factors	HIV infection	HIV infection

regarding their clinical characteristics, distribution in populations, and risk factors. BCC is much more common than SCC; the ratio of BCC to SCC, respectively, varies across populations from 2:1 to 5:1 (Weinstock, 1994). A brief description of each histologic type is provided below.

2.2.1 Basal Cell Carcinoma of the Skin

BCCs originate in the basal skin cells, the lowest layer of the epidermis, and generally manifest as open sores, red patches, or pink growths. BCC itself is classified into four major subtypes: (1) superficial (10−30% of BCCs), (2) nodular-ulcerative (60—80% of BCCs), (3) pigmented (7% of BCCs), and (4) morpheaform (5% of BCCs) (Weedon & Strutton, 2002). They most commonly occur on areas with frequent sun exposure such as the head/ scalp, face, hands, and neck. In the United States, BCC accounts for approximately 80% of all new KC diagnoses (Raasch, Buettner, & Garbe, 2006).

If left untreated BCC can invade surrounding tissue and bone. Despite its ability to invade surrounding tissue, BCC has a very low likelihood of metastasizing. In the time between the first documented case in 1894 and 2011, fewer than 400 cases of metastatic BCC have been recorded. This exceedingly small number of documented cases with metastases in relation to the enormous number of cases diagnosed demonstrates that the probability of developing metastatic BCC is extremely low, but precisely quantifying this probability is challenging. Currently, the estimated likelihood of metastasis for BCCs is 0.003—0.55% (Roewert-Huber, Lange-Asschenfeldt, Stockfleth, & Kerl, 2007; Von Hoff et al., 2009; Wadhera, Fazio, Bricca, & Stanton, 2006).

2.2.2 Squamous Cell Carcinoma of the Skin

SCCs originate in the squamous skin cells, which compose the upper layers of the epidermis. SCC manifests as scaly red patches, open sores, elevated growths with a central depression, or warts; these lesions may crust or bleed. Approximately 700,000 SCC diagnoses are made annually in the United States, accounting for approximately 20% of all KC cases (Karia et al., 2013). Approximately 70—80% of all SCCs occur on the head or neck due to the frequency at which these areas are exposed to sunlight (Acartürk & Edington, 2005). The likelihood of metastatic SCC is estimated to be 2—3%—orders of magnitude greater than for BCC, indicative of the greater invasiveness and metastatic potential of SCC (Czarnecki, Staples, Mar, Giles, & Meehan, 1994; Joseph, Zulueta, & Kennedy, 1992); this increased propensity to metastasize explains why nearly all KC fatalities are attributable to SCC.

While invasive SCC may develop de novo, it has two premalignant forms: Bowen's disease (BD) and actinic keratosis. BD, the in situ stage of SCC, is a slow-growing erythematous plaque that exhibits histological changes similar to those seen in malignant SCC, including cellular atypia confined within the full thickness of the epidermis. It is estimated that 3—5% of BD patients progress to malignant SCC (Burge & Wallis, 2011).

The other premalignant form of SCC is actinic keratosis. Actinic keratosis presents as rough, scaly patches (keratosis) on the epidermis caused by years of exposure to the sun's ultraviolet rays (actinic) (Burge & Wallis, 2011). Actinic keratosis is the most common form of premalignant cancer, affecting more than 58 million people in the United States (Bickers et al., 2006). It is estimated that 20% of untreated actinic keratoses progress to SCC (Burge & Wallis, 2011).

2.3 The Occurrence of KC According to Person, Place, and Time

A challenge for characterizing the occurrence of KC in populations is that the only type of skin cancer that cancer registries typically ascertain is melanoma. The lack of inclusion of KC in most cancer registries leads to a dearth of high-quality population-level data necessary to track its occurrence in populations. The data that has been gathered on KC indicates that there are distinct differences in KC prevalence and incidence across different populations, geographic locations, and time periods.

2.3.1 Person: Demographic Characteristics

The data that are available reveal very clear patterns in the occurrence of KC with respect to sex, age, and racial/ethnic group. One of the most robust predictors of KC risk is older age. The risk of being diagnosed with KC strongly increases with age, which can be attributed to the corresponding increase in cumulative sun exposure for every year of life. One in every five Americans will develop KC in their lifetime, and 40–50% of Americans who live to the age of 65 will have at least one KC (Robinson, 2005).

In general, men experience KC at rates twice that of women (Staples, Elwood, Giles, Burton, et al., 2006). This gender differential applies to both KC subtypes, as men have a twofold increased risk of BCC and threefold increased risk of SCC compared to women. This male predominance in KC risk is unlikely to be due to differences in inherent susceptibility to KC, but is instead attributable to the higher prevalence of exposure to solar UVR in men compared with women.

The important role of sun-sensitive skin as a susceptibility factor for KC naturally leads to marked racial/ethnic differences in the occurrence of KC in populations. KC is most common in Caucasians, and even among Caucasians differentials in risk are present according to skin color and sun-sensitivity. Comparisons have shown that compared to Caucasians, rates in Hispanics were as low as 1/14 lower and African Americans as low as 1/190 lower (Karagas et al., 2006).

This variation in risk is thought to be attributable to inherent differences in melanin levels between racial/ethnic groups. Since light-skinned Caucasians have low levels of melanin in their skin—the equivalent of 3.4 Sun Protection Factor (SPF)—they are inherently more susceptible to UVR damage. Conversely, dark-skinned African Americans are less susceptible to UVR damage due to the high levels of melanin in their skin, the equivalent of approximately 13.4 SPF (Gloster & Neal, 2006; Halder & Bridgeman-Shah, 1995; Montagna, Prota, & Kenney, 1993).

The occurrence of KC by histologic type has been observed to vary across racial/ethnic groups; BCC is the most common skin cancer among Caucasian, Hispanic, and Asian individuals, whereas SCC is the most common skin cancer in African Americans and Asian Indians (Agbai et al., 2014). This form of KC tends to be more aggressive in individuals of African origin, resulting in a risk of metastasis that is higher than seen in other racial/ethnic groups (Gloster & Neal, 2006).

2.3.2 Geographic Distribution of KC

Strong geographic gradients in the occurrence have KC have been described, with KC incidence rates observed to increase with increasing proximity to the equator due to the increase in the dose of UVR from sunlight (Holmes, Malinovszky, & Roberts, 2000; Marks & Staples, 1993). One example that highlights the importance of both latitude of residence and the interaction of sun-sensitive phenotypes with solar UVR exposure is a comparison of the occurrence of KC in Australia compared with the United Kingdom. While the populations of both regions are predominantly of UK ancestry, Australia is much nearer to the equator than the United Kingdom. Some of the highest SCC incidence rates in the world occur in Australia, with an incidence of 330 per 100,000 person-years (PY); this is a 10-fold greater rate than observed in the United Kingdom (23/100,000 PY) (Lomas, Leonardi-Bee, & Bath-Hextall, 2012). Similarly for BCC, Australia's incidence rate ranges from 726 to 1600 cases per 100,000 person-years which is greater than sixfold higher than rates observed in the United Kingdom (Holmes et al., 2000; Marks & Staples, 1993). To provide a frame of reference, BCC rates noted in other geographic regions are 40–80/100,000 PY in Northern Europe; 146/100,000 PY in Minnesota, USA; and 300/100,000 PY in Southern USA. This variation in incidence across geographic regions correlates with the dose of solar UVR (Holmes et al., 2000; Marks & Staples, 1993).

2.3.3 Time Trends

The incidence of KC is increasing in North America, Europe, and Australia. In the United States, KC has been increasing at a rate of 3–8% per year since the 1960s (Diepgen & Mahler, 2002; Ramos, Villa, Ruiz, Armstrong, & Matta, 2004). An estimated 3.5 million cases of KC were diagnosed in 2012, much higher than the 1 million cases of KC diagnosed in 1994 (Miller & Weinstock, 1994). An increasing trend in the incidence of both SCC and BCC has been noted for those younger than 40 years of age, with BCC rates increasing more rapidly in young women than in young men (Christenson, Borrowman, Vachon, et al., 2005). Such increases in younger age populations foreshadow subsequent population-level increases because KC occurrence increases with age. In the period between 1963 and 2011, the incidence of SCC in increased sixfold in males and ninefold in females in Norway (Robsahm, Helsing, & Veierød, 2015). Particularly dramatic upward trends in the incidence of KC have been seen in Australia. Between 1985 and 2002, BCC incidence increased by 35%, from 657 to 884 per 100,000, and SCC incidence increased 133%, from 166 to 387 per 100,000 people (Staples et al., 2006).

3. DETERMINANTS OF KC

The primary environmental cause of KC is exposure to solar UVR (Balk, 2011). Solar UVR exposure is such a strong determinant of KC in populations, that the occurrence of KC in populations can be tracked according to UVR exposure at the population level.

Individual risk for KC is largely determined by cumulative exposure to solar radiation, in combination with individual susceptibility (Fig. 1). Skin characteristics, such as ability to tan and pigmentation, largely determine

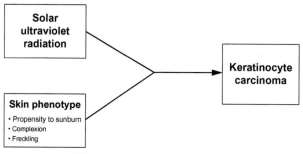

Fig. 1 Conceptual model of the major factors driving risk of keratinocyte carcinoma in populations.

host susceptibility to UVR. Thus, the major determinants of KC risk are best conceptualized as the interaction between UVR exposure and sun-sensitive skin phenotype.

3.1 Host Factors Associated with KC

3.1.1 Skin Type

The risk associated with UVR exposure is primarily concentrated among individuals with sun-sensitive skin phenotypes. Skin type is determined by genetic disposition (hair color, skin color, eye color) and how skin responds to prolonged periods of sun exposure (freckle, burn/peel, tan). Skin types that are particularly sensitive to UVR, and therefore at an increased risk of developing KC, are the Fitzpatrick skin types I, II, and III. These fair skin types lack the ability to tan and have a propensity to sunburn and freckle when exposed to UVR; these qualities exponentially increase the risk of skin cancer. To illustrate, the World Health Organization (WHO) estimated that approximately 98% of all KC cases occur in patients with sun-sensitive skin types (Fitzpatrick skin types I, II, III) (World Health Organization, 2006).

Upon unprotected exposure UVR those with fair skin typically burn or blister whereas dark-skinned individuals typically tan. Even tanning is associated with sun damage, but sunburns have far more deleterious effects with respect to increasing KC risk. High doses of UVR exposure lead to sunburn and cause DNA damage via cyclobutane pyrimidine dimers (Cadet, Sage, & Douki, 2005). Mild sunburns manifests as a slight reddening of the skin, whereas more intense sunburns can cause the skin to blister and peel, leaving the underlying, less pigmented layer of skin more vulnerable to UVR damage. The UVR-induced DNA damage accumulates with increased solar UVR exposure, especially sunburns, thus increasing the risk of developing KC.

In a population-based study in a single community of predominantly European ancestry, the majority of individuals with KC had a sunburn-prone skin type: 14.6% had a "blistering sunburn" skin type, 38.3% had a "sunburn without blistering" skin type, 33.8% had a "mild sunburn that turns tan" skin type, 10.4% had a "tan without sunburn" skin type, and 2.9% had a "no change in skin color" skin type (Wheless et al., 2009).

3.1.2 Genetic Susceptibility

Genetic susceptibility to KC can be conceptualized as rare but high-penetrant mutations and common, low-penetrant genetic variants. Both of these categories are described below, with examples of major inherited predisposition being xeroderma pigmentosum (XP) and epidermodysplasia verruciformis (EV).

3.1.2.1 Xeroderma Pigmentosum

XP is a very rare autosomal recessive disorder that occurs in 1 in 250,000 births in the United States (Lehmann, Mcgibbon, & Stefanini, 2011; Menck & Munford, 2014). It is caused by rare, high-penetrant mutations in nucleotide excision repair (NER) genes. The NER gene mutations prevent the patient from repairing DNA damage caused by UVR, rendering XP patients with extreme photosensitivity. The severity of XP depends on the extent to which NER genes are defective; in extreme cases XP patients are rendered incapable of repairing DNA damage, wherein even small doses of UVR have deleterious effects on health (Lehmann et al., 2011; Menck & Munford, 2014). Due to the inability to repair DNA damage, these patients more rapidly accumulate the sequence of genetic mutations necessary for skin carcinogenesis to occur. Patients with XP have a >2000-fold increased risk of KC before age 20 years and are estimated to be 10,000 times more likely to develop KC in their lifetimes (Cleaver, 2005). XP patients also have a significant excess risk of other types of cancer early in life (Cleaver, 2005).

3.1.2.2 Epidermodysplasia Verruciformis

EV is an extremely rare autosomal recessive genodermatosis that is characterized by chronic human papillomavirus (HPV) infection, primarily β-HPV types 5 and 8, caused by a defect in the cell-mediated immune response to HPV infection. The chronic HPV infection results in polymorphic cutaneous lesions, including verrucae (flat wart-like lesions) and rough pigmented plaques, and a higher risk of in situ or invasive KC (Patel, Morrison, Rady, & Tyring, 2010).

EV is thought to be a result of mutations in the *EVER1* or *EVER2* genes located on chromosome 17q25.3. These genes code for the EVER proteins that form a complex with zinc transporter protein ZnT-1 in the endoplasmic reticulum (ER) of human keratinocytes. It is hypothesized that this complex defends against HPV by maintaining intracellular Zn^{2+} homeostasis and thereby interfering with viral replication (Lazarczyk et al., 2008). Zn^{2+} inhibits the RNA-synthesizing activity of the replication and transcription complex (RCT) of the HPV virus (te Velthuis et al., 2010). Mutations in the *EVER1* or *EVER2* genes inhibit the formation of the EVER/ZnT-1 complex, leading to a zinc imbalance within the cell and thus facilitating replication of the HPV virus (Lazarczyk & Favre, 2008; Lazarczyk et al., 2008).

Research suggests that HPV acts in concert with UVR to produce KC. While the exact mechanisms responsible for the malignant transformation of keratinocytes in skin lesions of EV patients remain to be elucidated, evidence indicates that HPV interacts with antioncogene proteins, including p53, in a way that interferes with proper DNA repair and apoptosis. Defective apoptosis causes cell immortalization wherein cells with UVR-induced DNA damage accumulate, thereby causing normal human keratinocytes to transform into malignant KC (Kao et al., 1997). Defective DNA repair, coupled with the oncogenic HPV infection, is likely responsible for the propensity toward KC observed in patients with EV.

The association between HPV and KC was first documented in EV patients, who frequently develop SCC on areas prone to UVR exposure, such as the head and neck (Accardi & Gheit, 2014). It is estimated that 30–70% of EV patients develop KC, with SCC accounting for a majority of those diagnoses. While most of the SCCs remain in situ (BD), some are invasive; metastasis is rare (Emsen & Kabalar, 2010).

3.1.3 Common, Low-Penetrant Genetic Variants Associated with KC Risk

Biologic pathways of clear relevance to the pathogenesis of KC include those related to melanin synthesis and DNA repair, namely, NER. This raises the index of suspicion that polymorphisms in genes in these pathways are associated with risk of developing KC; in fact, there is supportive evidence that variants in genes in these pathways are associated with the pathogenesis of KC. Specific variants in pigmentation pathway genes have been observed to be associated with risk of KC (Binstock, Hafeez, Metchnikoff, & Arron, 2014). The melanocortin 1 receptor gene (*MC1R*) has emerged as a particularly important gene in this regard (Binstock et al., 2014). A vast array of evidence (Reichrath & Rass, 2014), including that from epidemiologic studies (Wheless et al., 2012), has characterized the important role of DNA repair, with NER as a focal point, in skin carcinogenesis.

3.1.4 Immunosuppression

Immunosuppression is another significant risk factor for KC. Patients who have undergone an organ transplant, and therefore received immunosuppressive therapy, are at a 10- to 250-fold increased risk of developing KC (Athar, Walsh, Kopelovich, & Elmets, 2011). Immunosuppressed individuals experience KC at higher rates than the general population because immunosuppressant drugs used to prevent organ rejection impairs the immune system's ability to repair DNA damaged by UVR. A study conducted by Gallagher and colleagues investigated the long-term impact of immunosuppressants on renal transplant patients. Of the 489 kidney transplant recipients included in the study, 171 (35%) developed at least 1 KC, with approximately 60% of those KC diagnoses being SCC and 40% being BCC (Gallagher et al., 2010).

While BCC is the predominant form of KC in the general population, SCC is more common than BCC among immunosuppressed patients (Brin, Zubair, & Brewer, 2014). Even so, the KC incidence rates are so high in immunosuppressed patients even BCC occurs at much higher frequency than in the general population; for example, one study found that approximately 16% of renal transplant recipients developed a BCC postoperatively, a 10-fold increased risk compared with the general population (Rajpara & Ormerod, 2008).

Those on immunosuppressive therapy have a 50% risk of developing SCC within 20 years posttransplantation (Webb, Compton, Andrews, et al., 1997), with 30% of such SCCs being highly aggressive. SCC diagnoses in immunosuppressed patients are more likely to be aggressive, invasive, and poorly differentiated. Immunosuppressed patients have higher rates of SCC metastasis, approximately 5−8% (Athar et al., 2011; Martinez et al., 2003), and therefore greater mortality rates than the immunocompetent population (Zavos et al., 2011). The risk of KC associated with immunosuppressants has been noted to vary considerably according to the specific therapy, with calcinuerin inhibitors associated with greatest risk, which is postulated to be due to its interfering with NER, and lesser risk associated with mTOR inhibitors (Kuschal et al., 2011).

3.1.5 Infections

Individuals infected with the human immunodeficiency virus (HIV) have a greater risk of KC compared with the general population. Those who are HIV-positive have an incidence rate of KC that is twice the rate observed in HIV-negative individuals (odds ratio (OR) 2.1, 95% CI 1.9−2.3) (Silverberg et al., 2013). This is thought to be due to the HIV virus infecting the host's $CD4^+$ T cells, macrophages, and dendritic cells, and to relate to compromised immune status.

3.2 Environmental Risk Factors for KC

3.2.1 Solar Ultraviolet Radiation

The major environmental cause of skin cancer is epidermal exposure to solar UVR (Scotto et al., 1996). The three categories of UVR are ultraviolet A (UVA; 315−400 nm), ultraviolet B (UVB; 280−315 nm), and ultraviolet

C (UVC; 100−280 nm). Most of the population burden of skin cancer is due to UVA and/or UVB exposure (Rigel, Burnett, & Lim, 2011). UVA induces pyrimidine dimerization and damages DNA through the production of reactive oxygen and nitrogen species. UVB, the most mutagenic and carcinogenic category of solar UVR, is the principal cause of KC. UVB-induced DNA damage includes lesions, primarily cyclobutane pyrimidine dimers and pyrimidine(6-4)pyrimidone photoproducts (Cadet et al., 2005; Halliday, 2005) which can result in oncogenic DNA mutations. UVC contains the most energy and therefore has the greatest potential to damage biological systems, but fortunately it is completely blocked by the ozone layer. The ozone layer also partially impedes the transmission of UVB and, to a lesser extent, UVA (Rigel et al., 2011). Thus any environmental insult that results in depletion of the ozone layer would be expected to increase the population risk of KC.

UVR exposure is associated with significantly increased risk of both SCC and BCC in a dose-dependent manner (Karagas et al., 2006). For example, a meta-analysis of outdoor work and BCC risk found a pooled OR of 1.43 (95% CI 1.23−1.66; $p = 0.0001$) when comparing cases to controls; this result remained significant after adjusting for sex and nonoccupational sun exposure (Bauer, Diepgen, & Schmitt, 2011; Schmitt, Seidler, Diepgen, & Bauer, 2011).

For a given duration of UVR exposure there are several factors that influence the biologically effective dose, such as latitude, altitude, and time of day. Latitude is important because those who live near the equator receive higher UVR doses due to greater proximity to the sun. Altitude also influences the level of UVR exposure, with higher altitude associated with higher UVR dose. UVR dose also varies according to the sun's position in the sky, hence why solar UVR doses are greatest during the afternoon and in summer months (World Health Organization, 2015).

3.2.2 Artificial Ultraviolet Radiation Exposure: Indoor Tanning

Indoor tanning use in the United States is most prevalent among adolescents and young adults with an estimated 15–19% of high school students and 55% of university students engaging in indoor tanning (Guy et al., 2014; Wehner et al., 2014). Artificial UVR is of greater intensity than solar UVR due to the fact that tanning lamps primarily emit UVA radiation, which penetrates deeper into the skin than exposure to any other UVR sources. While the UVR dose from indoor tanning devices varies considerably by device type, an investigation of 62 different tanning beds found that tanning beds had roughly fourfold greater UVA and twofold greater UVB output than the summer noonday sun (Hornung, Magee, & Lee, 2003).

As expected based on the robust role of solar UVR in the causation of KC, artificial UVR exposure delivered via tanning beds is also a strong determinant of KC risk. A meta-analysis of 12 studies observed that after adjusting for potential confounding factors, ever vs never use of tanning beds was associated with a significantly increased risk of both SCC (summary RR 1.67, 95% CI 1.29–2.17) and BCC (summary RR 1.29, 95% CI 1.08–1.53) (Wehner et al., 2012). This level of risk combined with the high prevalence of use resulted in estimates that 170,000 cases of KC per year are attributable to indoor tanning (Wehner et al., 2012). A prospective study of indoor tanning observed a clear dose−response relationship with SCC and BCC risk (Zhang et al., 2012).

3.2.3 Cigarette Smoking

Cigarette smoking has been investigated as a potential risk factor for KC, but has yet to emerge as a clear risk factor. The evidence in favor of an association is stronger for SCC than for BCC, but even for SCC the evidence is inconsistent. Several case−control studies found an increased risk for SCC among smokers that ranged from approximately 1.5 to 3 times that of nonsmokers (Aubry & Macgibbon, 1985; Bajdik, Gallagher, Hill, & Fincham, 1995; De Hertog, Wensveen, Bastiaens, et al., 2001). These associations have been observed in both current smokers (OR 2.9, 95% CI 1.5–5.6) and former smokers (OR 1.8, 95% CI 1.0–3.0) (De Hertog et al., 2001). SCC risk has been observed to increase with greater levels of exposure, with a statistically significant positive correlation between SCC risk and number of pack-years (Lear et al., 1998).

While case−control studies clearly indicate that cigarette smoking is associated with increased risk of SCC, cohort studies have produced varied results. A cohort study conducted by Karagas, Stukel, Greenberg, et al. (1992) found an increased risk of SCC in both current (RR 2.01, 95% CI 1.21–3.34) and former smokers (RR 1.62, 95% CI 1.07–2.47), whereas other cohort studies have not observed an association (Lindelöf, Odenbro, Bellocco, Boffetta, & Adami, 2005).

The current body of evidence does not provide support for an association between cigarette smoking and BCC risk. Of the four cohort studies (Freedman, Sigurdson, Doody, Mabuchi, & Linet, 2003; Hunter et al., 1990; Karagas et al., 1992; van Dam et al., 1999) and three case−control studies (De Hertog et al., 2001; Gamble, Lerman, Holder, Nicolich, &

Yarborough, 1996; Milan, Verkasalo, Kaprio, et al., 2003) that have examined the association between smoking and risk of BCC, none have reported that smoking is significantly associated with increased risk of BCC.

4. KC AS A MARKER OF INCREASED RISK OF OTHER FORMS OF CANCER

A personal history of KC is predictive of other or recurrent KC (Cantwell, Murray, Catney, et al., 2009). It is also a risk factor for malignant melanoma, likely due to the shared risk factors of sun-sensitive skin types and exposure to UVR (Marcil & Stern, 2000). In individuals with a previous KC diagnosis the risk of other malignancies may not be limited to skin cancers. The potential association between KC and risk of noncutaneous malignancies is schematically depicted in Fig. 2. Based on this conceptualization, there is no obvious reason to expect that KC would be associated with excess risk of noncutaneous malignancies; neither solar UVR exposure nor skin type is known to be associated with risk of internal cancers. Notwithstanding this lack of expectation, a substantial body of evidence, reviewed below, supports the notion that individuals with a previous diagnosis of KC also have an increased risk of developing subsequent noncutaneous primary malignancies.

The most informative body of evidence on this topic is based on prospective studies that entail follow-up of those with KC and those without KC for the occurrence of other forms of cancer. These prospective studies tend to fall into one of two categories: large-scale population registry linkage studies that tend to have limited covariate data or prospective cohort studies with smaller sample sizes but more detailed individual-level data.

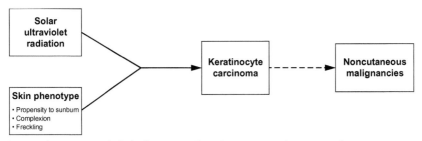

Fig. 2 The potential link between keratinocyte carcinoma and noncutaneous malignancies.

4.1 Registry Studies

Registry linkage studies have been conducted in nations with population registries that have ascertained data on both KC and other malignancies and have the capacity to link these data. Strengths of these studies include the relative ease of implementation with existing data and often very large sample sizes, but a limitation is that they usually can only account for age, sex, and region of residence and sometimes socioeconomic status but typically little else.

A systematic review and meta-analysis synthesized the results of 12 registry-based studies (Wheless, Black, & Alberg, 2010). Across the 12 studies, the summary relative risk (SRR) estimates indicated that there was a significantly elevated risk of other types of malignancy following the diagnosis of KC (SRR 1.12, 95% CI 1.07−1.17). The excess risk of other cancers was significant for both SCC (SRR 1.17, 95% CI 1.12−1.23, $n=7$ studies) and BCC (SRR 1.09, 95% CI 1.01−1.17, $n=7$ studies). Since the systematic review and meta-analysis was published, evidence from registry-based studies documenting the association between KC and increased risk of noncutaneous malignancies has continued to accrue (Jung, Dover, & Salopek, 2014; Ong, Goldacre, Hoang, Sinclair, & Goldacre, 2014; Robsahm, Karagas, Rees, & Syse, 2014; Sitas et al., 2011).

The results observed in a study of more than nine million patients conducted by Ong and colleagues using the record-linked hospital and mortality databases in England reinforce the patterns seen in the larger body of evidence on this topic. Individuals with a personal history of KC were 1.27 (95% CI 1.26−1.28) times more likely to develop a noncutaneous malignancy compared with those with a negative history of KC. This study is notable for its large study population of >500,000 patients with KC and a comparison cohort of >8.7 million individuals without KC. This large sample size enabled many different specific types of cancer to be assessed with adequate statistical precision. The data clearly demonstrated the cross-cutting nature of the association between KC and different types of cancer, as 28 of the 29 cancer type-specific risk ratios were in the direction of increased risk, with 26 of those 28 RRs being statistically significant (Ong et al., 2014). The results were consistent in both men and women and the association was stronger the younger the age of onset of KC (Ong et al., 2014).

A study using Alberta Cancer Registry data that included almost 86,000 cases of KC observed that a personal history of KC was associated with 1.4-fold (95% CI 1.3−1.5) increased risk of noncutaneous malignancies (Jung et al., 2014). The standardized incidence ratios (SIR) were consistently elevated in both men (1.7, 95% CI 1.6−1.7) and women (1.5, 95% CI 1.4−1.5). The association between KC and internal malignancies was strongest in younger ages, with SIRs of 2.4 (95% CI 2.0−3.0), 1.8 (95% CI 1.7−1.9), and 1.6 (95% CI 1.5−1.6) for ages <40, 40−59, and ≥60 years, respectively. Of the 40 different types of cancer for which data were presented, 36 had SIRs in the direction of increased risk (i.e., >1.0) and the excess risk was statistically significant for 28 different types of cancer (Jung et al., 2014).

Australian Cancer Registry data, comprised of >9000 cases of SCC and >20,000 cases of BCC diagnosed from 1980 to 2003, were used to characterize the association between KCs and risk specific to lung cancer and all smoking-caused cancers (Sitas et al., 2011). For the variable of all smoking-caused cancers, the associations were in the direction of increased risk, but were stronger for SCC (males 1.38, females 1.78) than for BCC (males 1.09, females 1.10) and were statistically significant only for SCC. The association with any subgroup of cancers would be expected based on the broad spectrum of malignancies associated with KC; associations of a similar magnitude would be also expected for cancers other than smoking-caused cancers but these data were not presented.

A study in Norway focused exclusively on SCC and observed SIRs for noncutaneous malignancies of 1.33 (95% CI 1.28−1.39) in males and 1.22 (95% CI 1.15−1.31) in females (Robsahm et al., 2014). Associations were in the direction of increased risk for 22 of 27 comparisons with 16 of the 22 being statistically significant.

This additional evidence published since the 2010 meta-analysis indicates that associations consistently run in the direction of increased risk and the magnitude of the associations in the more recent studies is larger than measured in the meta-analysis. Due to their substantial sample sizes, these studies are of unique value in having the capacity to characterize the association between KC and risk of noncutaneous malignancies by cancer site and the evidence clearly illustrates that the association cuts across a very broad range of cancers. Further, some of these studies documented a stronger association in younger age groups.

4.2 Prospective Cohort Studies with Individual-Level Data

While the registry-based studies described above are typically comprised of sample sizes of more than 100,000, they usually do not include thorough covariate data needed to investigate the association between KC and noncutaneous malignancies while accounting for potential confounding variables. Prospective cohort studies provide evidence from smaller populations, usually tens of thousands, and are likely to have enhanced internal validity. In a systematic review and meta-analysis those with a personal history of KC had a statistically significant 49% greater risk (SRR 1.49, 95% CI 1.12−1.98, $n=3$ studies) of developing a noncutaneous cancer than those with no personal history of KC (Chen et al., 2008; Efird, Friedman, Habel, Tekawa, & Nelson, 2002; Friedman & Tekawa, 2000; Wheless et al., 2010). Evidence on this topic has continued to accrue with the publication of six additional prospective cohort studies with individual-level data since the meta-analysis and systematic review was published (Hsu et al., 2013; Lindelöf et al., 2000; Pressler et al., 2013; Rees et al., 2014; Roh, Shin, Lee, & Chung, 2012; Song et al., 2013).

This question was addressed within two large US cohorts, the Health Professionals Follow-up Study (46,237 males) and Nurses' Health Study (107,339 females) (Song et al., 2013). In both men (RR 1.11, 95% CI 1.05−1.18) and women (RR 1.20, 95% CI 1.15−1.25) a personal history of KC was significantly associated with excess of noncutaneous malignancies. When stratified by histologic type, the associations with both BCC and SCC were nearly identical in women but in men the association was largely confined to SCC. When the analyses were stratified by specific types of cancer, the associations were in the direction of increased risk for 21 of the 26 comparisons.

The Women's Health Initiative study data were used to specifically examine the association between KC and risk of subsequent breast cancer (Pressler et al., 2013). The relative risk adjusted for age and ethnicity was 1.13 (95% CI 1.01−1.25); this association was weaker when adjusted for a more complete set of variables (RR 1.07, 95% CI 0.95−1.20).

The New Hampshire Skin Cancer Study ($n=3584$) is a skin cancer case−control study in which follow-up of the cases and controls revealed that a personal history of KC was associated with increased risk of noncutaneous malignancies. The association was statistically significant for BCC (RR 1.40, 95% CI 1.15−1.71) but not for SCC (RR 1.18, 95% CI 0.94−1.46); these results were adjusted for age, sex, and smoking status (Rees et al., 2014). When the analyses were stratified by age, the risk for SCC was confined to those <60 years of age (RR 1.96, 95% CI 1.24−3.12; $p < 0.003$), whereas the association for BCC was consistent across age categories.

In a study carried out in a high arsenic exposure area in Taiwan, skin lesions including KC were used as a marker of arsenic exposure and studied in relation to the risk of subsequent internal malignancies (Hsu et al., 2013). Compared to those with no skin lesions, study participants with KC were more than twice as likely to be diagnosed with a subsequent internal malignancy; this association was consistent regardless of whether hyperkeratosis was present (RR 2.36, 95% CI 1.65−3.37) or absent (RR 2.17, 95% CI 1.66−2.85). The magnitude of the relative risks observed by Hsu et al. is somewhat stronger than previously observed in other prospective cohort studies with individual-level data. In addition to the impact of the arsenic exposure, another possible explanation for the stronger association than seen in previous studies is that the entire study population was assessed by dermatologists. This study by Hsu and colleagues is one of the few studies to employ this unique study design feature that has the potential to substantially reduce misclassification of KC status.

Almost all studies related to this topic have focused on Caucasian populations, which is appropriate because this ethnic group has the highest KC incidence rates by far. Against this backdrop, a notable feature of the study conducted by Hsu et al. is the Asian ethnicity of the study population. Another study was carried out in Korea wherein a follow-up of 532 patients with KC was compared to cancer rates in the general population. The KC cohort was observed to have a significantly higher risk of cancer than the general population (SIR 1.38, 95% CI 1.10−1.90); however, this was likely an overestimate because skin cancers were included as an outcome (Roh et al., 2012). These are the first studies to document the excess risk of noncutaneous malignancies associated with a personal history of KC in populations of Asian ancestry.

4.3 Is the Association Between KC and Noncutaneous Malignancies Direct or Indirect?

A large body of prospective epidemiologic evidence consistently points toward a personal history of KC being associated with an excess risk of noncutaneous malignancies. An important next question then becomes whether this association is direct and therefore etiologically relevant or, alternatively, if the association is indirect and thus simply due to shared risk factors for both KC and other malignancies. In assessing this issue, it is worth noting that the likelihood of a shared risk factor explaining away the association between KC and risk of other cancers is extremely remote because the predominant risk factor for KC is solar UVR, which is not known to be linked to risk of internal malignancies. Further, the diverse suite of malignancies associated with KC have such heterogeneous risk factor profiles that this makes it difficult to conceive of a common set of confounding variables that could account for the consistent body of evidence reviewed above.

The types of environmental or lifestyle risk factors for cancer that could most likely be implicated are those that are involved in the etiology of many malignancies, like cigarette smoking and obesity. Even cancer risk factors such as smoking and obesity are extremely unlikely to be major confounding factors due to the lack of a clear-cut link between these potential confounders and risk of developing KC. Nevertheless, in attempting to discern the relevance of the statistical association between KC and risk of cutaneous malignancies, this is an important issue to consider.

In all four of the studies that adjusted for cigarette smoking (Chen et al., 2008, Efird et al., 2002; Rees et al., 2014; Song et al., 2013), the association between KC and risk of other cancer persisted after adjusting for smoking status. Similarly, in three studies that adjusted for body mass index (BMI) (Chen et al., 2008; Efird et al., 2002; Song et al., 2013), the association between KC and risk of other cancer persisted after statistically controlling for BMI. To illustrate, in the study by Chen et al. (2008) the relative risk of other types of cancer in those with a personal history of KC compared to those without KC was 1.96 (95% CI 1.68–2.31) in analyses only adjusted for age and 1.98 (95% CI 1.69–2.31) in analyses also adjusted for sex, smoking status, BMI and years of education. In the Health Professionals Follow-up Study and Nurses' Health Study, not only were smoking and BMI adjusted for in the primary analyses, but the investigators presented the results of analyses stratified by these factors and the associations persisted in the direction of increased risk in the subcategories for cigarette smoking status and BMI (Song et al., 2013). The fact that the association persists even after adjusting for smoking and BMI indicates that the association is not an artifact of confounding by these factors; rather, this provides evidence that the association is direct.

In the prior meta-analysis, the strength of the association was notably stronger in cohort studies with individual-level data than in the registry-based studies (Wheless et al., 2010), and even though this gap appears to have diminished in the more recently published studies, this general pattern is still evident. One possibility for this discrepancy is that more refined control for confounding in studies with individual-level data produces more accurate determination of risks. Direct support for this hypothesis was generated in the study by Robsahm et al. (2014) wherein the registry-based approach was directly compared with the individual-level approach with the same prospective data and found a relative risk estimate of 1.5 with the individual-level data approach and 1.2–1.3 with the registry-based approach.

4.3.1 The Strength of the Evidence that KC is Associated with Increased Risk of Other Cancers

In many studies carried out in various settings, KC has consistently been observed to be a marker of increased risk of other cancers. The results of a meta-analysis (Wheless et al., 2010) that noted that a prior KC diagnosis was associated with significantly greater risk of developing another type of cancer continues to be reinforced with the results of both registry-based studies and prospective cohort studies with individual-level data. Although there is variation in the results from study to study, the association between KC and risk of other cancers is consistently seen in both males and females and for both major histologic types of KC, BCC and SCC. The more recent results demonstrate even more clearly that this association is not limited to just one or a few types of malignancy but rather applies to essentially almost all malignancies. The association has now even been documented in Asian populations, indicating that the association holds relevance beyond Caucasian populations.

A relatively clear indication continues to emerge that the association is stronger in younger age groups. In several studies the excess overall risk of noncutaneous malignancies has been observed to be stronger in individuals with earlier age of onset KC or in younger age groups (Chen et al., 2008; Jung et al., 2014; Ong et al., 2014; Rees et al., 2014; Song et al., 2013). This observation is consistent with enhanced genetic susceptibility.

Even in kidney transplant recipients, who are at higher risk of both SCC and internal malignancies, those who developed an SCC were three times (95% CI 1.9–4.7) as likely to go on to develop an internal malignancy than those with no SCC (Wisgerhof, Wolterbeek, de Fijter, Willemze, & Bouwes Bavinck, 2012). This observation of KC as a marker of increased cancer risk in transplant recipients provides strong evidence to validate KC as a marker of risk of noncutaneous second primary cancers.

With respect to the overall consistency of the evidence, it is worth highlighting a small group of studies viewed as discrepant findings. Due to the suspected anti-cancer properties of vitamin D, several studies have been conducted to investigate the hypothesis that KC, as a biomarker of vitamin D status, is inversely correlated with risk of developing cancers other than KC. All four of the studies to use this approach have reported a statistically significant inverse association in at least one subgroup (de Vries, Soerjomataram, Houterman, Louwman, & Coebergh, 2007; Grant, 2007; Soerjomataram, Louwman, Lemmens, Coebergh, & de Vries, 2008; Tuohimaa et al., 2007). For example, an inverse association was observed between SCC and colorectal cancer (SIR 0.69, 95% CI 0.50–0.94) (Soerjomataram et al., 2008), as well as between KC and advanced prostate cancer (SIR 0.73, 95% CI 0.56–0.95) (de Vries et al., 2007). Tuohimaa et al. (2007) observed that KC was associated with a significantly elevated risk of other cancers (SIR 1.39, 95% CI 1.38–1.41). After stratifying by sunny vs less sunny countries and excluding skin and lip cancers, the association of BCC with other cancers was determined to be concentrated in less sunny countries (SIR 1.35, 95% CI 1.32–1.37), whereas an inverse association was present in sunny countries (SIR 0.86, 95% CI 0.80–0.92) (Tuohimaa et al., 2007). While the hypothesis that as a biomarker of high vitamin D status KC is inversely associated with risk of other cancers is conceptually appealing, it has only been supported in selected subgroups of a few studies and is therefore not substantiated by the evidence (Alberg & Fischer, 2014). A nested case–control study in Sweden provided further evidence against this hypothesis as they found that BCC risk was significantly elevated (RR 1.37, 95% CI 1.35–1.39) after a first primary cancer that was a noncutaneous malignancy (Lindelöf et al., 2012).

For many reasons, the association between KC and risk of other cancers is likely to represent a true etiologic association. First, the evidence synthesized above was limited to studies reporting follow-up after KC unequivocally establishes that the KC diagnosis preceded the occurrence of other malignancies. Second, the large number of studies produced remarkably consistent results; almost all studies showed a significantly increased risk for all other cancers.

When viewed in its totality, the evidence clearly indicates that those with a personal history of KC experience a statistically significant higher subsequent risk of developing noncutaneous malignancies and that this association is of large enough magnitude to be clinically meaningful. While KC is associated with excess cancer risk across almost all types of malignancy, risk factors tend to vary across malignancies so that there are no known shared environmental exposures that increase risk for both KC and noncutaneous malignancies. The predominant cause of KC, UVR, is not known to be linked with risk of noncutaneous malignancies. In the apparent absence of any viable alternative explanations that could account for the increased risk of multiple cancers, the possibility that KC is a marker of enhanced susceptibility to cancer merits attention.

4.3.2 KC and Risk of Other Cancers in Relation to the Multiple Primary Cancer Model

How does the association between a personal history of KC and increased risk of noncutaneous malignancies align within the context of cancer research? The root of this research may be found in the longstanding hypothesis that individuals who experience multiple primary cancers (MPCs) represent a population subset with enhanced susceptibility to cancer. This has been referred to as the "multiple primary cancer model." The hypothesis regarding enhanced host susceptibility in patients with MPCs has been difficult to test in practice for multiple reasons.

The opportunity to study the risk of second cancers is dependent upon the prognosis of the first primary cancer, as the feasibility of characterizing the risk of a second primary is greater for cancers with excellent survival than for cancers that are rapidly fatal; in the latter scenario patients do not live long enough to develop second primary cancers. Survival differentials across cancer sites introduce challenges; for example, studying risk of MPCs in pancreatic cancer patients is difficult because it is often rapidly fatal (Curtis et al., 2006). In contrast, studying second cancers is much easier in cancer sites with favorable prognoses such as cancers of the breast and prostate (Curtis et al., 2006).

Another issue is that cancer treatments themselves can alter future cancer risk (Newhauser & Durante, 2011; Travis, 2006; Wood et al., 2012). Treatments such as radiotherapy and select types of chemotherapy increase second cancer risk. Complicating matters further, some treatments can both decrease and increase risk of other cancers; for example, adjuvant tamoxifen therapy decreases the risk of contralateral breast cancer but increases the risk of endometrial cancer (Grilli, 2006). Additionally, the impact of these issues varies by the site, stage and tumor subtype of the first cancer. Factors such as survival bias and treatment-related risks will interfere with valid inferences in studies where the goal is to study susceptibility to MPCs.

The excess risk of noncutaneous malignancies among those with a personal history of KC is in close alignment with multiple primary cancer model. In fact, the study of KCs in relation to noncutaneous malignancies overcomes the obstacles mentioned above and therefore leads to more clearcut inferences. KC acts as an excellent sentinel first cancer to study risk of multiple primary cancers because most KCs are non-fatal, allowing for follow-up sufficiently long to detect second primary cancers. Two reasons that KC is an excellent model for studying the etiology of MPCs are that it is the most common form of cancer (Karagas et al., 2006; Rogers et al., 2010) so it can be readily studied and the survival rate is so high that survivor bias is not an issue. Another characteristic that makes KC a good model is that it overcomes the problem of increased risk introduced by cancer treatments because it can be cured by surgical excision, eliminating the need for systemic chemotherapy, radiation, and their concomitant side effects. Regardless of the underlying mechanisms that lead to KC acting as a marker of increased risk of other noncutaneous malignancies, this combination of characteristics indicate that KCs provide an excellent model for studying MPCs.

Given these considerations, a comparison of the risk of MPCs using KC vs other types of cancer as the sentinel cancer is of interest. Ignoring KC, those with one primary cancer have a 14% (SIR 1.14, 95% CI 1.14−1.15) greater age- and sex-adjusted risk of subsequent cancer than the general population (Fraumeni, Curtis, Edwards, & Tucker, 2006). The risk is stronger the younger the first primary is diagnosed (Fraumeni et al., 2006). In comparison, the risk of second cancers after a KC diagnosis is at least as strong and likely stronger. Further, as reviewed above the stronger association at younger ages for KC is in keeping with what has been observed for the MPC model in general. Regardless of the underlying mechanistic explanations for the excess risk of noncutaneous malignancies among those with a personal history of KC, the alignment of this observation with the multiple primary cancer model provides a strong rationale to speculate that KC may be a marker of a cancer-prone phenotype.

4.3.3 Why would KC be Associated with Increased Risk of Noncutaneous Malignancies?

The multiple primary cancer model provides a context to think about this topic, raising the question of what underlying mechanisms could explain why KC is a marker of a high cancer-risk phenotype. The fact that the excess risk of noncutaneous cancers seen in those with a personal history of KC applies to so many different types of cancer suggests that determining the mechanisms underlying this relationship could potentially yield valuable clues regarding human carcinogenesis across multiple tissues.

The lack of environmental and lifestyle risk factors to explain this association shifts the focus to factors associated with inter-individual differences in cancer susceptibility. There are several plausible biological mechanisms that could explain the association between KC and risk of other cancers. Among the many potential explanations, two particularly intriguing mechanisms that may explain why those with a personal history of KC experience an overall excess risk of cancer are highlighted: DNA repair and inflammatory/immune response pathways.

4.3.3.1 DNA Repair Gene Variants

Major DNA repair defects cause cancer-prone phenotypes. For example, mutated DNA repair genes cause cancer-prone syndromes that involve multiple cancers, such as XP (Cleaver, 2000, 2005). As clearly demonstrated by XP, defective NER is a robust determinant of genetic predisposition to risk of both KC as well as noncutaneous malignancies (Cleaver, 2005). The fact that rare mutations in DNA repair genes cause increased cancer susceptibility in XP patients suggests that even common, low-penetrant DNA repair gene variants may jointly affect susceptibility to KC and other malignancies in the general population (Halliday, 2005; Vineis et al., 2009). XP is caused by mutations in genes in the NER pathway. Ultraviolet radiation can cause skin cancer by inducing mutations in the DNA of skin cells; NER genes are responsible for repairing this damage.

Brewster and colleagues used a candidate gene approach to test the hypothesis that the *XPD* Lys751Gln polymorphism is associated with the likelihood that a participant with a personal history of KC ($n = 481$, $n = 80$ second primary cancers) would go on to develop a second primary cancer (Brewster, Alberg, Strickland, Hoffman, & Helzlsouer, 2004). The findings showed that compared with the homozygous wild-type (Lys/Lys) genotype, those with at least one variant (Gln) allele had an increased risk of a second primary cancer (adjusted RR 2.22, 95% CI 1.30−3.76). These findings support the hypothesis that NER gene variants may contribute to the KC cancer-prone phenotype.

The findings of Brewster et al. (2004) were followed up by a larger scale study nested within the community-based CLUE II Cohort that used a candidate gene pathway approach (Jorgensen et al., 2009) to test the hypothesis that DNA repair gene variants contribute to the increased cancer risk associated with a personal history of KC. The frequency of minor alleles in 759 DNA repair single nucleotide polymorphisms (SNPs) among those with KC plus another type of cancer compared with a cancer-free control group, 10 SNPs had allelic trend p values < 0.01 (Ruczinski et al., 2012). The third and seventh ranked SNPs were from NER genes, rs1038144 (*ERCC8*) and rs4150454 (*ERCC3*). However, SNPS from other DNA repair pathways such as base excision repair, homologous recombination and mismatch repair were also represented. The results pinpoint the DNA repair genes most likely to contribute to the KC cancer-prone phenotype suggesting that associations are not limited solely to NER but rather extend to other DNA repair pathways, and provide proof-of-principle evidence to document the value of this line of inquiry (Ruczinski et al., 2012). In this same study population, but limited to BCC, variants in Hedgehog pathway-related genes were studied with null results (Jorgensen et al., 2012).

4.3.3.2 Inflammation and Immune Status

The strong link between immunosuppression and KC reviewed previously very clearly demonstrates that immune status plays a prominent role in susceptibility to KC. The ubiquitous role of immune dysregulation in carcinogenesis is becoming increasingly clear (Finn, 2012); this makes it plausible to speculate that suboptimal inflammatory/immune response may be associated with the risk of both KC and other types of cancer. Despite a strong scientific rationale, currently there is no evidence to address this hypothesis. This reflects the overall status of this field at present, with a paucity of hypothesis-driven research to advance understanding of why KC is linked with excess risk of noncutaneous malignancies.

5. KERATINOCYTE CARCINOMA AND FATAL OUTCOMES

A personal history of KC is clearly linked to increased risk of developing other forms of cancer. Further, there is an emerging body of evidence to suggest that a personal history of KC may be associated with excess risk of fatal outcomes. Multiple reports have been published on each of the following outcomes: (1) higher overall mortality rates, (2) higher cancer-specific mortality rates, and (3) poorer survival after a diagnosis of another form of cancer.

Studies of the association between a personal history of KC and these fatal endpoints have been carried out in various populations, including the general population and cohorts of cancer patients. These reports have been centered largely on registry-based data in Denmark and Sweden (Frisch, Hjalgrim, Olsen, & Melbye, 1996; Frisch & Melbye, 1995; Hemminki & Dong, 2000; Hemminki, Jiang, & Dong, 2001; Hemminki, Jiang, & Steineck, 2003; Jaeger, Gramkow, Hjalgrim, Melbye, & Frisch, 1999), as well as studies in North America (Chen et al., 2008; Efird et al., 2002; Friedman & Tekawa, 2000). The North American studies include the American Cancer Society's Cancer Prevention Study II, New Hampshire Skin Cancer Study, New Hampshire State Cancer Registry, and Manitoba Cancer Registry.

Overall, the results tend to support the notion that those with a personal history of KC have higher mortality rates than those with no personal history of KC. The results are heterogeneous according to histologic type. SCC has been consistently observed to be associated with increased all-cause mortality, with relative risks that range from 1.11 (95% CI 1.07−1.15) to 1.54 (95% CI 1.41−1.68). In contrast, the results for BCC tend to run in the opposite direction. A personal history of BCC has consistently been associated with a slight decrease in all-cause mortality, with relative risks ranging from 0.89 (95% CI 0.83−0.95) to 0.97 (95% CI 0.96−0.98). The reasons for the observed inverse association between BCC and all-cause mortality are unclear, but this observation persists even after adjustments for potential confounding factors such as comorbidities and socioeconomic status. Results of studies that did not stratify by histologic subtype but rather looked at overall KC thus represent the combination of increased mortality risk for SCC but decreased risk for BCC, thus a relative risk close to 1.0 is to be expected; this is what was observed in one study with a RR of 0.96 (95% CI 0.84−0.98) (Jensen et al., 2007).

In addition to all-cause mortality, KC has also been studied in relation to cancer-specific mortality. In a study of overall KC, a significantly increased risk of cancer-specific mortality was observed for both males (RR 1.30, 95% CI 1.23−1.36) and females (RR 1.26, 95% CI 1.17−1.35) (Kahn, Tatham, Patel, Thun, & Heath, 1998). These associations are much stronger than those for all-cause mortality (RR 1.03 in men, RR 1.04 in women) (Kahn et al., 1998), which could be interpreted as further evidence of KC acting as a marker of a cancer-prone phenotype. A stronger association with mortality from malignancy was seen in patients with SCC (standardized mortality ratio (SMR): 1.18 in men, 1.55 in women) compared with BCC patients (SMR 1.09 in men, 1.24 in women) (Nugent, Demers, Wiseman, Mihalcioiu, & Kliewer, 2005).

There are also several studies that evaluated the impact of a personal history of KC on survival after a diagnosis with another type of cancer. The prognosis of cancer patients with a history of KC was compared to cancer patients with no history of KC for multiple types of malignancies. The most common malignancies included non-Hodgkin's lymphoma (NHL) and the chronic lymphocytic leukemia (CLL) subtype, due to the suspected association with decreased immune function, as well as the four most common cancers: colon, lung, breast and prostate cancer. Recent studies have yielded relative mortality risk estimates to suggest that cancer patients with a prior history SCC have a significantly higher risk of dying from CLL (RR 1.86, 95% CI 1.46−2.36) (Toro et al., 2009), lung cancer (RR 1.29, 95% CI 1.01−1.65), and NHL (RR 1.33, 95% CI 1.14−1.54). Relative risks in the direction of increased risk were also observed for colon cancer (RR 1.24, 95% CI 1.09−1.41), breast cancer (RR 1.19, 95% CI 1.00−1.42), and prostate cancer (RR 1.17, 95% CI 1.06−1.28) (Askling et al., 1999). While there are few comparable studies for BCC, the existing estimates indicate that mortality risk is not significantly altered after a BCC (RR 0.96, 95% CI 0.77−1.19) (Rees et al., 2015).

This more recently emerging body of evidence on the association between a personal history of KC and fatal outcome tends to support the notion that KC may also be linked with fatal outcomes; given that KC itself is so rarely fatal, this is an unexpected finding. The fact that fatal outcomes tend to be more strongly associated with SCC than with BCC and that SCC is the more invasive form of KC that is more likely to metastasize may provide clues to the nature of this association. The relatively small number of studies providing evidence for the association between KC and these fatal outcomes hinders the ability to make any concrete conclusions on the subject at this time. However, the provocative results to date provide strong justification for further research on this topic to better clarify the nature of these associations.

6. OVERALL SUMMARY AND WRAP-UP

A review of the epidemiology of KC gave little foreshadowing that KC would be linked to an increased risk of noncutaneous malignancies. Nevertheless, a solid body of epidemiologic evidence clearly indicates that a personal history of KC is associated with excess risk of a broad spectrum of noncutaneous malignancies. KC has consistently been observed to be a marker of increased risk of other cancers in many studies carried out in various settings. This association applies to both major histologic types of KC (SCC and BCC) and to both men and women. The association is stronger when KC is diagnosed at younger ages. The association between KC and increased risk of noncutaneous malignancies has been observed in Caucasian and Asian populations.

The association cannot be readily explained by any environmental or lifestyle factor. Viewed in their totality, these observations support the notion that KC may be a marker of a cancer-prone phenotype; this is consistent with the multiple primary cancer model. Currently, the underlying mechanisms for this association are poorly understood. The fact that KC is so common amplifies the importance of research to advance understanding of why KC is a marker of increased risk for other cancers. Research to advance this line of inquiry holds promise to provide novel insights into the determinants of susceptibility to human cancer across all types of malignancy.

REFERENCES

Acartürk, T., & Edington, H. (2005). Nonmelanoma skin cancer. *Clinics in Plastic Surgery, 32,* 237–248.

Accardi, R., & Gheit, T. (2014). Cutaneous HPV and skin cancer. *Presse Medicale, 43,* e435–e443.

Agbai, O., Buster, K., Sanchez, M., Hernandez, C., Kundu, R., Chiu, M., et al. (2014). Skin cancer and photoprotection in people of color: A review and recommendations for physicians and the public. *Journal of the American Academy of Dermatology, 70*(4), 748–762.

Alberg, A. J., & Fischer, A. (2014). Is a personal history of nonmelanoma skin cancer associated with increased or decreased risk of other cancers? *Cancer Epidemiology, Biomarkers & Prevention, 23*(3), 433–436.

American Cancer Society. (2007). *Cancer facts and figures 2007.* Atlanta: American Cancer Society.

Askling, J., Sørensen, P., Ekbom, A., Melbye, M., Glimelius, G., & Hjalgrim, H. (1999). Is history of squamous-cell skin cancer a marker of poor prognosis in patients with cancer? *Annals of Internal Medicine, 131,* 655–659.

Athar, M., Walsh, S., Kopelovich, L., & Elmets, C. (2011). Pathogenesis of nonmelanoma skin cancers in organ transplant recipients. *Archives of Biochemistry and Biophysics, 508*(2), 159–163.

Aubry, F., & Macgibbon, B. (1985). Risk factors of squamous cell carcinoma of the skin: A case-control study in the Montreal region. *Cancer, 55,* 907–911.

Australian Institute of Health and Welfare and Cancer Australia (2008). *Non-melanoma skin cancer: general practice considerations, hospitalization and mortality.* Cancer series no. 43. Cat. no. 39. Canberra: AIHW.

Bajdik, C., Gallagher, R., Hill, G., & Fincham, S. (1995). Sunlight exposure, pigmentation factors, and risk of nonmelanocytic skin cancer. II. Squamous cell carcinoma. *Archives of Dermatology, 3*(2), 164–169.

Balk, S. (2011). Ultraviolet radiation: A hazard to children and adolescents. *Pediatrics, 127*(3), e791–e817.

Bauer, A., Diepgen, T. L., & Schmitt, J. (2011). Is occupational solar ultraviolet irradiation a relevant risk factor for basal cell carcinoma? A systematic review and meta-analysis of the epidemiological literature. *British Journal of Dermatology, 165,* 612–625.

Binstock, M., Hafeez, F., Metchnikoff, C., & Arron, S. (2014). Single-nucleotide polymorphisms in pigment genes and nonmelanoma skin cancer predisposition: A systematic review. *British Journal of Dermatology, 171*(4), 713–721.

Bickers, D. R., Lim, H. W., Margolis, D., Weinstock, M. A., Goodman, C., Faulkner, E., et al. (2006). The burden of skin diseases: 2004. *Journal of the American Academy of Dermatology, 55*(3), 490–500.

Brewster, A., Alberg, A. J., Strickland, P., Hoffman, S., & Helzlsouer, K. (2004). XPD polymorphism and risk of subsequent cancer in individuals with nonmelanoma skin cancer. *Cancer Epidemiology, Biomarkers & Prevention, 13*(8), 1271–1275.

Brin, L., Zubair, A., & Brewer, J. (2014). Optimal management of skin cancer in immunosuppressed patients. *American Journal of Clinical Dermatology, 15*(4), 339–356.

Burge, S., & Wallis, D. (2011). *Oxford handbook of medical dermatology.* New York: Oxford University Press.

Cadet, J., Sage, E., & Douki, T. (2005). Ultraviolet radiation-mediated damage to cellular DNA. *Mutation Research, 571*, 3–17.

Cantwell, M. M., Murray, L. J., Catney, D., et al. (2009). Second primary cancers in patients with skin cancer: A population-based study in Northern Ireland. *British Journal of Cancer, 100*, 174–177.

Centers for Disease Control and Prevention. (2015). Vital signs: Melanoma incidence and mortality trends and projections—United States, 1982–2030. *Morbidity and Mortality Weekly Report, 64*, 591–596.

Chen, J., Ruczinski, I., Jorgensen, T. J., Yenokyan, G., Yao, Y., Alani, R., et al. (2008). Nonmelanoma skin cancer and risk for subsequent malignancy. *Journal of the National Cancer Institute, 100*, 1215–1222.

Christenson, L. J., Borrowman, T. A., Vachon, C. M., et al. (2005). Incidence of basal cell and squamous cell carcinomas in a population younger than 40 years. *JAMA, 294*(6), 681–690.

Cleaver, J. E. (2000). Common pathways for ultraviolet skin carcinogenesis in the repair and replication defective groups of xeroderma pigmentosum. *Journal of Dermatological Science, 23*, 1–11.

Cleaver, J. E. (2005). Cancer in xeroderma pigmentosum and related disorders of DNA repair. *Nature Reviews. Cancer, 5*, 564–573.

Curtis, R. E., Freedman, D. M., Ron, E., Ries, L. A. G., Hacker, D. G., & Edwards, B. K. et al. (Eds.), (2006). *New malignancies among cancer survivors: SEER Cancer Registries, 1973-2000.* Bethesda, MD: National Cancer Institute. NIH Publ. No. 0505302.

Czarnecki, D., Staples, M., Mar, A., Giles, G., & Meehan, C. (1994). Metastases from squamous cell carcinoma of the skin in southern Australia. *Dermatology, 189*(1), 52–54.

De Hertog, S., Wensveen, C., Bastiaens, M., et al. (2001). Relation between smoking and skin cancer. *Journal of Clinical Oncology, 19*(1), 231–238.

de Vries, E., Soerjomataram, I., Houterman, S., Louwman, M. W., & Coebergh, J. W. (2007). Decreased risk of prostate cancer after skin cancer diagnosis: A protective role of ultraviolet radiation? *American Journal of Epidemiology, 165*, 966–972.

Diepgen, T. L., & Mahler, V. (2002). The epidemiology of skin cancer. *British Journal of Dermatology, 146*, 1–6.

Efird, J. T., Friedman, G. D., Habel, L., Tekawa, I. S., & Nelson, L. M. (2002). Risk of subsequent cancer following invasive or in situ squamous cell skin cancer. *Annals of Epidemiology, 12*, 469–475.

Emsen, I. M., & Kabalar, M. E. (2010). Epidermodysplasia verruciformis: An early and unusual presentation. *The Canadian Journal of Plastic Surgery, 18*(1), 21–24.

Finn, O. (2012). Immuno-oncology: Understanding the function and dysfunction of the immune system in cancer. *Annals of Oncology, 23*(Suppl. 8), viii6–viii9.

Fraumeni, J. F., Jr., Curtis, R. E., Edwards, B. K., & Tucker, M. A. (2006). Chapter 1: Introduction. In R. E. Curtis, D. M. Freedman, E. Ron, L. A. G. Ries, D. G. Hacker, & B. K. Edwards, et al. (Eds.), *New malignancies among cancer survivors: SEER Cancer Registries, 1973-2000.* Bethesda, MD: National Cancer Institute. NIH Publ. No. 0505302.

Freedman, D. M., Sigurdson, A., Doody, M. M., Mabuchi, K., & Linet, M. S. (2003). Risk of basal cell carcinoma in relation to alcohol intake and smoking. *Cancer Epidemiology, Biomarkers & Prevention, 12*, 1540–1543.

Friedman, G. D., & Tekawa, I. S. (2000). Association of basal cell skin cancers with other cancers (United States). *Cancer Causes & Control, 11*, 891–897.

Frisch, M., Hjalgrim, H., Olsen, J. H., & Melbye, M. (1996). Risk for subsequent cancer after diagnosis of basal cell carcinoma. *Annals of Internal Medicine, 125*, 815–821.

Frisch, M., & Melbye, M. (1995). New primary cancers after squamous cell skin cancer. *American Journal of Epidemiology, 141*, 916–922.

Gallagher, M., Kelly, P., Jardine, M., Perkovic, V., Cass, A., Craig, J., et al. (2010). Long-term cancer risk of immunosuppressive regimens after kidney transplantation. *Journal of the American Society of Nephrology, 21*(5), 852–858.

Gamble, J., Lerman, S., Holder, W., Nicolich, M., & Yarborough, C. (1996). Physician-based case-control study of non-melanoma skin cancer in Baytown, Texas. *Occupational Medicine, 46*, 186–196.

Gloster, H. M., & Neal, K. (2006). Skin cancer in skin of color. *Journal of the American Academy of Dermatology, 55*, 741–760.

Grant, W. B. (2007). A meta-analysis of second cancers after a diagnosis of nonmelanoma skin cancer: Additional evidence that solar ultraviolet-B irradiance reduces the risk of internal cancers. *The Journal of Steroid Biochemistry and Molecular Biology, 103*, 668–674.

Grilli, S. (2006). Tamoxifen (TAM): The dispute goes on. *Annali dell'Istituto Superiore Di Sanità, 42*(2), 170–173.

Guy, G. P., Berkowitz, Z., Tai, E., Holman, D. M., Everett Jones, S., & Richardson, L. C. (2014). Indoor tanning among high school students in the United States, 2009 and 2011. *JAMA Dermatology, 30341*(5), 1–11.

Halder, R. M., & Bridgeman-Shah, S. (1995). Skin cancer in African Americans. *Cancer, 75*, 667–673.

Halliday, G. M. (2005). Inflammation, gene mutation and photoimmunosupression in response to UVR-induced oxidative damage contributes to photocarcinogensis. *Mutation Research, 571*, 107–120.

Hemminki, K., & Dong, C. (2000). Subsequent cancers after in situ and invasive squamous cell carcinoma of the skin. *Archives of Dermatology, 136*, 647–651.

Hemminki, K., Jiang, Y., & Dong, C. (2001). Second primary cancers after anogenital, skin, oral, esophageal, and rectal cancers: Etiological links? *International Journal of Cancer, 93*, 294–298.

Hemminki, K., Jiang, Y., & Steineck, G. (2003). Skin cancer and non-Hodgkin's lymphoma as second malignancies: Markers of impaired immune function? *European Journal of Cancer, 39*, 223–229.

Holmes, S. A., Malinovszky, K., & Roberts, D. L. (2000). Changing trends in non-melanoma skin cancer in South Wales, 1988–1998. *The British Journal of Dermatology, 143*, 1224–1229.

Hornung, R. L., Magee, K. H., & Lee, W. J. (2003). Tanning facility use: Are we exceeding food and drug administration limits? *American Academy of Dermatology, 49*, 655–661.

Hsu, L. I., Chen, G. S., Lee, C. H., Yang, T. Y., Chen, Y. H., Wang, Y. H., et al. (2013). Use of arsenic-induced palmoplantar hyperkeratosis and skin cancers to predict risk of subsequent internal malignancy. *American Journal of Epidemiology, 177*, 202–212.

Hunter, D. J., Colditz, G. A., Stampfer, M. J., Rosner, B., Willett, W. C., & Speizer, F. E. (1990). Risk factors for basal cell carcinoma in a prospective cohort of women. *Annals of Epidemiology, 1*(1), 13–23.

Jaeger, A. B., Gramkow, A., Hjalgrim, H., Melbye, M., & Frisch, M. (1999). Bowen disease and risk of subsequent malignant neoplasms. *Archives of Dermatology, 135*, 790–793.

Jensen, A. O., et al. (2007). Do incident and new subsequent cases of non-melanoma skin cancer registered in a Danish prospective cohort study have different 10-year mortality? *Cancer Detection and Prevention, 31*(5), 352–358.

Jorgensen, T. J., Ruczinski, I., Kessing, B., Smith, M., Shugart, Y., & Alberg, A. J. (2009). Hypothesis-driven candidate gene association studies: Practical design and analytical considerations. *American Journal of Epidemiology*, *170*(8), 986–993.

Jorgensen, T., Ruczinski, I., Shugart, Y., Wheless, L., Schaad, Y., Kessing, B., et al. (2012). A population-based study of hedgehog pathway gene variants in relation to the dual risk of basal cell carcinoma plus another cancer. *Cancer Epidemiology*, *36*(5), e288–e293.

Joseph, M. G., Zulueta, W. P., & Kennedy, P. J. (1992). Squamous cell carcinoma of the skin of the trunk and limbs: The incidence of metastases and their outcome. *Australian and New Zealand Journal of Surgery*, *62*(9), 697–701.

Jung, G., Dover, D., & Salopek, T. (2014). Risk of second primary malignancies following a diagnosis of malignant melanoma or non-melanoma skin cancer in Alberta, Canada from 1979 to 2009. *British Journal of Dermatology*, *170*, 136–143.

Kahn, H. S., Tatham, L. M., Patel, A. V., Thun, M. J., & Heath, C. W. (1998). Increased cancer mortality following a history of nonmelanoma skin cancer. *JAMA*, *280*(10), 910–912.

Kao, G., et al. (1997). Cutaneous carcinogenesis: Etiologic factors-viruses. In S. Miller & M. Mahoney (Eds.), *Cutaneous oncology: Pathophysiology, diagnosis, and treatment* (pp. 148–157). London, England: Blackwell Science.

Karagas, M. R., Stukel, T. A., Greenberg, E. R., et al. (1992). Risk of subsequent basal cell carcinoma and squamous cell carcinoma of the skin among patients with prior skin cancer. Skin Cancer Prevention Study Group. *JAMA*, *267*, 3305–3310.

Karagas, M., Weinstock, M., & Nelson, H. (2006). Keratinocyte carcinomas (basal and squamous cell carcinomas of the skin) 1230-50. In *Cancer epidemiology and prevention* (3rd ed.). New York: Oxford University Press.

Karia, P. S., Han, J., & Schmults, C. D. (2013). Cutaneous squamous cell carcinoma: Estimated incidence of disease, nodal metastasis, and deaths from disease in the United States, 2012. *Journal of the American Academy of Dermatology*, *68*(6), 957–966.

Kuschal, C., Thoms, K., Schubert, S., Schäfer, A., Boeckmann, L., Schön, M., et al. (2011). Skin cancer in organ transplant recipients: Effects of immunosuppressive medications on DNA repair. *Experimental Dermatology*, *21*(1), 2–6.

Lazarczyk, M., & Favre, M. (2008). Role of Zn2+ ions in host-virus interactions. *Journal of Virology*, *82*(23), 11486–11494.

Lazarczyk, M., Pons, C., Mendoza, J. A., Cassonnet, P., Jacob, Y., & Favre, M. (2008). Regulation of cellular zinc balance as a potential mechanism of EVER-mediated protection against pathogenesis by cutaneous oncogenic human papillomaviruses. *The Journal of Experimental Medicine*, *205*(1), 35–42.

Lear, J., Tan, B., Smith, A., Jones, P., Heagerty, A., Strange, R., et al. (1998). A comparison of risk factors for malignant melanoma, squamous cell carcinoma and basal cell carcinoma in the UK. *International Journal of Clinical Practice*, *52*(3), 145–149.

Lehmann, A., Mcgibbon, D., & Stefanini, M. (2011). Xeroderma pigmentosum. *Orphanet Journal of Rare Diseases*, *6*, 70.

Lewis, K., & Weinstock, M. (2007). Trends in nonmelanoma skin cancer mortality rates in the United States, 1969 through 2000. *Journal of Investigative Dermatology*, *127*(10), 2323–2327.

Lindelöf, B., Krynitz, B., Ayoubi, S., Martschin, C., Wiegleb-Edström, D., & Wiklund, K. (2012). Previous extensive sun exposure and subsequent vitamin D production in patients with basal cell carcinoma of the skin, has no protective effect on internal cancers. *European Journal of Cancer*, *48*(8), 1154–1158.

Lindelöf, B., Odenbro, A., Bellocco, R., Boffetta, P., & Adami, J. (2005). Tobacco smoking, snuff dipping and the risk of cutaneous squamous cell carcinoma: A nationwide cohort study in Sweden. *British Journal of Cancer*, *92*, 1326–1328.

Lindelöf, B., et al. (2000). Incidence of skin cancer in 5356 patients following organ transplantation. *British Journal of Dermatology*, *143*(3), 513–519.

Lomas, A., Leonardi-Bee, J., & Bath-Hextall, F. (2012). A systematic review of worldwide incidence of nonmelanoma skin cancer. *British Journal of Dermatology*, *166*(5), 1069–1080.

Marcil, I., & Stern, R. (2000). Risk of developing a subsequent nonmelanoma skin cancer in patients with a history of nonmelanoma skin cancer. *Archives of Dermatology*, *136*, 1524–1530.

Marks, R., & Staples, M. (1993). Trends in non-melanocytic skin cancer treated in Australia: The second national survey. *International Journal of Cancer*, *53*, 585–590.

Martinez, J., Otley, C., Stasko, T., Euvrard, S., Weaver, A., & Brown, C. (2003). Defining the clinical course of metastatic skin cancer in organ transplant recipients. *Archives of Dermatology*, *139*(3), 301–306.

Menck, C., & Munford, V. (2014). DNA repair diseases: What do they tell us about cancer and aging? *Genetics and Molecular Biology*, *37*, 220–233.

Milan, T., Verkasalo, P. K., Kaprio, J., et al. (2003). Lifestyle differences in twin pairs discordant for basal cell carcinoma of the skin. *British Journal of Dermatology*, *149*, 115–123.

Miller, D., & Weinstock, M. (1994). Nonmelanoma skin cancer in the United States: Incidence. *Journal of the American Academy of Dermatology*, *30*(5), 774–778.

Montagna, W., Prota, G., & Kenney, J. A., Jr. (1993). *Black skin structure and function*. London: Academic Press. pp. 55–60.

Newhauser, W. D., & Durante, M. (2011). Assessing the risk of second malignancies after modern radiotherapy. *Nature Reviews. Cancer*, *11*(6), 438–448.

Nugent, Z., Demers, A. A., Wiseman, M. C., Mihalcioiu, C., & Kliewer, E. V. (2005). Risk of second primary cancer and death following a diagnosis of nonmelanoma skin cancer. *Cancer Epidemiology, Biomarkers & Prevention*, *14*(11), 2584–2590.

Ong, E. L. H., Goldacre, R., Hoang, U., Sinclair, R., & Goldacre, M. (2014). Subsequent primary malignancies in patients with non-melanoma skin cancer in England: A national record linkage study. *Cancer Epidemiology, Biomarkers & Prevention*, *23*, 490–498.

Patel, T., Morrison, L. K., Rady, P., & Tyring, S. (2010). Epidermodysplasia verruciformis and susceptibility to HPV. *Disease Markers*, *29*(3–4), 199–206.

Perera, E., Gnaneswaran, N., Staines, C., Win, A. K., & Sinclair, R. (2015). Incidence and prevalence of non-melanoma skin cancer in Australia: A systematic review. *The Australasian Journal of Dermatology*, *56*, 258–267.

Pressler, M., Rosenberg, C., Derman, B., Greenland, P., Khandekar, J., Rodabough, R., et al. (2013). Breast cancer in postmenopausal women after non-melanomatous skin cancer: The Women's Health Initiative observational study. *Breast Cancer Research and Treatment*, *139*(3), 821–831.

Raasch, B. A., Buettner, P. G., & Garbe, C. (2006). Basal cell carcinoma: Histological classification and body-site distribution. *British Journal of Dermatology*, *155*(2), 401–407.

Rajpara, S., & Ormerod, A. (2008). *Clinical evidence handbook*. London: BMJ Publishing Group.

Ramos, J., Villa, J., Ruiz, A., Armstrong, R., & Matta, J. (2004). UV dose determines key characteristics of nonmelanoma skin cancer. *Cancer Epidemiology, Biomarkers & Prevention*, *13*, 2006–2011.

Rees, J. R., Zens, M. S., Celaya, M. O., Riddle, B. L., Karagas, M. R., & Peacock, J. L. (2015). Survival after squamous cell and basal cell carcinoma of the skin: A retrospective cohort analysis. *International Journal of Cancer*, *137*(4), 878–884.

Rees, J. R., Zens, M. S., Gui, J., Celaya, M. O., Riddle, B. L., & Karagas, M. R. (2014). Non melanoma skin cancer and subsequent cancer risk. *PLoS One*, *9*(6), e99674.

Reichrath, J., & Rass, K. (2014). UV damage and DNA repair in malignant melanoma and nonmelanoma skin cancer. Sunlight, vitamin D and skin cancer. *Advances in Experimental Medicine and Biology*, *810*, 162–178.

Rigel, D., Burnett, C., & Lim, H. (2011). Current concepts in photoprotection. In *Cancer of the skin expert consult* (2nd ed.). London: Elsevier Health Sciences.

Robinson, J. K. (2005). Sun exposure, sun protection, and vitamin D. *JAMA*, *294*, 1541–1543.

Robsahm, T., Helsing, P., & Veierød, M. (2015). Cutaneous squamous cell carcinoma in Norway 1963–2011: Increasing incidence and stable mortality. *Cancer Medicine*, *4*(3), 472–480.

Robsahm, T. E., Karagas, M. R., Rees, J. R., & Syse, A. (2014). New malignancies after squamous cell carcinoma and melanomas: A population-based study from Norway. *BMC Cancer*, *14*(1), 210. http://doi.org/10.1186/1471-2407-14-210.

Roewert-Huber, J., Lange-Asschenfeldt, B., Stockfleth, E., & Kerl, H. (2007). Epidemiology and etiology of basal cell carcinoma. *The British Journal of Dermatology*, *157*, 47–51.

Rogers, H. W., Weinstock, M. A., Harris, A. R., Hinckley, M. R., Feldman, S. R., Fleischer, A. B., et al. (2010). Incidence estimate of nonmelanoma skin cancer in the United States, 2006. *Archives of Dermatology*, *146*, 283–287.

Roh, M. R., Shin, H. J., Lee, S. H., & Chung, K. Y. (2012). Risk of second cancers after the diagnosis of non-melanoma skin cancer in Korean patients. *The Journal of Dermatology*, *39*, 541–544.

Ruczinski, I., Jorgensen, T. J., Shugart, Y. Y., Berthier-Schaad, Y., Kessing, B., Hoffman-Bolton, J., et al. (2012). A population-based study of DNA repair gene variants in relation to nonmelanoma skin cancer as a marker of a cancer-prone phenotype. *Carcinogenesis*, *33*, 1692–1698.

Schmitt, J., Seidler, A., Diepgen, T. L., & Bauer, A. (2011). Occupational ultraviolet light exposure increases the risk for the development of cutaneous squamous cell carcinoma: A systematic review and meta-analysis. *The British Journal of Dermatology*, *164*, 291–307.

Scotto, J., Fears, T. R., Kraemer, K. H., & Fraumeni, J. F., Jr. (1996). Nonmelanoma skin cancer. In *Cancer epidemiology and prevention*. New York: Oxford University Press.

Silverberg, M., Leyden, W., Warton, E., Quesenberry, C., Engels, E., & Asgari, M. (2013). HIV infection status, immunodeficiency, and the incidence of non-melanoma skin cancer. *Journal of the National Cancer Institute*, *105*(5), 350–360.

Sitas, F., Yu, X. Q., O'Connell, D. L., Blizzard, L., Otahal, P., Newman, L., et al. (2011). The relationship between basal and squamous cell skin cancer and smoking related cancers. *BMC Research Notes*, *4*, 556.

Soerjomataram, I., Louwman, W. J., Lemmens, V. E., Coebergh, J. W., & de Vries, E. (2008). Are patients with skin cancer at lower risk of developing colorectal or breast cancer? *American Journal of Epidemiology*, *167*, 1421–1429.

Song, F., Qureshi, A. A., Giovannucci, E. L., Fuchs, C. S., Chen, W. Y., Stampfer, M. J., et al. (2013). Risk of a second primary cancer after non-melanoma skin cancer in white men and women: A prospective cohort study. *PLoS Medicine*, *10*(4), e1001433.

Staples, M., Elwood, M., Giles, G., Burton, R., et al. (2006). Non-melanoma skin cancer in Australia the 2002 national survey and trends since 1985. *The Medical Journal of Australia*, *184*(1), 6–10.

te Velthuis, A. J. W., van den Worm, S. H. E., Sims, A. C., Baric, R. S., Snijder, E. J., & van Hemert, M. J. (2010). Zn^{2+} inhibits coronavirus and arterivirus RNA polymerase activity *in vitro* and zinc ionophores block the replication of these viruses in cell culture. *PLoS Pathogens*, *6*(11), e1001176.

Toro, J. R., Blake, P. W., Björkholm, M., Kristinsson, S. Y., Wang, Z., & Landgren, O. (2009). Prior history of non-melanoma skin cancer is associated with increased mortality in patients with chronic lymphocytic leukemia. *Haematologica*, *94*(10), 1460–1464.

Travis, L. B. (2006). The epidemiology of second primary cancers. *Cancer Epidemiology, Biomarkers & Prevention*, *15*, 2020–2026.

Tuohimaa, P., Pukkala, E., Scélo, G., Olsen, J. H., Brewster, D. H., Hemminki, K., et al. (2007). Does solar exposure, as indicated by the non-melanoma skin cancers, protect from solid cancers: Vitamin D as a possible explanation. *European Journal of Cancer*, *43*, 1701–1712.

van Dam, R. M., Huang, Z., Rimm, E. B., Weinstock, M. A., Spiegelman, D., Colditz, G. A., et al. (1999). Risk factors for basal cell carcinoma of the skin in men: Results from the health professionals follow-up study. *American Journal of Epidemiology*, *150*(5), 459–468.

Vineis, P., Manuguerra, M., Kavvoura, F. K., Guarrera, S., Allione, A., Rosa, F., et al. (2009). A field synopsis on low-penetrance variants in DNA repair genes and cancer susceptibility. *Journal of the National Cancer Institute*, *101*, 24–36.

Von Hoff, D. D., LoRusso, P. M., Rudin, C. M., Reddy, J. C., Yauch, R. L., Tibes, R., et al. (2009). Inhibition of the hedgehog pathway in advanced basal-cell carcinoma. *The New England Journal of Medicine*, *361*, 1164–1172.

Wadhera, A., Fazio, M., Bricca, G., & Stanton, O. (2006). Metastatic basal cell carcinoma: A case report and literature review. How accurate is our incidence data? *Dermatology Online Journal*, *12*, 7.

Webb, M. C., Compton, F., Andrews, P. A., et al. (1997). Skin tumours posttransplantation: A retrospective analysis of 28 years experience at a single centre. *Transplantation Proceedings*, *29*, 828–830.

Weedon, D., & Strutton, G. (2002). *Skin pathology*. Edinburgh: Churchill livingstone. pp. 765–772.

Wehner, M. R., Chren, M. M., Nameth, D., Choudhry, A., Gaskins, M., Nead, K. T., et al. (2014). International prevalence of indoor tanning: A systematic review and meta-analysis. *JAMA Dermatology*, *150*(4), 390–400.

Wehner, M. R., Shive, M. L., Chren, M. M., Han, J., Qureshi, A. A., & Linos, E. (2012). Indoor tanning and non-melanoma skin cancer: Systematic review and meta-analysis. *BMJ*, *345*, e5909.

Weinstock, M. A. (1994). Epidemiologic investigation of nonmelanoma skin cancer mortality: The Rhode Island Follow Back Study. *Journal of Investigative Dermatology*, *102*(6), 6S–9S.

Wheless, L., Black, J., & Alberg, A. J. (2010). Nonmelanoma skin cancer and the risk of second primary cancers: A systematic review. *Cancer Epidemiology, Biomarkers & Prevention*, *19*(7), 1686–1695.

Wheless, L., Kistner-Griffin, E., Jorgensen, T. J., Ruczinski, I., Berthier-Schaad, Y., Kessing, B., et al. (2012). A community-based study of nucleotide excision repair polymorphisms in relation to the risk of non-melanoma skin cancer. *The Journal of Investigative Dermatology*, *132*(5), 1354–1362.

Wheless, L., Ruczinski, I., Alani, R. M., Clipp, S., Hoffman-Bolton, J., Jorgensen, T. J., et al. (2009). The association between skin characteristics and skin cancer prevention behaviors. *Cancer Epidemiology, Biomarkers & Prevention*, *18*(10), 2613–2619.

Wisgerhof, H. C., Wolterbeek, R., de Fijter, J. W., Willemze, R., & Bouwes Bavinck, J. N. (2012). Kidney transplant recipients with cutaneous squamous cell carcinoma have an increased risk of internal malignancy. *The Journal of Investigative Dermatology*, *132*, 2176–2183.

Wood, M. E., Vogel, V., Ng, A., Foxhall, L., Goodwin, P., & Travis, L. B. (2012). Second malignant neoplasms: Assessment and strategies for risk reduction. *Journal of Clinical Oncology*, *30*(30), 3734–3745.

World Health Organization. (2006). Solar ultraviolet radiation: Global burden of disease from solar ultraviolet radiation. *Environmental burden of disease series*: Vol. 13.

World Health Organization. (2015). *Ultraviolet radiation and health*. http://www.who.int/uv/uv_and_health/en/.

Zavos, G., Karidis, N., Tsourouflis, G., Bokos, J., Diles, K., Sotirchos, G., et al. (2011). Nonmelanoma skin cancer after renal transplantation: A single-center experience in 1736 transplantations. *International Journal of Dermatology*, *50*(12), 1496–1500.

Zhang, M., Qureshi, A., Geller, A., Frazier, L., Hunter, D., & Han, J. (2012). Use of tanning beds and incidence of skin cancer. *Journal of Clinical Oncology*, *30*(14), 1588–1593.

INDEX

Note: Page numbers followed by "*f*" indicate figures, and "*t*" indicate tables.

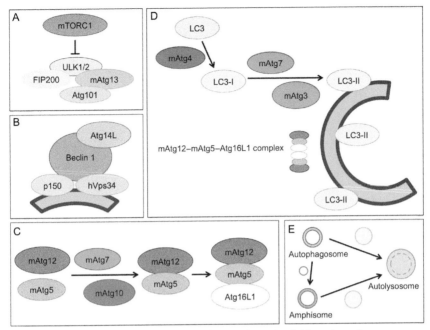

Fig. 1, J. Liu and J. Debnath (See Page 4 of this volume.)

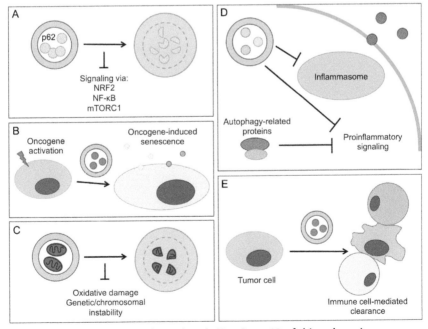

Fig. 2, J. Liu and J. Debnath (See Page 13 of this volume.)

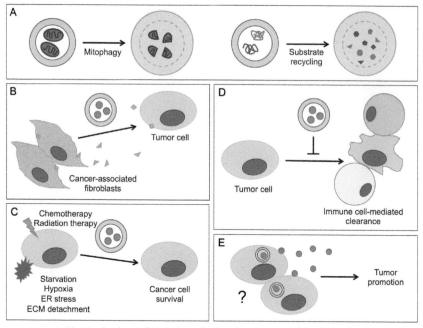

Fig. 3, J. Liu and J. Debnath (See Page 21 of this volume.)

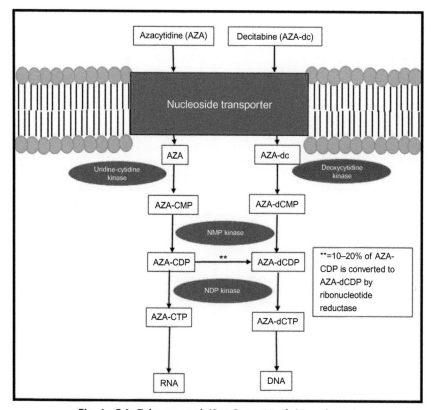

Fig. 1, C.A. Zahnow *et al.* (See Page 60 of this volume.)

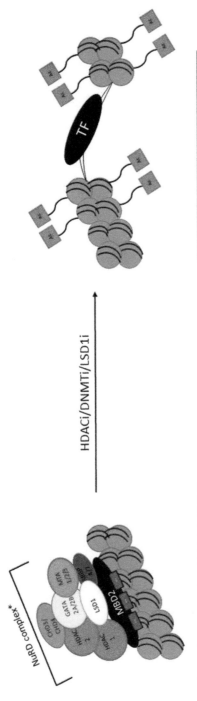

Closed chromatin: transcriptionally inactive

NuRD complex*

HDAC 2
HDAC 1
CHD3/ CHD4
GATA 2A/2B
LSD1
MTA 1/2/3
RBBP 4/7
MBD2

HDACi/DNMTi/LSD1i

Open chromatin: transcriptionally permissive

TF

NuRD complex*=sample repressor complex, other complexes include Sin3, NCoR, CoREST

■ =DNA methylation

Ac =Histone lysine acetylation

TF =Transcription factor

Fig. 2, C.A. Zahnow et al. (See Page 70 of this volume.)

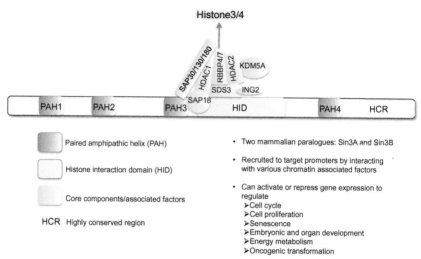

Fig. 1, N. Bansal *et al.* (See Page 115 of this volume.)

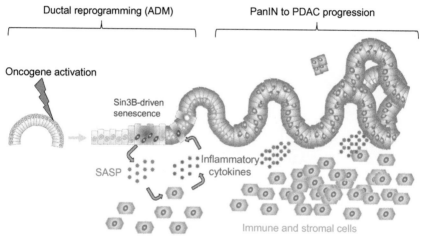

Fig. 2, N. Bansal *et al.* (See Page 123 of this volume.)

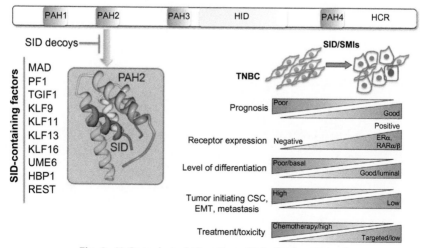

Fig. 3, N. Bansal *et al.* (See Page 124 of this volume.)

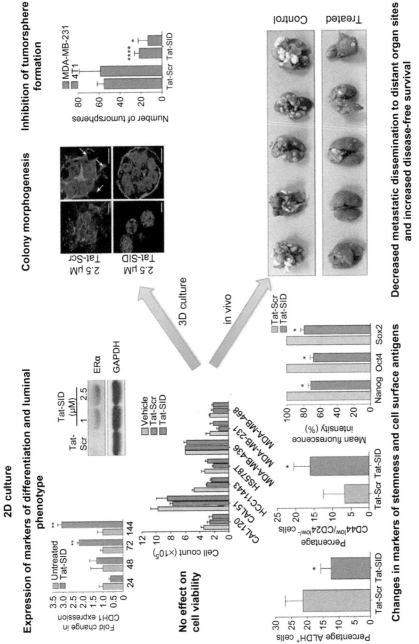

Fig. 4, N. Bansal et al. (See Page 129 of this volume.)

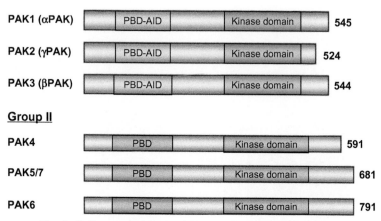

Fig. 1, R. Kumar and D.-Q. Li (See Page 139 of this volume.)

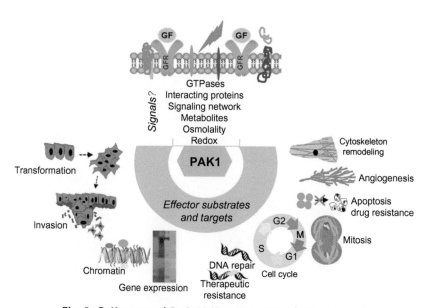

Fig. 2, R. Kumar and D.-Q. Li (See Page 154 of this volume.)

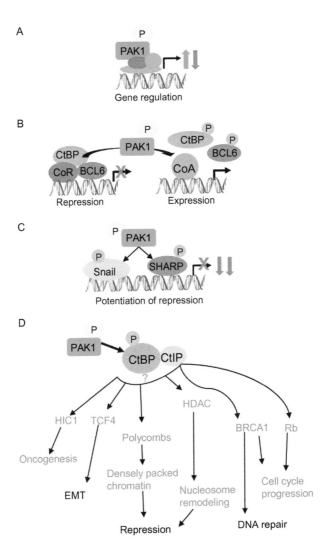

Fig. 3, R. Kumar and D.-Q. Li (See Page 164 of this volume.)

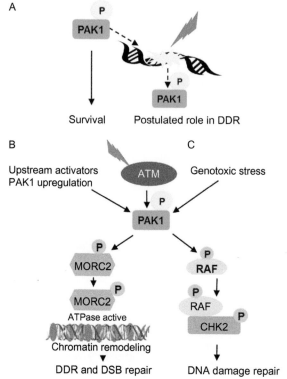

Fig. 4, R. Kumar and D.-Q. Li (See Page 170 of this volume.)

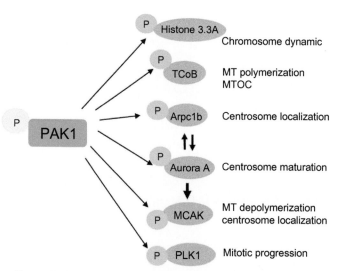

Fig. 5, R. Kumar and D.-Q. Li (See Page 173 of this volume.)

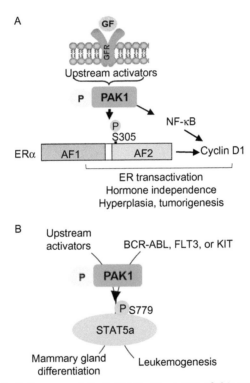

Fig. 6, R. Kumar and D.-Q. Li (See Page 177 of this volume.)

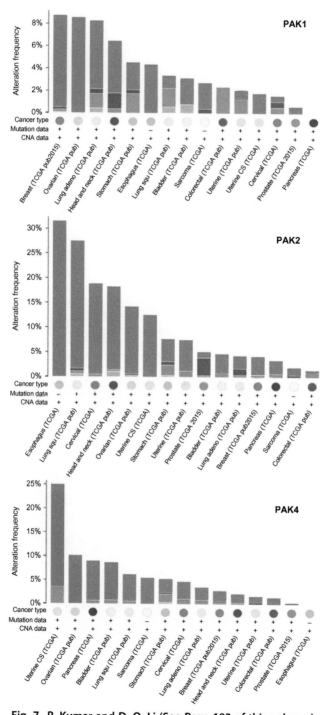

Fig. 7, R. Kumar and D.-Q. Li (See Page 183 of this volume.)

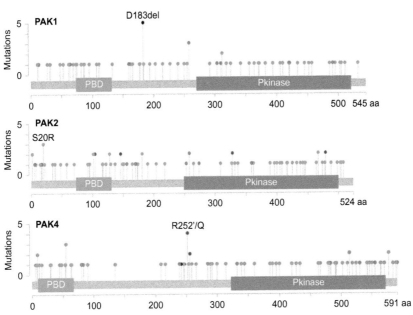

Fig. 8, R. Kumar and D.-Q. Li (See Page 184 of this volume.)

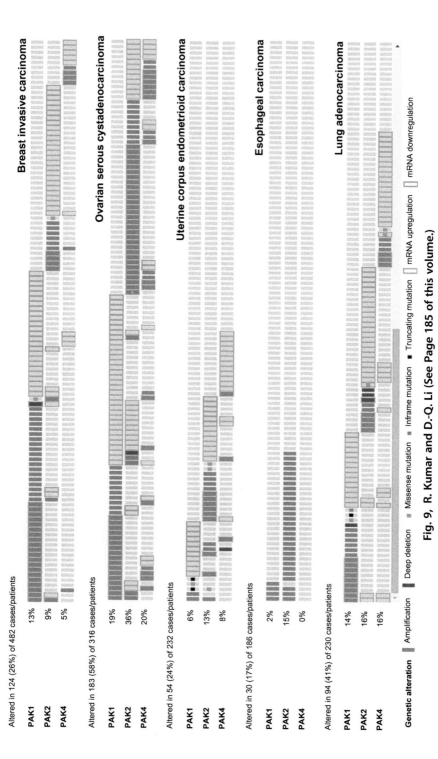

Fig. 9, R. Kumar and D.-Q. Li (See Page 185 of this volume.)

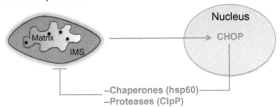

**: Misfolded proteins

Fig. 1, D. Germain (See Page 213 of this volume.)

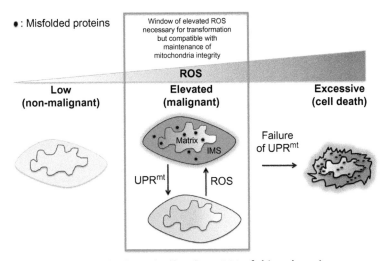

**: Misfolded proteins

Fig. 2, D. Germain (See Page 221 of this volume.)

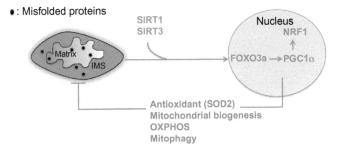

**: Misfolded proteins

Fig. 3, D. Germain (See Page 224 of this volume.)

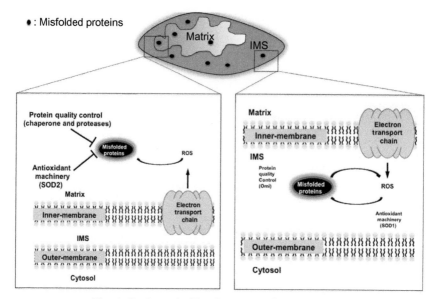

Fig. 4, D. Germain (See Page 228 of this volume.)

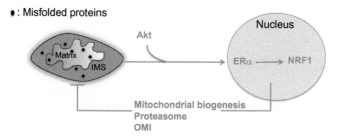

Fig. 5, D. Germain (See Page 229 of this volume.)